EMBRYO POLITICS

EMBRYO POLITICS

ETHICS AND POLICY IN ATLANTIC DEMOCRACIES

THOMAS BANCHOFF

CORNELL UNIVERSITY PRESS
Ithaca and London

First published 2011 by Cornell University Press
First printing, Cornell Paperbacks, 2013

Library of Congress Cataloging-in-Publication Data

Banchoff, Thomas F., 1964–
Embryo politics : ethics and policy in Atlantic democracies / Thomas Banchoff.
        p. cm.
    Includes bibliographical references and index.
    ISBN 978-0-8014-4957-4 (cloth : alk. paper)
    ISBN 978-0-8014-7881-9 (paper : alk. paper)
    1. Human embryo—Research—Moral and ethical aspects—United States. 2. Human embryo—Research—Moral and ethical aspects—Europe. 3. Human embryo—Research—Political aspects—United States. 4. Human embryo—Research—Political aspects—Europe. I. Title.
    QM608.B36   2011
    174.2'8—dc22   2010052639

❧ Contents

✌ PREFACE

Embryo research is one of the few political issues with no historical precedent. When does human life in the laboratory begin and deserve protection? When may embryos be destroyed to advance biomedical progress? These ethical and policy questions are only four decades old, but they will remain with us for a long time to come.

In this book I explore how the United States, the United Kingdom, Germany, and France have grappled with these questions so far. In setting out an argument about the intersection of politics, ethics, and policy, I focus on national bioethics committees, elected leaders, and their efforts to reconcile the moral status of the embryo and the imperative of biomedical progress in practice. In order to streamline the presentation, I have had to limit the treatment given to other aspects of embryo politics, including controversy within the scientific community over research priorities; social conflicts over sexuality, the family, and gender roles linked with in-vitro fertilization; and clashes over embryo donation and equal access to infertility and stem cell therapies.

I have labored not to make this a work of advocacy. In keeping with the ideal of a value-free social science as articulated by the great German sociologist Max Weber (1864–1920), I seek to describe and explain the views and actions of participants in embryo politics, not to inject my own. In one fundamental sense, however, I admit to a normative agenda. I believe that the moral status of the embryo and the promise of biomedical research to reduce human suffering are critical and complex ethical issues. And I favor a politics that grapples openly with those issues over one that ignores or obfuscates them. Given the stakes, we should aspire to a high level of public ethical discourse that draws on the resources of our philosophical and religious traditions.

I have incurred many debts in the writing of this book. Research leaves in 2000–2001 and 2004–5, supported by an Alexander von Humboldt Fellowship, gave me as a scholar of German foreign policy and European integration an opportunity to delve into a new topic area. A series of in-depth interviews with experts and policymakers in the United States, United Kingdom, Germany, and France proved an invaluable source of information and insight.

Many colleagues at Georgetown University and elsewhere have read all or part of the manuscript and contributed very helpful comments and criticism. Peter Engelke, Amy Vander Vliet, and Chris Vukicevich provided invaluable research assistance. I am particularly grateful to Roger Haydon of Cornell University Press, who encouraged the project early on and shepherded it expertly to completion.

Most of all I would like to express thanks to my wife Anja and our three daughters, Emma, Luisa, and Sophie. Their love and understanding have been an enduring source of strength and support throughout my work on this book. It is dedicated to them.

❧ EMBRYO POLITICS

Introduction

Nineteen sixty-eight was a pivotal year. On both sides of the Atlantic, youth protest and civil unrest shook the foundations of the social and political order, marking an end to the postwar era. This book traces the legacy of another 1968 event, less noticed at the time but no less revolutionary in the long run: the first successful fertilization of a human egg outside the womb. That feat, accomplished by the team of Robert Edwards and Patrick Steptoe in Cambridge, England, launched a scientific and biomedical revolution with far-reaching consequences that continue to unfold. Key milestones have included the birth of the first child born of in-vitro fertilization (IVF) in 1978; the derivation of human embryonic stem cells in 1998; and the first verified cloning of a human embryo in 2008. The first four decades of embryo research created new vistas for reproduction and regenerative medicine and, perhaps ultimately, for human genetic selection and enhancement. The path is open to a very different future.[1]

Politics, as much as science and technology, will determine that path. By action or inaction, governments make rules that govern the creation, utilization, and destruction of embryos in the laboratory. They support research

---

1. Throughout this book, "embryo research" refers to the creation, observation and/or manipulation, and eventual destruction of embryos in the laboratory as part of an effort to advance biomedical knowledge. The terms "proresearch" and "antiresearch" refer to embryo research.

through funding and restrict it through regulation—in diverse ways. Among leading Atlantic democracies, the United States banned federal funding for embryo research through the first decade of the twenty-first century, while allowing experiments in the private sector. The United Kingdom permitted research funded both publicly and privately. Germany imposed criminal penalties for all research involving the deliberate production or destruction of embryos. And France moved, gradually and unevenly, away from a similarly restrictive research regime in a more liberal direction.[2]

What explains these different political responses to the same scientific and technological revolution? This book focuses on the intersection of ethical contestation, historical and institutional legacies, and electoral and interest group competition. Over the four post–1968 decades, national ethics committees and elected leaders wrestled over the moral status of the embryo and the promise of biomedical research. They addressed moral conundrums against the backdrop of historical legacies including Nazi eugenics and more recent battles over the legalization of abortion. Backed by shifting coalitions of parties and interest groups, governments hammered out divergent policy regimes.

The centrality of ethics gave embryo politics its particular character. New questions about when life begins, deserves protection, and can be utilized in experiments posed challenges for old religious and philosophical traditions. Through the early 1990s, ethics committees and elected leaders wrestled with how to combine respect for the embryo and solidarity with those suffering from infertility and other ailments. In the decade after the cloning and stem cell breakthroughs of 1997–98 public debate grew more polarized. Research proponents, enthusiastic about the prospect of a new era of regenerative medicine, increasingly dismissed the problem of the moral status of the embryo. And research opponents tended to deny the promise of embryonic stem

---

2. On connections between science, ethics, and politics see, in particular, Sheila Jasanoff, *Designs on Nature: Science and Democracy in Europe and the United States* (Princeton: Princeton University Press, 2005); and John Hyde Evans, *Playing God?: Human Genetic Engineering and the Rationalization of Public Bioethical Debate* (Chicago: University of Chicago Press, 2002). Embryo politics are addressed in a growing literature, including Cynthia B. Cohen, *Renewing the Stuff of Life: Stem Cells, Ethics, and Public Policy* (Oxford: Oxford University Press, 2007); Herbert Gottweis, Brian Salter, and Catherine Waldby, *The Global Politics of Human Embryonic Stem Cell Science: Regenerative Medicine in Transition* (Basingstoke, UK: Palgrave Macmillan, 2009); Lori P. Knowles and Gregory E. Kaebnick, *Reprogenetics: Law, Policy, and Ethical Issues* (Baltimore: Johns Hopkins University Press, 2007); and Russell Korobkin and Stephen R. Munzer, *Stem Cell Century: Law and Policy for a Breakthrough Technology* (New Haven: Yale University Press, 2007). A useful global overview is Rosario M. Isasi and Bartha Knoppers, "Mind the Gap: Policy Approaches to Embryonic Stem Cell and Cloning Research in 50 Countries," *European Journal of Health Law* 13, no. 1 (2006): 9–25.

cell research altogether. Each side accused the other of pursuing a narrow ideological agenda.

Wherever one comes down on the moral status of the embryo and the healing promise of research, the intersection of science with perennial questions of human life, death, and suffering should be occasion for critical reflection and debate—not polemics or accusations of bad faith. As research moves into frontier areas, including human genetic selection and enhancement, we should draw on our religious and philosophical traditions to engage diverse arguments, aware of the incompleteness of our own knowledge and of the unprecedented nature of the ethical challenges. We should also look backward. A better understanding of the history of embryo politics over four decades can better prepare us for the critical policy decisions that lie ahead.

Paths of Embryo Politics

Political struggles over embryo, stem cell, and cloning research, like all politics, have an interest-driven dimension. They feature coalitions of interest groups, civil servants, parties, and politicians seeking to maximize their power and resources and implement their preferred agendas. In the context of embryo politics, however, building majorities and shaping policy in Atlantic democracies has also involved advancing and defending competing arguments about the protection of human life and the alleviation of human suffering. Those arguments, informed by contrasting religious and philosophical traditions, evolved in response to a series of technological breakthroughs after 1968.

Why did certain ethical arguments prevail in some national policy struggles but not in others? The internal logic and coherence of the arguments mattered, as did the power and resources of those advancing them. But historical legacies also played a critical role. During a first phase of embryo politics, from 1968 through the mid–1990s, contrasting historical experiences shaped national responses to the fundamentally new problem of how to treat embryos outside the womb. In the United States and the United Kingdom recent clashes over abortion informed the struggle over embryo research. In Germany and France, the historical legacy of Nazism and eugenics provided a more salient frame. The clash of ethical arguments against these historical backdrops culminated in the period from 1990 to 1995 in four different research regimes, ranging from most liberal in Britain to most restrictive in Germany.

During a second phase of embryo politics, inaugurated by the cloning of Dolly the sheep and the isolation of human embryonic stem cells in 1997–98, abortion and eugenics legacies continued to frame political controversy. More decisive, however, were the policy institutions that had been created between 1990 and 1995, which provided a shared point of reference for the forces arrayed for and against research in each country. The subsequent liberalization of restrictions, carried forward by arguments about an ethic of healing and the promise of regenerative medicine, did not break sharply with the national institutional and policy framework forged by the mid-1990s, despite the increasingly polarized terms of public ethical debate. A further breakthrough in 2006—induced pluripotent stem cells (IPS) created by reprogramming body cells to act like embryonic stem cells—shifted but did not transform the terms of controversy. Embryo research advocates backed continued work on multiple fronts, including with surplus IVF and cloned embryos, while opponents supported an exclusive focus on IPS and adult stem cell research.

In decades to come the speed of development of tissue replacement therapies with embryonic, adult, and IPS cells will shape embryo politics, as will advances in preimplantation genetic diagnosis (PGD), which involves the selection of embryos on different criteria before implantation, and the possible advent of genetic enhancement technologies. National policy outcomes will turn on the force of historical and institutional legacies and on configurations of electoral and interest group politics. They will also depend on whether and how leaders and citizens deploy religious and philosophical resources in an effort to puzzle through difficult ethical dilemmas.

Main Contours of Ethical Controversy

Public controversy about the ethics of scientific conduct is relatively recent. As late as the early 1960s Michael Polanyi could extol the "Republic of Science" as a free and collaborative enterprise with its own independent procedures and values.[3] Whatever its merits as an ideal, this absolute view of scientific freedom had already been undermined by revelations about inhuman Nazi eugenics and medical experiments first exposed at the 1946 Nuremberg Trials. The Nazi legacy made clear the necessity of external ethical standards to govern the practice of science, as did subsequent revelations into the postwar decades, which exposed experiments like those inflicted on black American airmen in Tuskegee, Alabama.[4] A series of

---

3. Michael Polanyi, "The Republic of Science: Its Political and Economic Theory," *Minerva* 1, no. 1 (1962), 54–73.

4. See, for example, Ruth Ellen Bulger, Elizabeth Heitman, and Stanley Joel Reiser, *The Ethical Dimensions of the Biological Sciences* (New York: Cambridge University Press, 1993); Jacques J. Rozenberg, *Bioethical and Ethical Issues Surrounding the Trials and Code of Nuremberg: Nuremberg Revisited*

scientific and medical breakthroughs in the 1960s and 1970s, including organ transplants, artificial life support, and recombinant DNA, raised further ethical questions about research bearing on human life, suffering, and death. By the 1980s, public awareness of such questions had grown, and the mainly U.S.-based discipline of bioethics had emerged in an effort to make sense of them.[5]

Embryo research was part of this broader trend. The first fertilization of a human egg in 1968 and the culturing of human embryos in the years that followed raised a host of ethical questions.[6] Controversy first centered on the dangers of genetic engineering and eugenic manipulation, the safety of transferring embryos from the laboratory to the womb, and the implications of IVF for traditional family and gender roles. Only after 1978, when Edwards and Steptoe facilitated the first IVF child, Louise Brown, did controversy focus on the question of the moral status of the embryo and its use in research. Two core questions were at issue: When does fully human life begin and deserve protection? And under what conditions can embryos be created and destroyed to advance biomedical knowledge that might alleviate human suffering?

The scientific method alone cannot answer these questions. Embryology has provided an increasingly complete account of the growth of the embryo from fertilization onward, but it cannot settle the issue of when the embryo deserves to be protected or how its moral status should be weighed against the promise of life saving research. Supporters and opponents of embryo research have both invoked scientific findings to support their views. For example, opponents tend to emphasize a unique genetic identity of the human organism from fertilization, while supporters often maintain that an individual embryo exists only at about two weeks, when it can no longer split and form twins. But empirical facts alone cannot settle these ethical disputes. The facts considered relevant, and their moral significance, are framed by ethical claims drawn, explicitly or implicitly, from religious or philosophical

---

(Lewiston, NY: Edwin Mellen Press, 2003); and Harold Y. Vanderpool, ed., *The Ethics of Research Involving Human Subjects: Facing the 21st Century* (Frederick, MD: University Pub. Group, 1996).

5. On the rise of bioethics, see Albert R. Jonsen, *The Birth of Bioethics* (New York: Oxford University Press, 1998); Jennifer K. Walter and Eran P. Klein, *The Story of Bioethics: From Seminal Works to Contemporary Explorations* (Washington, DC: Georgetown University Press, 2003); and Renée C. Fox, Judith P. Swazey, and Judith C. Watkins, *Observing Bioethics* (Oxford: Oxford University Press, 2008).

6. For Edwards's own account, see Robert G. Edwards and Patrick Christopher Steptoe, *A Matter of Life: The Story of a Medical Breakthrough* (New York: Morrow, 1980); and Robert G. Edwards, *Life before Birth: Reflections on the Embryo Debate* (New York: Basic Books, 1989).

traditions. As one leading researcher has noted, the "crux of the question is when life begins, a debate that cannot be settled by science."[7]

That debate took on definable contours during the post-1968 decades. Whether they drew on religious or philosophical resources—or some combination of them—participants in embryo research debates in Atlantic democracies converged around two core values by the 1980s: the protection of human life and the alleviation of suffering.[8] During most of the period, a degree of general consensus held across government and the academy, the scientific and medical community, faith leaders, the media, and public opinion. Most of those who did not view the embryo as fully human nevertheless acknowledged the question of when it becomes human and deserves protection as an important one. And those who asserted the full humanity of the early embryo generally affirmed the value of biomedical research as a means of reducing human suffering. If a dual concern with life and health was the object of broad consensus in Atlantic democracies, the implications for embryo research and its proper limits were open to sharply different religious and philosophical interpretations.

At a religious level the belief that individual human life is sacred and that healing is a duty has roots in Christianity, the dominant religious tradition on both sides of the Atlantic, as well as in Judaism and Islam, the most significant minority communities. Humanity has ultimate value because God created human beings in His image. Men and women are called to love and serve one another as fellow children of God. This basic approach to human life and healing set down in scripture and developed in theological and legal reflection has gone through historic variations. It has been most fully articulated over the past century in the three major branches of Atlantic Christianity—Catholic, evangelical, and mainline Protestant—in the context of the rise of the idea of individual rights in liberal democratic thought.

---

7. Irving L. Weissman,"Medicine: Politic Stem Cells," *Nature* 439 (2006): 148.

8. There is a vast and growing literature on the ethics of embryo, stem cell, and cloning research, and divergent philosophical and religious perspectives. Important collections of essays include Kristen R. Monroe, Ronald Baker Miller, and Jerome S. Tobis, *Fundamentals of the Stem Cell Debate: The Scientific, Religious, Ethical, and Political Issues* (Berkeley: University of California Press, 2008); Suzanne Holland, Karen Lebacqz, and Laurie Zoloth, *The Human Embryonic Stem Cell Debate: Science, Ethics, and Public Policy* (Cambridge: MIT Press, 2001); Michael Ruse and Christopher A. Pynes, *The Stem Cell Controversy: Debating the Issues* (Amherst, NY: Prometheus Books, 2003); and Brent Waters and Ronald Cole-Turner, *God and the Embryo: Religious Voices on Stem Cells and Cloning* (Washington, DC: Georgetown University Press, 2003). On links between the scientific and ethical issues, see Jane Maienschein, *Whose View of Life?: Embryos, Cloning, and Stem Cells* (Cambridge: Harvard University Press, 2003).

Claims about the inviolability of human life and an ethic of healing can also be espoused in a secular idiom. Whatever their historical debt to biblical religion, leading secular thinkers since the Enlightenment have articulated the importance of protecting life and alleviating suffering without recourse to scripture or religious authority, often drawing on classical Greek and Roman thought. Two philosophical currents have provided dominant nonreligious points of departure. Utilitarianism, first developed by Jeremy Bentham and John Stuart Mill, emphasizes the greatest good for the greatest number. Its main concern is minimizing overall human suffering and maximizing overall human happiness. Deontological ethics, by contrast, begin with the right thing to do, regardless of consequences. In this tradition, Immanuel Kant emphasized the inviolability of rational persons, not any utilitarian calculus. Leading contemporary philosophers such as John Rawls and Martha Nussbaum have drawn elements of both utilitarianism and Kantianism into a vision of human flourishing that combines the pursuit of happiness with respect for basic human dignity.[9]

The main arguments for and against embryo research that emerged by the 1980s drew on these religious and philosophical resources, in different combinations. The core antiresearch argument was grounded in *respect for the embryo* as a human individual at the earliest stage of existence. In the religious variant, the embryo is *sacred*. As a human life it is a gift of God, to be treated as a person and never willfully killed. To experiment with embryos is to violate a divine command and to destroy humanity's weakest members. From a philosophical antiresearch perspective, the embryo is *inviolable*. Because it is a genetic individual with the potential to develop into a human person, it deserves absolute respect. In this view, research that destroys it falls under the deontological prohibition against treating any human life solely as a means to an end, no matter how young the life or noble the end. These antiresearch views, most forcefully articulated by Roman Catholic and evangelical leaders, have also been espoused by a small minority of scientists, secular bioethicists, and mainline Protestant moral theologians.

The central proresearch argument is centered on an *ethic of healing*. In this view the embryo is an early form of human life, but not a human individual or a person. It can therefore be utilized under some circumstances to advance

---

9. See, for example, John Rawls, *A Theory of Justice* (Cambridge: Harvard University Press, 1971); Martha Craven Nussbaum, *Frontiers of Justice: Disability, Nationality, Species Membership* (Cambridge: Harvard University Press, 2006); Amartya Kumar Sen and Bernard Arthur Owen Williams, *Utilitarianism and Beyond* (Cambridge: Cambridge University Press, 1982); and Thomas E. Hill, *Respect, Pluralism, and Justice: Kantian Perspectives* (Oxford: Oxford University Press, 2000).

knowledge that can reduce human suffering. In a religious idiom, God, the giver of life, calls on humanity to use its reason to heal the sick and give hope to those in need. Given this call to heal and the enormous biomedical potential of research, the embryo may be destroyed for worthy ends under certain conditions. From a philosophical perspective centered on human flourishing, the reduction of suffering is an ethical imperative. Embryos are not fully formed or autonomous individuals and cannot feel pain; they can therefore be used as a means to valid biomedical ends, such as combating infertility or advancing regenerative medicine. These proresearch views predominate among leading secular bioethicists and scientists as well as among most mainline Protestant, Jewish, and Muslim thinkers and a minority of Catholic and evangelical moral theologians.

The Evolution of Ethical Conflict

The core tension between the moral status of the embryo and an ethic of healing evolved in complex ways in response to successive scientific and technological breakthroughs. During the first phase of embryo politics, through the mid-1990s, basic pro- and antiresearch arguments adapted across three key thresholds: the fertilization of an egg in the laboratory (1968), the birth of a child through IVF (1978), and the freezing of surplus IVF embryos (1983). The announcement of the cloning of Dolly (1997) and the isolation of human embryonic stem cells (1998) were the critical breakthroughs that launched a second phase of embryo politics. And the discovery of IPS cells (2006) proved a further important juncture. Each scientific and technological development introduced new variations on existing ethical themes. In tracing those variations—in outline here, and in the chapters that follow—this book focuses on the work of ethics bodies convened at the national level to bring critical reflection to bear on new developments and to frame the policy alternatives facing political leaders.

Between 1968 and the birth of Louise Brown a decade later, Edwards and Steptoe produced, observed, and implanted hundreds of embryos.[10] In their race to the same goal of the first "test-tube" baby, other international teams, mainly in the United States and Australia, also worked with embryos in the laboratory. At this early stage, the ethical fronts were more fluid than in subsequent decades. Within the Catholic Church of the early 1970s, for

---

10. Robert G. Edwards, Barry D. Bavister, and Patrick C. Steptoe, "Early Stages of Fertilization In Vitro of Human Oocytes Matured In Vitro," *Nature* 221, no. 5181 (1969): 632–35.

example, there was no official position on the legitimacy of IVF for married couples or on whether the early embryo had the same moral standing as a developing fetus. During that same period, scientists and bioethicists differed sharply on the appropriate cutoff point for embryo experiments, with some arguing for research up to four to six weeks after fertilization. By the late 1970s, the debate started to narrow. The Vatican insisted more forcefully that the embryo should be treated as a person from conception, and scientists and ethicists converged around the idea that experiments should be allowed only up to the implantation stage, at around fourteen days. The work of the U.S. Ethics Advisory Board (EAB, 1978–79), the first national bioethics committee to address embryo research, illustrated this trend. The board backed research only through the implantation stage and solely in order to improve IVF as an infertility treatment.[11]

The birth of Louise Brown and the subsequent spread of IVF technology added a new twist to established lines of ethical controversy. As the new infertility treatment became more routine, some scientists turned their attention to wider research agendas involving embryo research. Edwards was among those who pointed out its potential to unlock secrets of early human development in areas from cancer to congenital disease. His public statements helped to spark a national debate in the United Kingdom about the purpose and limits of embryo research that culminated in the 1984 recommendations of the government's Committee of Inquiry into Human Fertilisation and Embryology, commonly known as the Warnock committee. The committee majority agreed that embryo experimentation should remain legal as long as it focused on the development of IVF and related ends. The Warnock committee also supported the deliberate creation of embryos for research in some cases.[12]

By the time the first national ethics committees began to address these issues in Germany and France in 1985–86, a further technological development had altered the backdrop for ethical debate: the routine freezing of embryos left over from IVF treatments. In 1983 Australian fertility specialists had achieved the cryopreservation and thawing of human embryos; a first child

---

11. Ethics Advisory Board, *Report and Conclusions: HEW Support of Research Involving Human In Vitro Fertilization and Embryo Transfer* (Washington, DC: Department of Health, Education, and Welfare, 1979). There is a considerable literature on these committees, their composition, work habits, and effectiveness. See, for example, Robert H. Blank, *Regulating Reproduction* (New York: Columbia University Press, 1990); and Bulger et al., *Society's Choices: Social and Ethical Decision Making in Biomedicine.*

12. United Kingdom, Department of Health and Social Security, *Report of the Committee of Inquiry into Human Fertilisation and Embryology* (London: Her Majesty's Stationery Office, 1984).

born from a frozen surplus IVF embryo was announced in February 1984.[13] From that point on, embryos created for IVF but not implanted could, with parents' permission, be preserved for later fertility treatments or, eventually, scientific research. In 1985 a first national German ethics committee, the Benda Commission, opposed research in principle but made exceptions for such surplus IVF embryos. Since they were destined to perish in any case, it was argued, they might be used up for "medical findings of great value." The French National Consultative Ethics Committee (CCNE) arrived at a similar conclusion. Its major 1986 report described embryos as "potential human persons" worthy of protection but supported research with those no longer part of any "parental project." In contrast to the Warnock committee, the German and French bodies rejected any deliberate creation of embryos for research as an illicit instrumentalization of human life.[14]

Two major technological breakthroughs in 1997–98 launched a new phase in embryo politics and added variations to established ethical debates. The first was the February 1997 announcement of Dolly the sheep, the first mammal to be cloned from an adult body cell. While public controversy centered on the almost universally condemned prospect of human reproductive cloning, a quiet ethical debate gradually emerged around cloning for research purposes. At the time, scientists were racing to isolate pluripotent stem cells from embryos, which would have the capacity to grow into the different tissue types and to multiply indefinitely in vitro. (Stem cells in adults and in umbilical cord blood did not have the same versatility.) The cloning of embryos, it was hoped, might permit the derivation of stem cells that matched a particular patient, enabling transplant therapies with a lower risk of immune rejection. The Dolly breakthrough and the prospect of such "therapeutic cloning" introduced a new wrinkle into existing embryo research debates. Research opponents tended to attack therapeutic cloning as the deliberate creation of embryos in order to destroy them, while supporters focused almost exclusively on the technique's eventual promise to deliver immune-compatible cells for therapy.

The November 1998 announcement of the derivation of human embryonic stem cells in a Wisconsin laboratory proved an even more critical juncture

---

13. The existence of the pregnancy was announced in July 1983. See Alan Trounson and Linda Mohr, "Human Pregnancy Following Cryopreservation, Thawing and Transfer of an Eight-Cell Embryo," *Nature* 305, no. 5936 (1983): 707–9.

14. Benda Commission, *Working Group on In Vitro Fertilisation, Genom Analysis, and Gene Therapy Report* (Bonn: Federal Ministry for Research and Technology, 1985); Comité Consultatif National d'Ethique, "Opinion on Research and Use of In-Vitro Human Embryos for Scientific and Medical Purposes," December 15, 1986, http://www.ccne-ethique.fr/docs/en/avis008.pdf.

in embryo politics.[15] It demonstrated the plausibility of a new era of regenerative medicine, sharpened the therapeutic cloning debate, and shifted the terms of controversy about the proper ends of research with surplus IVF embryos. Almost overnight ethic-of-healing arguments shifted from a focus on infertility to a wider emphasis on the potential to alleviate the suffering of millions of victims of Parkinson's, Alzheimer's, and other debilitating diseases. The rise of an ethic of healing did not drown out the voices of those categorically opposed to the deliberate destruction of embryos. But the prospect of a new era of regenerative medicine threw those research opponents on the defensive. With few exceptions, national bioethics committees that tackled embryonic stem cell issues in the United States, the United Kingdom, Germany, and France during the post-1998 decade advocated some changes in existing research regimes to allow either for the derivation of stem cells from embryos or for experiments with such cells derived abroad or in the private sector.

The ethical fronts shifted somewhat in the years from 2006 to 2008, a period that saw the approval of the first clinical trials for embryonic stem cell therapy, the first verified cloning of a human embryo from a human body cell, and—most significantly—the emergence of IPS cells.[16] A Japan-based team demonstrated in 2006 that the adult body cells of a mouse could be reprogrammed to take on the flexibility of embryonic stem cells; the experiment was extended to human cells in 2007–8.[17] Opponents of embryonic stem cell research could now more plausibly point to promising research paths that would not involve embryo destruction. Overall, though, established patterns of ethical contestation persisted. One side now held up IPS cells, alongside adult stem cells, as the most promising path to regenerative medicine. The other insisted that embryonic stem cell research be pursued alongside other research programs, as their relative therapeutic promise was yet to be determined.

The ethical debates that framed policy decisions during the second phase of embryo politics differed from those of the earlier phase not only in substance but in tone. There was generally less deliberation at the intersection of the moral status of the embryo and the promise of biomedical research and more polarization between fixed positions centered on one or the other. Research advocates, flush with excitement about the promise of a new era

---

15. James A. Thomson, "Embryonic Stem Cell Lines Derived from Human Blastocysts," *Science* 282, no. 5391 (1998): 1145–47.

16. Andrew J. French et al., "Development of Human Cloned Blastocysts Following Somatic Cell Nuclear Transfer with Adult Fibroblasts," *Stem Cells* 26, no. 2 (2008): 485–93.

17. Constance Holden and Gretchen Vogel, "Cell Biology: A Seismic Shift for Stem Cell Research," *Science* 319, no. 5863 (2008): 560–63.

of regenerative medicine, often dismissed the moral status of the embryo as irrelevant, while opponents of embryo destruction were often loath to acknowledge that promise or address the fate of hundreds of thousands of frozen IVF embryos destined to perish in any case. The polarization of ethical discourse would be magnified once political leaders took up the issues.

From Ethical Contestation to Policy Struggle

How did ethical controversy shape policy struggles and outcomes over four decades? Why did some ethical arguments prevail over others in the political process?

Contests for power and resources provide part of the answer. Around embryo research, as with other issue areas, policy emerges out of competition among interest groups, civil servants, and party leaders seeking to maximize their control over the state and its material resources. In the United States and Europe, scientific and religious organizations, biotechnology companies, patient-advocacy groups, and others with a stake in embryo research and its outcomes sought to translate their policy preferences into government action over the post-1968 decades. They interacted with one another and with parties and politicians to build winning coalitions within the legislature and the executive branch. Electoral cycles and trends in the mobilization of interest groups favored the rise and fall of different ethical arguments, as the political fortunes of different camps shifted.

The changing constellation of political power did not tell the whole story. Around value-driven issues such as embryo research, abortion, and euthanasia ethical arguments have an independent impact alongside material interests. Because they touch on questions of life and death, sexuality, and suffering, such issues have a strong emotional and normative dimension.[18] Arguments about right and wrong do more than legitimate policies pursued out of material self-interest. They are critical in building and sustaining coalitions that encompass political actors without a material stake.

In the case of embryo research, difficult ethical tradeoffs left room for political debate over how best to protect life and alleviate suffering in practice.

---

18. On the politics of ethics-driven issues see, for example, Christopher Z. Mooney, ed., *The Public Clash of Private Values: The Politics of Morality Policy* (New York: Chatham House, 2001); and Raymond Tatalovich and Byron W. Daynes, eds., *Moral Controversies in American Politics: Cases in Social Regulatory Policy* (Armonk, NY: M. E. Sharpe, 1998). On the limits of interest-driven accounts of embryo politics, see Simon Fink, "Politics as Usual or Bringing Religion Back In?: The Influence of Parties, Institutions, Economic Interests, and Religion on Embryo Research Laws," *Comparative Political Studies* 41, no. 12 (2008): 1631–56.

The ethics bodies set up by governments served to define the key issues, summarize options, and make recommendations. These committees were not insulated from political pressures or from trends in media coverage and elite and public opinion.[19] But they also were not simply reflections of their wider context. To varying degrees they did important work of translation and agenda setting, describing scientific and technological developments and ethical issues they raised, constructing policy alternatives, and thereby shaping the views of citizens and elected leaders uncertain of what to make of novel developments. The committees influenced—but did not determine—how leaders in legislatures and the executive conceived and sifted policy options from one country to the next. The EAB's recommendation in favor of federal funding for embryo research in 1979, while never adopted, became a focal point for decades of political conflict in the United States. The Warnock committee's seminal 1984 report recommending the creation of embryos for research defined the terms of the British debate. The Benda Commission's endorsement of research for "medical findings of great value" shaped the policy struggle in Germany. And key ideas put forward by the CCNE, including the embryo as a "potential human person" in the context of a "parental project," informed subsequent policy controversies in France.

National historical and institutional legacies, this book argues, can best explain considerable national variations in the policy struggles and their outcomes. The historical institutionalist approach to comparative politics explores the path-dependent effects of historical experience and established institutions on subsequent politics and policy.[20] It is most often applied to interest-driven issues, where critical junctures such as wars and depressions lead to institutional innovation such as alliances and social programs that generate supportive networks of politicians and interest groups who benefit from

---

19. For one of the few comparative surveys of public attitudes, see Sofres, *Les attitudes de l'opinion publique en France, Allemagne, Grande-Bretagne et aux Etats-Unis à l'égard de la science* (Paris: Sofres, 2001). A useful overview of U.S. polling data is Matthew C. Nisbet, "The Polls—Trends: Public Opinion about Stem Cell Research and Human Cloning," *Public Opinion Quarterly* 68, no. 1 (2004): 131–54.

20. See, for example, Peter A. Hall and Rosemary C. R. Taylor, "Political Science and the Three New Institutionalisms," *Political Studies* 44 (1996): 936–57; Paul Pierson and Theda Skocpol, "Historical Institutionalism in Contemporary Political Science," in *Political Science: The State of the Discipline*, ed. Ira Katznelson and Helen V. Milner (New York: Norton, 2002), 693–721; Ira Katznelson, "Structure and Configuration in Comparative Politics," in *Comparative Politics: Rationality, Culture, and Structure*, ed. Mark I. Lichbach and Alan S. Zuckerman (Cambridge: Cambridge University Press, 1997), 81–111; and Kathleen Thelen, "Historical Institutionalism in Comparative Politics," *Annual Review of Political Science* 2 (1999): 369–404. On the idea of path dependence in the social sciences, see James Mahoney, "Path Dependence in Historical Sociology," *Theory and Society* 29 (2000): 507–48; and Paul Pierson, "Increasing Returns, Path Dependence, and the Study of Politics," *American Political Science Review* 94, no. 2 (2000): 251–67.

and tend to preserve the status quo. Path-dependent dynamics also shape the politics of value-driven issues.[21] Even something as radically new as embryo research did not create its own radically new politics but flowed instead into established channels. During the first phase of embryo politics, through the mid-1990s, two historical legacies provided national frames for the policy struggle: the legalization of abortion in the United States and the United Kingdom, and Nazi eugenics in Germany and, to a lesser degree, in France. During the second phase, into the first decade of the new century, the policy institutions forged from 1990 to 1995 had a significant path-dependent impact on the subsequent evolution of policy.

The First Phase of Embryo Politics, 1968–96

The late 1960s and early 1970s saw a sweeping liberalization of restrictions on abortion, institutionalized in the United Kingdom with the 1967 Abortion Act and in the United States with the Supreme Court's 1973 *Roe v. Wade* decision. In both countries, the rolling back of prohibitions on abortion provoked a strong reaction, particularly from Catholics and later from evangelicals. An antiabortion movement gradually took shape in the 1970s and eventually took up the embryo research issue. The idea that life begins at conception, and that embryos as well as fetuses have a "right to life," served to mobilize principled opposition to embryo research where before there had been little organized resistance. There emerged pro- and antiresearch coalitions that roughly mirrored the balance of power on the abortion question in each country.

Throughout the 1980s, the administrations of Ronald Reagan and George H. W. Bush refused to approve funds for federally sponsored embryo research. Eager not to offend Catholics and evangelicals and their pro-life allies, they repeatedly ignored the entreaties of leading health officials and Democrats in Congress to revive the Ethics Advisory Board and take up its recommendations for federal funding of research. Bush's successor, the Democrat Bill Clinton, had a generally proresearch orientation. His administration created an ethics body, the Human Embryo Research Panel (HERP), which eventually advocated federal funding for work with surplus IVF embryos and for the deliberate creation of embryos for research. Under increasing pressure from Republicans, who swept the 1994 mid-term elections, President Clinton rejected the panel's recommendations on embryo creation. And in 1995 the Republican Congress, with the strong support and encouragement of an

---

21. For a discussion, see Thomas Banchoff, "Path Dependence and Value-Driven Issues: The Comparative Politics of Stem Cell Research," *World Politics* 57, no. 2 (2005): 200–30.

emboldened pro-life movement, attached the Dickey Amendment to an appropriations bill, which banned any expenditure of federal funds for research involving the destruction of embryos.

In the United Kingdom, too, the abortion issue provided a frame of reference for embryo politics. In the wake of the 1984 report of the Warnock committee, pro-life interest groups seized on the abortion parallel and, with the support of their allies in Parliament, sought to pass legislation that would have banned any and all embryo research in the country. In contrast to her conservative counterparts in the United States, however, Prime Minister Margaret Thatcher was less politically beholden to the pro-life movement. The government used its control over the legislative agenda to defeat the Unborn Children (Protection) Bill in 1985 and to delay parliamentary action on embryo research until 1990, by which time research advocates had effectively mobilized. The Human Fertilisation and Embryology (HFE) Act of 1990 set up a research regime allowing research with surplus IVF embryos and, in certain circumstances, the production of embryos for research.

Interestingly, the abortion legacy had almost no impact on French and German embryo politics. Strong legislative majorities had emerged by the early 1970s in favor of more liberal abortion regimes in both countries. Over the opposition of the Catholic Church, the French and German governments opted to legalize abortion, subject to some restrictions. Pointing to the human dignity provisions within their postwar constitutions, courts in both countries affirmed the principle of respect for human life at all stages in its development. At the same time, they upheld new, more liberal legislation, acknowledging the tragic nature of the abortion decision and refusing to countenance the prosecution of women and doctors who acted within the new law. This compromise solution—principled opposition to abortion and pragmatic acceptance of it in most cases—served to defuse political controversy. The divisive policy legacy that polarized politics in the United States, and to a lesser extent in the United Kingdom, failed to materialize. In France and Germany pro-life arguments against embryo research informed by the abortion parallel did not have the same resonance.[22]

In the case of Germany, and to a lesser extent, France, the most important historical backdrop for embryo politics was Nazi eugenics and the Holocaust. In Germany revulsion at the horrors of Nazism found its expression in

22. On contrasting abortion regimes in Atlantic democracies see Melanie Latham, *Regulating Reproduction: A Century of Conflict in Britain and France* (Manchester, U.K.: University of Manchester Press, 2002); and Myra Marx Ferree et al., *Shaping Abortion Discourse: Democracy and the Public Sphere in Germany and the United States* (Cambridge: Cambridge University Press, 2002).

Article 1 of the Basic Law of the Federal Republic of Germany (the constitution of 1949): "Human dignity is inviolable." From the early postwar decades onward, Christian Democrats and the more secular Social Democrats and Liberals articulated a shared commitment to the principle of human dignity and a determination to break with a terrible past. In light of the horrors of Nazi eugenics, German scientific and medical associations acknowledged the central importance of ethical considerations in the research setting. When embryo experimentation emerged as a political issue in the late 1980s, this legacy proved a resource for antiresearch forces. A cross-party coalition, supported by the Catholic and Lutheran churches, moved to legislate in a restrictive manner. The force of the Nazi legacy, the mobilization of the churches, and skepticism of technology among Social Democrats and in the new Green Party overrode the cautious proresearch stance articulated by the Benda Commission in 1985. The 1990 Embryo Protection Law (EPL) made all destructive embryo research a criminal offense.

A related pattern was evident in France. Against the backdrop of the war and occupation, the preamble to the 1946 constitution of the Fourth Republic, drafted under Christian Democratic and Social Democratic direction, underscored the value of human dignity. Here, recent history intersected with the deeper historical legacy: the French Revolution and its secular emphasis on the sanctity of human rights. The Constitutional Council under the Fifth Republic, founded in 1958, made human dignity one of the bases of its jurisprudence. Concern about the misuse of scientific power, shaped both by the Nazi experience and by a humanist revolutionary legacy, favored secular arguments skeptical of embryo research and its possible abuses, while the Catholic Church, a marginal force in French politics, had a limited impact on the debate. In early 1992 President François Mitterrand's Socialist Party majority in the National Assembly initially endorsed bioethics legislation that would have allowed research limited to surplus IVF embryos, along the lines advocated by the CCNE. But a conservative sweep in legislative elections later that year produced a new majority and a more restrictive research regime. The comprehensive Bioethics Laws passed in 1994 banned all research in France involving the destruction of embryos.

The Second Phase of Embryo Politics, 1997–2008

The ethical and policy controversies of the second phase of embryo politics, like those of the first, were shaped by the historical legacies of abortion and eugenics. But they were more immediately impacted by the policy institutions put in place between 1990 and 1995. Those research regimes provided a shared framework for national political struggles, an institutional configuration to be adapted to the new technological developments. Their staying power was a function of the political forces arrayed behind them and of an awareness that they represented the legitimate outcome of earlier political battles over divisive ethical questions. Some principled supporters and opponents of embryo research did seek to use the stem cell and cloning issues to fundamentally revisit those institutional outcomes. But most national leaders supportive of liberalization sought to adapt the policy status quo only incrementally.

In the United States, the abortion issue continued to shape embryo politics into the new century. Pro-life forces found a supporter in President George W. Bush, who took office in 2001. The Dickey Amendment remained in place. But, in the decade after 1997–98, hopes for a new era of regenerative medicine and the rise of ethic-of-healing arguments changed the political constellation. Efforts in Congress to ban therapeutic and not just reproductive cloning failed. And in August 2001 President Bush disappointed many of his Catholic and evangelical supporters by allowing federal funding for embryonic stem cell research with cells that had already been derived by that date. For a proresearch majority in Congress that grew after the 2006 mid-term elections, Bush had not gone far enough. Bills pressing for the elimination of the August 2001 cutoff date for approved stem cell lines provoked two presidential vetoes. Only after the 2008 elections was the new president, Barack Obama, able to lift Bush's restrictions. Despite the urging of many supporters, however, Obama did not seek to overturn the Dickey Amendment. The 1995 research regime, with its sharp dichotomy between prohibited federal and permitted private embryo research, remained.

In the United Kingdom the political marginalization of the pro-life movement, evident in resounding parliamentary support for the HFE Act of 1990, all but eliminated the abortion issue as a subsequent backdrop for embryo politics. Catholic leaders, the evangelical wing of the Church of England, and some members of the All-Party Pro-Life Parliamentary Group sought to use the 2000–02 struggle over embryonic stem cell and cloning research to revisit the established liberal policy regime. But Prime Minister Tony Blair—like Thatcher before him, sympathetic to the scientific community— successfully forged a coalition to adapt established policy institutions for both new technologies. Parliamentary supporters of embryonic stem cell and cloning research could argue persuasively that if experiments involving the destruction of embryos were already allowed in order to combat human infertility and related ailments, they should be extended to new areas with the potential to reduce human suffering on a much broader scale. Years after final approval of these changes in 2002, Blair and his successor, Gordon Brown, won parliamentary approval in 2008 for a further adaptation of the existing regime designed to get around a shortage of human eggs: the creation of animal-human hybrid embryos as a source of stem cells.

In Germany and France, where the abortion issue had never framed the debate, the historical shadow of eugenics had a more limited impact on stem cell and cloning policy than did the restrictive policy regimes put in place in 1990 and 1994. The German Embryo Protection Law of 1990 had outlawed cloning and all embryo research as an affront to human dignity, but it had not anticipated the possibility of embryonic stem cell research. In the German policy struggle that began in 2000 and 2001, only small minorities, centered on the Liberal Free Democratic Party, suggested amending the EPL to allow for the derivation of cells in Germany or the possibility of therapeutic cloning. As in the United States, national political controversy centered on the ethics of research with stem cells already derived from embryos. (In Germany the cells would have to be imported, while in the United States they were available in the private sector.) Within these constraints, arguments about an ethic of healing prevailed in the Bundestag twice, once under the chancellorship of Social Democrat Gerhard Schröder, and again under his successor, the Christian Democrat Angela Merkel. In 2002 the Bundestag voted to allow the import of embryonic stem cells derived before a cutoff date of that January. In 2007, by a stronger margin, the Bundestag moved the cutoff date ahead five more years. Even as political support for embryonic stem cell imports grew, the EPL, with its absolute ban on embryo destruction, cloning, and hybrids, remained the focus of broad political consensus.

In France there was more movement away from the established institutional foundation. In the initial debate about updating the Bioethics Laws in 2000–01, the Socialist government under Lionel Jospin backed not just the import of embryonic stem cells but also their derivation in France from surplus IVF embryos, and even the possibility of therapeutic cloning. Under fire from conservative French President Jacques Chirac—a rival to the prime minister in France's dual executive framework—Jospin dropped cloning from the proposed legislation. The government's support for research with stem cells derived from surplus IVF embryos won broad support in an initial vote in the National Assembly in early 2002, only to be annulled by a conservative sweep in national elections several months later. The revision of the Bioethics Laws that eventually passed in 2004 banned the destruction of embryos to derive stem cells in principle, but allowed for some exceptions over a period of five years. In the run-up to the next revision of bioethics legislation, envisioned for 2010–11, controversy centered on therapeutic cloning and on whether research with surplus IVF embryos should be approved in principle, and not just as an exception.

These national patterns of embryo politics have not unfolded in isolation. The chapters that follow point to cross-border connections among scientific communities and in the deliberations of ethics committees. They show how those arrayed for and against research, ranging from pro-life activists to patient-advocacy groups, have seen themselves as part of transnational movements and sought to learn from the experience of other countries. But the comparison also shows how, in the end, embryo politics has played out on a national stage and has been shaped most powerfully by agendas and politics with particular historical and institutional roots. International institutions at the level of the United Nations and the European Union have had limited impact. Ethical controversies bearing on sensitive questions have been decided within the political institutions that bound the nation state, the enduring focus of collective identity and locus of democratic politics into the twenty-first century.

The Way Forward

A comparison of embryo politics in four leading Atlantic scientific powers obviously has geographic limitations. Researchers based in other countries, including Australia, Japan, South Korea, Singapore, and Israel, have made significant contributions to embryo, stem cell, and cloning research. China and India have entered the arena and loom as future biotechnological superpowers. And as the science and technology have spread, ethical debates and policy contestation has emerged not just in Europe and North America but also in the former Soviet Union, Latin America, Asia, and the Middle East. In the context of globalization, different combinations of national histories, institutions, politics, and religious and philosophical traditions will shape multiple paths of embryo politics worldwide.

The focus on the United States, United Kingdom, Germany, and France undertaken here allows for a careful comparison and analysis of the shifting politics of embryo research across four decades and four countries. It also holds two main lessons for the future. First, the variety of different national responses to the same scientific and technological breakthroughs underscores the existence of choices going forward. Prohibition is an option, as the German and French experience suggests, as is a more permissive regime along U.S. and U.K. lines. Political decisions matter. Second, serious ethical reflection and deliberation can have an independent impact on those decisions. Concern about how to combine the protection of life and the alleviation of suffering can inform ethical contestation and the policy struggle, as it did into the 1990s. Or a polarized confrontation that obscures core ethical dilemmas can dominate embryo politics, the trend during the first part of the new century. A willingness to confront and debate new issues through constructive dialogue will not guarantee wise policy decisions going forward. But it will make them more likely.

❧ CHAPTER 1

The Emergence of Ethical Controversy

The human embryo only slowly emerged as an object of ethical controversy. A first alleged account of human in vitro fertilization, reported by the *New York Times* in 1944, occasioned little public reaction. News stories about work with embryos appeared intermittently during the early 1960s but, in the absence of scientific confirmation, generated very little notice. Even after the first confirmed fertilization of a human egg in the laboratory in Cambridge, England, in 1968, questions surrounding the moral status of the embryo and the promise of biomedical research sparked little public controversy. Groups later embroiled in embryo politics, including scientific associations, patient-advocacy organizations, and even the Catholic Church, took up the moral quandaries of embryo research only slowly.

An important catalyst was a series of national ethics committees convened on both sides of the Atlantic to advise governments on how to govern IVF and embryo research. Reports by the Ethics Advisory Board (1979) and the Human Embryo Research Panel (1994) in the United States, the Warnock committee (1984) in the United Kingdom, the Benda Commission in Germany (1985), and the National Consultative Ethics Committee (1986) in France translated rapid scientific developments for a wider audience, identified some of the key moral dilemmas, and made a set of convergent policy recommendations.

The relatively slow emergence of controversy was due in part to the pace of scientific and technological development. Before the February 1969 publication of Robert Edwards's breakthrough the previous year, experiments with human fertilization were rare and poorly documented. Even after the breakthrough, *Le Monde* could comment, nonchalantly, that it was "still too early to see anything in this experiment beyond an interesting technological prowess now only of interest to scientists."[1] In the years after 1969 only a handful of teams were active in the IVF field worldwide, mainly in the United Kingdom, the United States, and Australia. Through the late 1970s, estimates of the number of eggs fertilized, observed, or manipulated, and then discarded in the laboratory, ran into the hundreds rather than the thousands.[2] With the birth of the first "test-tube" baby, Louise Brown, in 1978, this picture changed. Work with embryos in the laboratory spread as IVF treatments moved around the world. Embryo freezing techniques introduced in 1983–84 made a growing number of surplus IVF embryos available for experiments. Scientists gradually turned greater attention to research questions beyond infertility.

It was not just the pace of technology but the existence of other, competing ethical concerns that crowded out concern with the moral status of the embryo early on. Anxiety about a eugenic "brave new world"—an allusion to the dystopian future evoked by Aldous Huxley's 1932 novel—dominated early media coverage of IVF research. The Catholic Church focused its ire on IVF as an unnatural form of artificial reproduction. Governments approached IVF primarily as a safety issue for both mothers and children. Gradually, however, the new discipline of bioethics did take up the issue of the moral status of the embryo and when it might be used up in research. As national ethics committees joined the debate, other social actors, including scientific organizations and churches, entered the fray. During the 1980s, Catholic and evangelical leaders discovered links between the abortion issue and embryo protection, while scientists and their allies in the bioethics field emphasized, not respect for the embryo, but the promise of research to address infertility and, potentially, other medical conditions. By the time governments moved to legislate embryo research regimes, from the late 1980s

---

1. "Recherche sur l'embryon," *Le Monde,* February 16–17, 1969.

2. The bioethicist Richard McCormick noted in 1978 that "Dr. Steptoe estimated that he had, in his research, gone through roughly 200 fertilized ova." A quarter-century later a widely cited survey concluded that about four hundred thousand surplus embryos had been stockpiled in the United States. See Richard A. McCormick, "Life in the Test Tube," *New York Times,* August 6, 1978, E17; and D. I. Hoffman et al., "Cryopreserved Embryos in the United States and Their Availability for Research," *Fertility and Sterility* 79, no. 5 (2003): 1063–69.

through the mid-1990s, terms of debate centered on the moral status of the embryo and the imperative of biomedical research were in place.

The Trajectory of Embryo Research

The late emergence of embryo debates during the final decades of the twentieth century was largely a function of the slow growth of scientific understanding. Through the nineteenth century, knowledge about human embryos and embryonic development was extraordinarily fragmentary. Long-running scientific, philosophical, and theological debates pitted two irreconcilable positions against each other: preformation and epigenesis. Without much evidence to go on, one side argued that the human being was preformed at the embryonic stage, while the other insisted that it gradually took shape in utero. During the late nineteenth and early twentieth centuries scientific discoveries gave a partial vindication to each side. The microscopic analysis of embryonic tissue revealed successive developmental stages, while advances in cell biology and genetics pointed to the existence of a hereditary program from fertilization onward. Embryologists turned increasingly to experiments with animal embryos kept alive in the laboratory to deepen their understanding. In 1935 Hans Spemann received the Nobel Prize for his work with amphibian embryos. A year later Gregory Pincus claimed to have achieved the first "test-tube" birth of a mammal—a rabbit.[3]

Initial efforts to culture human embryos in the laboratory date from this era. John Rock, a Harvard gynecologist with research support from the National Research Council and the Carnegie Foundation, began a series of human IVF experiments during the late 1930s. Over several years, he and his lab assistant, Miriam Menkin, exposed eggs removed from hysterectomy patients to sperm. In February 1944 they apparently achieved a breakthrough: fertilization and cleavage to the two- and three-cell stage. "We believe we have succeeded in these experiments," they wrote, somewhat tentatively, in the leading U.S. research journal, *Science*. Subsequent experts have argued that fertilization probably did not take place; the cells observed and photographed may have been the result of parthenogenesis, or egg division. At the time, the *Science* article and purported breakthrough drew only moderate media

---

3. For an overview of the history of the embryology controversy, see Jane Maienschein, *Whose View of Life?: Embryos, Cloning, and Stem Cells* (Cambridge: Harvard University Press, 2003); and Edward Yoxen, "Historical Perspectives on Human Embryo Research," in *Experiments on Embryos*, ed. Anthony Oakley Dyson and John Harris (London: Routledge, 1990), 27–41. On Pincus's claim, see "Life is Generated in Scientist's Tube," *New York Times,* March 27, 1936.

attention. In its end-of-year review of major scientific events of 1944, the *New York Times* reported the feat as fact but gave it only passing mention, noting simply that Rock and Menkin had "succeeded in fertilizing a human ovum (egg) in a glass flask for the first time in history."[4] There was no public outcry.

Human embryo experimentation did not make headlines again until the 1960s. Daniele Petrucci, an Italian gynecologist, claimed in 1961 to have successfully cultivated human embryos in the laboratory for twenty-nine days. He provided no evidence for his assertion but still garnered attention in the international press. While Petrucci made further fantastic claims—he alleged in 1964 that twenty-eight children had been born through IVF—a number of researchers in the United States and United Kingdom were pressing ahead with difficult and painstaking research designed to overcome two main obstacles: the extraction of eggs from infertility patients, and an effective culture medium for their union with sperm in the laboratory.[5] Among the researchers was Dr. Landrum Shettles of Columbia University, who claimed to have fertilized embryos that survived for up to six days during the 1950s and to have tried to initiate a pregnancy in the early 1960s. Shettles never published these early results and admitted years later that "fertilization was as rare as hen's teeth."[6] His self-description as a first IVF pioneer has never been convincingly corroborated.

By the mid-1960s, the U.K.-U.S. team of Robert Edwards of Cambridge University and Georgeanna and Howard Jones of Johns Hopkins University in the United States had made the most progress in overcoming the technological obstacles. Howard Jones maintains that their research led to the fertilization of at least one egg in Baltimore in the summer of 1965. Edwards dates the breakthrough later, after his subsequent return to the United Kingdom. In early 1968 he began to work with Patrick Steptoe, a gynecologist based in Oldham who had developed a successful laparoscopic technique for extracting eggs from patients.[7] With support from the Ford Foundation, a supply of

4. "Science in Review," *New York Times,* December 31, 1944; Loretta McLaughlin, *The Pill, John Rock, and the Church: The Biography of a Revolution* (Boston: Little, Brown, 1982), chap. 5. Rock later teamed up with Pincus to work on the successful development of oral contraceptives in the 1950s and 1960s.

5. On Petrucci, see Edward Grossman, "The Obsolescent Mother: A Scenario," *Atlantic 227, no. 5* (1971): 39–50. Strangely, a *New York Times* obituary gave credence to Petrucci's claims: "Dr. Daniele Petrucci, Kept Test Tube Embryo Alive," *New York Times,* October 16, 1973.

6. "Egg Fertilized Outside the Body; Aid to Infertile Women Foreseen," *New York Times,* March 4, 1966.

7. Ibid.; Robert G. Edwards and Patrick Christopher Steptoe, *A Matter of Life: The Story of a Medical Breakthrough* (New York: Morrow, 1980), chaps. 7–8.

eggs, and a newly developed culture solution, the Cambridge team achieved the first documented success of in vitro fertilization in March 1968. Edwards and Steptoe published their results in *Nature,* the leading British scientific journal, in February 1969. In a classic understatement, the article abstract referred to "certain clinical and scientific uses for human eggs fertilised by this procedure."[8]

The avowed goal of Edwards and Steptoe was the alleviation of infertility: the transfer of an embryo into a woman's uterus and the birth of a child. By 1970 they routinely succeeded in culturing embryos to the blastocyst stage—the phase several days after fertilization when implantation can take place—but they did not make their first, unsuccessful transfer attempts until the following year. Other international fertility specialists in pursuit of the same goal included the Joneses and Shettles in the United States and an Australian team under Carl Wood and John Leeton based in Melbourne. Two German teams working on infertility problems reportedly cultured early human embryos in Kiel and Hamburg in the mid-1970s, and a French team around Jacques Testart and René Frydman took up IVF work in 1977. While embryo transfer and the birth of healthy children was the primary goal of this research, Edwards and many of his colleagues also viewed work with embryos as a means to increase basic knowledge about infertility, human genetics, and congenital disease. Whatever the ultimate goal—infertility treatment, scientific knowledge, or some combination—this work involved the creation, observation, and subsequent discarding of embryos in the laboratory.[9]

The race to produce the world's first "test-tube baby" garnered world media attention intermittently during the decade after 1969. A 1970 series of news reports left the impression that Edwards and Steptoe were on the verge of a successful embryo transfer. In fact, they only began their transfer efforts in 1972. In 1973 reports of first, failed pregnancies surfaced in Australia and then the United Kingdom. In 1974 a British gynecologist, Douglas Bevis, claimed—falsely, as it turned out—to have facilitated the birth of twenty children by in vitro fertilization. It was not until July 1978, after years of effort and a series of failures, that Edwards and Steptoe first reached the goal. One of Steptoe's patients, Lesley Brown, gave birth to a child conceived in the laboratory, Louise. Her arrival sparked a global media sensation. Joy at

---

8. Edwards and Steptoe, *A Matter of Life,* 81–83; Robert G. Edwards, Barry D. Bavister, and Patrick C. Steptoe, "Early Stages of Fertilization In Vitro of Human Oocytes Matured In Vitro," *Nature* 221, no. 5181 (1969): 632.

9. For an early statement of these broader research agendas, including the possibility of preimplantation diagnosis for sex-linked diseases, see Robert G. Edwards and David J. Sharpe, "Social Values and Research in Human Embryology," *Nature* 231, no. 5298 (1971): 87–91.

the arrival of a healthy baby was joined with an initial surge of apprehension about the new technology's implications for "designer babies" and a eugenic future. Only with the rapid and successful march of IVF procedures around the world—first births in Australia in 1980, the United States in 1981, and France and Germany in 1982—and an awareness that genetic engineering was a far-off prospect did eugenic fears begin to fade.[10]

As the techniques spread, so did research with human embryos designed to improve the efficiency of IVF. The work was slow and painstaking, and limited by the short life span of embryos outside the uterus. Clinicians tended to transfer viable embryos to the patient, leaving mostly defective ones and perhaps some healthy ones for experimentation, with only a short window for research before they should perish. In this context embryo freezing techniques proved a revolutionary breakthrough. In the early 1980s, an Australia-based research team successfully applied cryopreservation methods recently developed with livestock to human embryos. By retrieving and fertilizing more eggs than were to be transferred to infertility patients, and freezing the remainder, doctors created a store of embryos for future treatments. The March 1984 birth of Zoe Leyland in Melbourne, the first child from a frozen and thawed embryo, generated worldwide attention.[11] Less remarked on at the time were the implications of freezing techniques for embryo research. A stock of frozen surplus IVF embryos was a potential bonanza for scientists interested not just in infertility research but in work on human genetics, embryonic development, congenital disease, and even stem cell and cloning research—horizons already visible to Edwards at the time.[12] The question of what might be done with embryos, under what conditions—first raised by the 1968 breakthrough—took on greater immediacy.

The Slow Emergence of Ethical Controversy

Given the rapid development of embryo and IVF research during the decade after 1968, it is striking how slowly the main contours of subsequent ethical controversies emerged. The idea that embryo research involves weighing the moral status of the embryo against the promise of biomedical research

---

10. On the IVF race of the 1970s, see Robin Marantz Henig, *Pandora's Baby: How the First Test Tube Babies Sparked the Reproductive Revolution* (Boston: Houghton Mifflin, 2004), 104–17.

11. Alan Trounson and Linda Mohr, "Human Pregnancy Following Cryopreservation, Thawing and Transfer of an Eight-Cell Embryo," *Nature* 305, no. 5936 (1983): 707–9.

12. Robert G. Edwards, "The Case for Studying Human Embryos and Their Constituent Tissues *In Vitro*," in *Human Conception In Vitro*, ed. Robert G. Edwards and Jean M. Purdy (London: Academic Press, 1982), 371–87.

was there at the outset, but the fledgling bioethics profession initially viewed embryo research mainly through the lens of eugenics, safety, and sexuality. Even the Catholic Church was slow to seize upon the moral status of the embryo and the parallel with the abortion issue. By the early 1980s, however, as IVF was spreading, public awareness was growing, and national bioethics committees had begun to take up the embryo research issue, arguments about the protection of life and the alleviation of suffering, later familiar, began to take shape.

Eugenic Anxieties

Through the 1970s, the tradeoff between the moral status of the embryo and the potential of biomedical research did not organize the ethical debate in Atlantic democracies. The first and most persistent frame was one of eugenic anxiety. A leading point of reference was Aldous Huxley's *Brave New World,* with its arresting image of ectogenesis—controlled gestation outside the womb. While the novel described selective breeding in a future, hierarchical society, it also evoked past myths about the danger of tampering with nature or "playing God"—the disobedience of Prometheus, the pride of Faust, or the hubris of Dr. Frankenstein.[13] As early as 1936, a *New York Times* editorial commented on Pincus's in vitro experiments with rabbit eggs under the heading "Brave New World." And in the wake of the Cambridge breakthrough three decades later, John Maddox, editor of *Nature,* acknowledged similar cultural anxieties. "These are not perverted men in white coats doing nasty experiments on human beings," he assured his readers, "but reasonable scientists carrying out perfectly justifiable research."[14]

Such anxieties were fed by breakthroughs in genetics and scientific and philosophical speculation about the genetic manipulation of human beings. During the 1920s biologist Stephen Haldane had mused about the possibility of "selective breeding"—and provided one of the main inspirations for Huxley's novel.[15] In the decades after World War II, technological progress suggested to many the imminent arrival of a new, truly scientific eugenics. Key breakthroughs—the discovery of the structure of DNA in 1953, the deciphering of its code in 1966, and its first successful recombination in the

---

13. On concerns about genetic engineering in connection with IVF, see Jon Turney, *Frankenstein's Footsteps: Science, Genetics, and Popular Culture* (New Haven: Yale University Press, 1998), 160–87.

14. "Brave New World," *New York Times,* March 28, 1936; "Human Egg Fertilized in Test Tube by Britons," *New York Times,* February 15, 1969.

15. J. B. S. Haldane, *Daedalus; or, Science and the Future* (New York: E. P. Dutton and Company, 1924).

laboratory in 1971—evoked the vision of a not-too-far-off future of human reproductive cloning and genetic enhancement. During the late 1960s, Joshua Lederberg, geneticist and Nobel laureate, spoke approvingly of the "engineering of human development," and a colleague, Robert Sinsheimer, saw "a turning point in the whole evolution of life." In ancient myths, Sinsheimer argued, "man was constrained by his essence. He could not rise above his destiny. This day we can envision that change and choice."[16] In the wake of the Cambridge IVF breakthrough, British DNA pioneer James Watson, in a widely cited 1971 article in the *Atlantic,* made the same point in a less celebratory tone. Now that "human embryological development need no longer be a process shrouded in secrecy," he argued, the possibility of genetic manipulation and enhancement in the laboratory—what he called "clonal man"—was on the horizon.[17]

Eugenic hopes and fears also characterized much of the response of the emergent bioethics profession to these scientific breakthroughs. During the late 1960s and early 1970s, moral theologians and philosophers increasingly focused their attention on the ethical implications of biomedical advances. New life-support technologies, for example, unleashed a debate about the definition of death and the morality of artificial means to extend it. The first successful organ transplants—particularly the first heart transplant in 1966—raised questions about the medical risk, cost, and the "naturalness" of the procedure. And safer abortion procedures, and the drive to legalize them, focused attention on the moral status of the fetus in relationship to the rights of the mother. Two new U.S.-based institutions served as focal points for scholars to debate these and other issues: the Hastings Center in New York (1969) and the Kennedy Institute of Ethics at Georgetown University (1971). As the bioethics profession gradually took shape, it remained a U.S.-dominated enterprise but also encompassed prominent scholars from around the world, including Hans Jonas, who had studied philosophy in Germany before emigrating to the United States, and Peter Singer in Australia.[18]

One initial response of bioethicists to the combination of IVF technology and recombinant DNA was a stress on the dangers of genetic manipulation.

---

16. Robert L. Sinsheimer, "Genetic Engineering: The Modification of Man," *Impact of Science on Society* 20, no. 4 (1970): 280.

17. James Watson, "Moving toward the Clonal Man," *Atlantic* 227, no. 5 (1971): 50–53.

18. Overviews of the emergence of bioethics as a profession include: Albert R. Jonsen, *The Birth of Bioethics* (New York: Oxford University Press, 1998); M. L. Tina Stevens, *Bioethics in America: Origins and Cultural Politics* (Baltimore: Johns Hopkins University Press, 2000); and Jennifer K. Walter and Eran P. Klein, *The Story of Bioethics: From Seminal Works to Contemporary Explorations* (Washington, DC: Georgetown University Press, 2003).

Paul Ramsey, a Protestant theologian based at Princeton University, launched a fierce attack on the dehumanizing potential of new reproductive technologies. In his book *Fabricated Man* (1970) he predicted that Huxley's vision of ectogenesis might "become a possibility within the next fifteen to fifty years." The book decried "the fascinating prospect of man's limitless self modification" as a catastrophic path to "species-suicide."[19] In a less apocalyptic and more secular register, another influential scholar, University of Chicago physician Leon Kass, made a related argument. Writing in *Science* in 1971, he saw the prospect "that man can for the first time recreate himself" and warned of the dehumanizing consequences of unfettered technological advance. C. S. Lewis's warning of the "abolition of man," he suggested, might become reality.[20]

Another group of bioethicists cast breakthroughs in embryo research and genetics in a thoroughly different light—not as a danger but as an opportunity. Echoing Lederberg and Sinsheimer, they celebrated what Ramsey and Kass feared: that mankind might take its evolution into its own hands. Joseph Fletcher of the University of Virginia was the most prominent and controversial. Unswervingly utilitarian in outlook, he conceived of genetic engineering, and any embryo research associated with it, as a means to root out birth defects and disease and improve the health of future generations. "We cannot accept the 'invisible hand' of blind natural chance or random nature in genetics," he argued in 1971. "To be men we must be in control. That is the first and last ethical word."[21]

The most comprehensive contemporary survey of the U.S. scene—and it was primarily in the United States that the debate took place in the early 1970s—underscored the prominence of the genetic manipulation theme. A report commissioned by Congress in 1972 made the remarkable prediction that "when the techniques for fertilization in the laboratory and genetic intervention can be combined with an effective artificial placenta, the potential for genetic engineering will have been achieved." The text identified "the major objection to in vitro experimentation" not as the moral status of the embryo but as "the ethics of performing experiments upon the 'unborn and unconceived'"—that is, the danger that science could damage children or alter human evolution. Of seven major publicly articulated concerns, the

---

19. Paul Ramsey, *Fabricated Man: The Ethics of Genetic Control* (New Haven: Yale University Press, 1970), 104–5, 151–60.

20. Leon R. Kass, "The New Biology: What Price Relieving Man's Estate?" *Science* 174, no. 4011 (1971): 779.

21. Joseph Fletcher, "Ethical Aspects of Genetic Controls: Designed Genetic Changes in Man," *New England Journal of Medicine* 285, no. 14 (1971): 83.

report highlighted three relating to genetic manipulation and dehumanization and three pertaining to better alternative technologies, informed consent, and safety issues. Only one referred to the moral status of the embryo. "Moral and legal questions about the disposition of defective experimental embryos," the report noted almost in passing, "are of serious concern."[22]

The new cadre of bioethicists did take up the problem of the moral status of the embryo, but it rarely figured centrally in their work during the early 1970s. In a widely cited 1972 article published in the *Journal of the American Medical Association,* Ramsey mentioned "zygote loss" as one of the potential objections to IVF. But in developing his own argument against IVF, he bracketed the question of "when the possible future human being is an actual human being."[23] In an overview of the state of the debate that same year, Kass also discussed the moral status of the embryo. "The embryos are clearly biologically alive," he argued. Given continuities in development in the early embryo, he maintained, "we had better face the question now and draw whatever lines need to be drawn." While he did raise the issue of the moral status of the embryo, Kass did not offer his own view of where the line should be drawn. He focused his attention on the potential for new technologies to distort our genetic makeup—the eugenic issue.[24] Ironically, Fletcher, who referred to the early embryo as simply "fallopian and uterine cell material," was among the first to raise the abortion parallel. He suggested in 1971 that if one believed that fully human life began with conception, embryo research amounted to the "killing of unborn babies."[25]

The Catholic Church and Human Sexuality

As it happened, the Catholic Church in the United States and around the world was slow to emphasize the link between embryo research and abortion. The Vatican did not openly censure John Rock, a practicing Catholic, for his in vitro experiments in the 1940s. It was his subsequent pioneering work developing oral contraceptives that drew ire from Rome. Similarly, when a Vatican spokesman attacked Petrucci's purported 1961 experiments as

---

22. Congressional Research Service, *Genetic Engineering: Evolution of a Technological Issue* (Washington, DC: Government Printing Office, 1972), 20, 34.

23. Paul Ramsey, "Shall We 'Reproduce'?: The Medical Ethics of In Vitro Fertilization," *Journal of the American Medical Association* 220, no. 20 (1972): 1347.

24. Leon Kass, "Making Babies: The New Biology and the 'Old' Morality," *Public Interest* 26 (1972): 32–33.

25. Fletcher, "Ethical Aspects of Genetic Controls." He developed his arguments more fully in *The Ethics of Genetic Control: Ending Reproductive Roulette* (Garden City, NJ: Anchor Books, 1974).

monstrous, he expressed more concern about a distortion of the natural process of procreation than about the fate of embryos. The official *L'Osservatore
Romano* opposed IVF research at the time because "God surrounded the act
of creation of a human being with the most supreme assistances of love, nature and conscience." A Vatican spokesman similarly condemned the news
of the first fertilization of an egg outside the womb, referring to "immoral
acts and absolutely illicit experiments." The fate of embryos created and discarded in IVF experiments garnered little attention or critique from Church
leaders.[26]

This initial, critical approach to efforts to combat infertility through IVF
reflected the Vatican's running concern with artificial technologies of procreation. The leading idea, hotly contested among Catholic moral theologians,
was that any intervention in the procreative process was against natural law
and God's will and deserved censure. IVF separated the unitive from the procreative dimensions of the sexual act—the joining of the flesh from openness
to conception. More broadly, it violated the sacred character of marriage as
an institution centered on, and open to, the gift of life. This logic was continuous with previous Church opposition to artificial insemination and artificial contraception. Pope Pius XII (1939–52) had campaigned vigorously
against artificial insemination, even within marriage. And, in 1968, Pope
Paul VI (1963–78) overrode his own theological commission and recon-
firmed the Church's traditional opposition to artificial birth control inside
as well as outside marriage. His 1968 encyclical *Humanae Vitae* condemned
human interference with "the laws that regulate the transmission of life."[27]
Moral theologians who had argued that marriage as a whole—and not every
physical act within it—should be open to life, suffered a sharp reversal.

Humanae Vitae had not explicitly ruled out IVF, a technology unknown
in 1968, and some Catholic moral theologians, including Charles Curran in
the United States and Franz Böckle in Germany, were open to new technologies that might help married couples to have healthy children. The birth of
Louise Brown demonstrated the diversity of views within the Church. The
bishops of England and Wales issued a supportive statement, as did the future
pope John Paul I, Cardinal Albino Luciani, who sent public congratulations
to the Brown family.[28] Openness to IVF for married couples was certainly

---

26. *L'Osservatore Romano,* quoted in Paul Ramsey, "Shall We 'Reproduce'?" 1347; "Vatican Scores
Experiments for Fertilizing Human Eggs," *New York Times,* February 16, 1969.

27. Paul VI, *Humanae Vitae: On the Regulation of Birth,* July 25, 1968, http://www.vatican.va/
holy_father/paul_vi/encyclicals/documents/hf_p-vi_enc_25071968_humanae-vitae_en.html.

28. Don O'Leary, *Roman Catholicism and Modern Science: A History* (London: Continuum,
2007): 223.

a minority position within the Church leadership. More typical was the response of Cardinal Joseph Höffner, president of the German bishops' conference, who insisted that "the Church rejects artificial fertilization most of all because such a manipulation mechanizes and depersonalizes marriage and marital love."[29] Through the 1970s, this anxiety about technology and sexuality, rather than a pro-life agenda and concern for the embryo, drove Catholic opposition to IVF. That would later change under Pope John Paul II (1978–2005).

Government, the Professions, and the Safety Issue

For government regulators, another set of key players in the emerging world of IVF, safety issues—not eugenics or sexuality—overshadowed the question of the moral status of the embryo. In contrast to speculation about future genetic manipulation or the ethics of human reproduction, safety posed a concrete governance challenge from an early stage. During the late 1960s and early 1970s, civil servants and professional associations following IVF developments were concerned, not with the fate of embryos created and discarded in the laboratory, but with the safety of embryo transfer for women and the health of any children resulting from the technique. Public funding agencies in the United Kingdom and the United States, the two early leaders in the field, proved initially skeptical. Their reflex was to urge caution and give precedence to animal experimentation. National medical associations in both countries were wary of the legal and public relations disaster that damaged IVF children might bring.

As embryo transfer appeared imminent in the early 1970s, Edwards and Steptoe found themselves under frequent attack from leaders within the nascent bioethics profession. Edwards relates a confrontation with Ramsey, Kass, and Watson at a September 1971 Washington, D.C., conference that brought matters to a head. Before a large audience Ramsey called IVF "unethical medical experimentation on possible future human beings" and therefore "subject to absolute moral prohibition." Kass argued that one could never be certain that babies "won't be born without defect." And Watson asked Edwards point blank: "What are we going to do with the mistakes?" A defiant Edwards emphasized the promise of IVF as an infertility treatment and, by his own account, won over the crowd.[30]

---

29. Quoted in *Frankfurter Rundschau,* August 20, 1978.
30. Edwards and Steptoe, *A Matter of Life,* 112–14.

The primacy of the safety issue was also evident within the governance structures of the medical profession. The American Medical Association and the British Medical Association expressed reservations about IVF as an infertility treatment, even as several international teams worked feverishly to accomplish it. In May 1972 the journal of the AMA called for "a moratorium on experiments that would attempt to implant an in-vitro conceptus into a woman's womb." The editors argued that the time was "clearly at hand" to convene experts across disciplines and professions to sort out thorny ethical issues.[31] The BMA was somewhat less cautious in its recommendations. It approved guidelines in March 1972 that allowed IVF experiments, but called for the formulation of safeguards to address safety concerns.[32] As in the United States, medical and scientific associations were open to public discussion but tended to oppose regulation or legislation that would abrogate professional self-governance. In France and Germany, where teams were also pursuing IVF research, no significant ethical and regulatory discussion had yet begun.

In the context of widespread concerns about safety, Edwards ran up against government regulation in a critical area—the provision of research funding. His work during the 1960s had been backed in large part by the U.S.-based Ford Foundation, a prominent supporter of infertility research. After the 1968 breakthrough, he submitted an application to the Medical Research Council (MRC), the main source for the public funding of science in the United Kingdom, to set up a laboratory and IVF clinic in Cambridge. The council turned down the proposal in April 1971, citing safety concerns. In his memoir, Edwards quotes from the rejection letter: "Serious doubts about ethical aspects of the proposed investigations in humans" made embryo transfer "premature in view of the lack of preliminary studies on primates and the present deficiency of detailed knowledge of the possible hazards involved." The MRC said nothing about the moral or legal status of human embryos; the safety issue was paramount. Edwards and Steptoe would have to continue to rely mainly on private research funds.[33]

---

31. "Genetic Engineering in Man: Ethical Considerations," *Journal of the American Medical Association* 220, no. 5 (1972): 721.

32. Alun Jones and Walter F. Bodmer, *Our Future Inheritance: Choice or Chance?* (London: Oxford University Press, 1974), 41.

33. Quoted in Edwards and Steptoe, *A Matter of Life,* 106. On the insignificance of the moral status of the embryo in these early controversies, see Jennifer Gunning and Veronica English, *Human In Vitro Fertilization: A Case Study in the Regulation of Medical Innovation* (Aldershot, UK: Dartmouth, 1993), 6. A historical analysis published in 2010 revealed that one of the outside reviewers did raise the embryo status issue, but his concerns did not drive the MRC decision. See Martin H. Johnson

IVF researchers seeking funds in the United States also ran up against the safety issue. As early as November 1970 the National Institutes of Health (NIH), the main source of public funding for research in the life sciences, were reportedly skeptical of the safety of embryo transfer.[34] In 1972 revelations about the abuses of black American airmen in a syphilis study in Tuskegee, Alabama, raised public and congressional concerns about human-subject protections to a new level.[35] Around the same time, a funding application from Vanderbilt University's Pierre Soupart to generate embryos in order to examine genetic abnormalities that might arise as a result of IVF provided a concrete occasion for the Department of Health, Education, and Welfare (HEW)—NIH's bureaucratic parent—to formulate regulatory guidelines. After consulting with some twenty ethical and scientific experts, HEW opted in November 1973 against "research involving the implantation of human ova fertilized in the laboratory" until animal experiments had demonstrated the safety of the technique. It further stipulated that "all proposals for research involving human in vitro fertilization" should be subject to ethical review. Revised in 1974 and made official in 1975, HEW guidelines made public funding of human embryo research dependent on approval by a future Ethics Advisory Board.[36]

The Embryo Comes into Focus

The first decade of research with embryos was not devoid of controversy surrounding their moral status. As early as February 1969 a *Times* of London editorial supportive of Edwards's work nevertheless noted "the possible objection that if life begins at fertilization" a "potential human being is being sacrificed." The editor of the *New Scientist,* one of the two most influential scientific publications in the United Kingdom, asked that same month: "What happens to the embryos which are discarded at the end of the day? Washed down the sink?"[37] In the years that followed, however, such

---

et al., "Why the Medical Research Council Refused Robert Edwards and Patrick Steptoe Support for Research on Human Conception in 1971," *Human Reproduction* 25, No. 9 (2010): 2166.

34. "A Step Nearer to the Test-Tube Baby," *New York Times,* November 1, 1970.

35. The scandal spurred Congress to set up the National Commission for the Protection of Human Subjects of Biomedical and Behavioral Research, which issued binding recommendations for human-subjects research legislation in 1975.

36. For an overview of early U.S. regulation of embryo and embryo-transfer research, see Albert R. Jonsen, Robert M. Veatch, and LeRoy Walters, eds., *Source Book in Bioethics: A Documentary History* (Washington, DC: Georgetown University Press, 1998), 88–102.

37. "Implications of the Test-Tube Embryo," *Times* (London), February 16, 1969; Donald Gould, quoted in "Britons Develop Test Tube Eggs," New York Times News Service, February 15, 1969.

questions were overshadowed by concerns about eugenics, procreation, and safety. Only as those concerns faded in relative importance did the embryo finally move to center stage. The greatest impetus for debate was the work of national ethics committees that assembled experts from different fields, took testimony from different points of view, studied the issues in depth, and published recommendations.

The Ethics Advisory Board

The first of these was the Ethics Advisory Board. President Jimmy Carter's first secretary of health, education, and welfare, Joseph Califano, constituted the EAB in September 1977 and charged it both with assessing Soupart's application and developing broader criteria for the approval of embryo-related research projects. Under the chairmanship of James Gaither, a San Francisco lawyer, the board took up its work without any public fanfare. It was made up of thirteen experts drawn mainly from the worlds of science and medicine, and included two influential bioethicists, Sissela Bok, a medical ethicist at Harvard, and Richard McCormick, SJ, a moral theologian based at Georgetown. Just as the EAB was quietly beginning its work the news of Louise Brown's birth in July 1978 transformed its mandate. In September Califano extended the committee's remit beyond developing criteria for re-search funding to include "scientific, ethical, legal and social issues surrounding human *in vitro* fertilization and embryo transfer in general." The reference to embryo "transfer" indicated a continued central concern with IVF as a reproductive technology and its implications for sexuality and the family. Califano also mentioned safety issues—whether IVF techniques could "damage the resulting fetus and lead to abnormal children"—and eugenic concerns about "selective breeding" and "attempts to control the genetic makeup of offspring."[38] Gradually, however, the moral status of the embryo would emerge as the paramount issue.

Between its meeting in May 1978 and its final report in May 1979, the EAB held eleven public hearings across the country. It received over two thousand letters and petitions from citizens and more than three hundred inquiries and statements from members of Congress. Its deliberations were informed by a series of expert presentations and commissioned papers that examined IVF from a variety of scientific and ethical perspectives. (Gaither

---

38. Joseph A. Califano, *Inside: A Public and Private Life* (New York: PublicAffairs, 2004), 350–51. Also quoted in "HEW Urged to Lift Ban on Test-Tube Birth Studies," *Washington Post,* September 16, 1978.

invited Edwards and Steptoe to appear before the board, but they declined, citing their desire not to get mixed up in the U.S. debate.)[39] In keeping with Califano's charge, the EAB focused many of its hearings and presentations on issues of surrogacy and family relations, safety, and genetic manipulation. But the specific task at hand—developing criteria for the approval of research projects—led the members inexorably to a discussion of when and under what conditions an embryo might be manipulated or destroyed in the laboratory.

On this central question, two broad arguments framed the EAB's deliberations, one utilitarian, the other deontological in inspiration. In line with the former, the philosopher Samuel Gorovitz used his testimony to develop an argument later made most famous by the Australian bioethicist Peter Singer—that the early embryo could not feel pain and could therefore be used up in useful research without moral qualms. For Gorovitz it was the "onset of the capacity for sentience" that marked the critical juncture, "sometime prior to quickening but well after the embryonic stage." He rejected the argument that embryos represented "potential persons," insisting that "any pair of sperm and egg have the potential, if all goes well, to become a genetically specific adult person."[40] Clifford Grobstein, a prominent professor of biological science and public policy, echoed this reasoning in his submission to the board, insisting that in the early weeks after fertilization "human cells, tissues or organs that have no reasonable prospect of possessing or developing sentient awareness" are "human materials rather than human beings or persons."[41]

In his testimony before the EAB, Leon Kass most clearly articulated a deontological view that the embryo should not be instrumentalized, whatever the social utility. He argued that "after fertilization is complete, there exists a new individual, with its unique genetic identity, fully potent for the self-initiated development into a mature human being, if circumstances are cooperative." Fertilization, for Kass, produced not just an early stage of human life but "potentially a mature human being, if all goes well." In their less-guarded moments, he pointed out, scientists supportive of research recognized that they were dealing with individual human lives. With some relish he cited an interview Edwards had given after the birth of Louise Brown: "The last time I saw *her, she* was just eight cells in a test tube. *She* was beautiful *then,* and she's still beautiful *now*"(emphasis added by Kass). Although not persuaded that the embryo was a person with human rights, Kass viewed it as

39. Gunning and English, *Human In Vitro Fertilization,* 18.
40. Ethics Advisory Board, *Report and Conclusions: HEW Support of Research,* chap. 3, 5–6.
41. Ibid., chap. 24, 4–5.

an individual human being worthy of protection. Noninvasive experiments were defensible, but the "most potentially interesting and useful," which would kill the embryo, were morally problematic. "Either we accept certain great restrictions on the permissible uses of embryos," he claimed, "or we deliberately decide to override—though I hope not deny—the respect due to embryos."[42]

In its deliberations, the board sought to navigate a path between these two contrasting philosophical perspectives. Its unanimous recommendations, published in May 1979, endorsed federal funding for research designed to further IVF. "The conduct of research involving human *in vitro* fertilization designed to establish the safety and effectiveness of the procedures," it asserted, "is ethically acceptable under certain conditions." Those conditions were fairly restrictive: donor consent from "lawfully married couples," appropriate human-subject protections, transparency, and provisions that the sought-after knowledge be "not reasonably attainable by other means." A further condition concerned the time frame: "No embryos will be sustained in vitro beyond the stage normally associated with the completion of implantation (14 days after fertilization)." In an effort to find a middle way between the permissive and restrictive perspectives articulated by Gorovitz and Kass, the board noted that "the human embryo is entitled to profound respect," but added that "this respect does not necessarily encompass the full legal and moral rights attributed to persons." While the board did not rule out funding embryo research not related to infertility, it refused to endorse such research in principle, calling for case-by-case review.[43]

Most striking about these recommendations was their unanimity, particularly the endorsement of McCormick, a leading Catholic moral theologian. His support for embryo research under some circumstances pointed to the relatively open nature of the Catholic debate through the 1970s. While the Church's teaching office or Magisterium had affirmed in a 1974 instruction on abortion that the embryo be treated as a person, it had not spoken definitively on whether it was in fact a person from the moment of conception. For centuries many in the Church had followed St. Thomas Aquinas in conceptualizing the development of the embryo and fetus through several phases, with ensoulment posited at around forty days. In 1869 new knowledge about continuity in early embryonic development contributed to Pius IX's insistence that the embryo was presumed to have a soul from its origins.

---

42. Ibid., chap. 2, 5–6, 10–11. The testimony was later reprinted in Leon R. Kass, *Toward a More Natural Science: Biology and Human Affairs* (New York: Free Press, 1985), chap. 4.

43. Ethics Advisory Board, *Report and Conclusions,* chap. 6, 101, 103, 107, 111.

But a century later, during the 1960s, another scientific discovery—that most embryos failed to implant and perished naturally—revived the debate. The prominent Jesuit scholar Karl Rahner asked in 1967 whether "today's moral theologian" could maintain that an individual human life begins at conception, given that "that 50 per cent of all fertilized female cells" fail to implant naturally. Would that theologian "be able to accept that 50 per cent of all 'human beings'—real human beings with 'immortal' souls and an eternal destiny—will never get beyond this first stage of human existence?" Given a "serious positive doubt about the human quality of the experimental material," Rahner cautiously suggested, "the reasons in favor of experimentation might carry more weight, if considered rationally, than the uncertain rights of a human being whose very existence is in doubt."[44] In 1972, leading Catholic moral theologian Bernard Häring responded to discoveries about twinning up to two weeks after conception with the suggestion that in the early embryo, "individualisation seems not yet to have reached that point which is indispensable to personhood."[45]

A critical issue for Catholic moral theology was not when the embryo becomes fully human, a person, or ensouled, but the point from which it deserved protection. The 1974 instruction on abortion expressly left aside "the question of the moment when the spiritual soul is infused," but nevertheless insisted that the embryo was a human individual not to be manipulated or destroyed: "From the time that the ovum is fertilized, a life is begun which is neither that of the father nor of the mother, it is rather the life of a new human being with his own growth." A life, in this argument, "would never be made human if it were not human already" from its beginnings. Vatican teaching, then, was that the embryo was not necessarily a person from conception, but that it should be *treated* as a person—because life is a gift of God and we cannot know for certain when ensoulment takes place. The conclusion followed from Church teaching against abortion from before St. Thomas through Pius IX to Paul VI—that it was wrong to deliberately destroy human life at any stage of its development.[46]

---

44. Karl Rahner, "The Problem of Genetic Manipulation," in *Theological Investigations: Writings of 1965–1967* (New York: Crossroad, 1976), 226, 236. On the evolution of the Church's position, see David Albert Jones, *The Soul of the Embryo: An Enquiry into the Status of the Human Embryo in the Christian Tradition* (New York: Continuum, 2004).

45. Bernard Häring and Gabrielle L. Jean, *Medical Ethics* (Slough, UK: St. Paul Publications, 1972), 80. For another influential contribution to the debate, see Joseph Donceel, "Immediate Animation and Delayed Hominization," *Theological Studies* 31, no. 1 (1970): 76–105.

46. Footnotes mentioned that Pius XII had insisted in 1944 on protection of life "in the embryonic stage" and that, two decades later, the Second Vatican Council had insisted that "life must be safeguarded with extreme care from conception." Sacred Congregation for the Doctrine of the Faith,

This official Catholic position was well known to McCormick and, at least in outline, to the other members of the EAB. But the board asked one of the Vatican's critics, Charles Curran, to provide testimony from a Catholic perspective. A well-known moral theologian and social liberal, Curran had publicly dissented on *Humanae Vitae,* affirming contraception within marriage and upholding the right of theologians to disagree with the Vatican. "In my judgment the Catholic moral theologian must always acknowledge the unique hierarchical teaching office and respect its teaching," he told the board, "but at times can and even should dissent from its teaching." Echoing Rahner's views on embryo loss and Häring's point about twinning, Curran argued that the early embryo was not, in fact, an individual deserving of protection. For him, "truly human life should be judged to be present two to three weeks after conception"—that is, after successful implantation. Curran did grant the early embryo "some value and importance," but did not consider it the equivalent of person with rights. It followed that embryo research for worthy ends was permissible.[47]

McCormick was sympathetic to Curran's general outlook. He, too, was a critic of *Humanae Vitae* and a supporter of the theologian's freedom to dissent in an effort to move the Church closer to the truth. But he also found himself in a difficult position as a Catholic clergyman on a committee making recommendations to the U.S. government. According to press reports about a critical two-day EAB meeting in February 1979, McCormick initially argued that all fertilized embryos be transferred into the uterus and that none be left for experiments. In language reminiscent of the Church's official position, he told reporters: "When we have doubts about the claim that life makes on us, we must give life the benefit." The following day, however, he found himself isolated on the committee and confronted with a powerful counterargument—that if one supported IVF one must also support research necessary to keep it safe. McCormick shifted his position, opting to support some research as a "necessary evil." He later wrote that he had made the switch "not without fear and trembling."[48] As it happened, McCormick did

---

"Declaration on Procured Abortion," November 18, 1974, http://www.vatican.va/roman_curia/congregations/cfaith/documents/rc_con_cfaith_doc_19741118_declaration-abortion_en.html.

47. Ethics Advisory Board, *Report and Conclusions,* chap. 4, 4–5, 15–16. For background on Curran's approach to ethics, see Charles E. Curran, *Moral Theology: A Continuing Journey* (Notre Dame, IN: University of Notre Dame Press, 1982).

48. "Test-Tube Baby Study Debated by HEW Panel," *Washington Post,* February 3, 1979; "Test-Tube Baby Study Wins Approval," *Washington Post,* February 4, 1979; Richard A. McCormick, *The Critical Calling: Reflections on Moral Dilemmas since Vatican II* (Washington, DC: Georgetown University Press, 2006), 206.

not earn any official Church censure, a sign of the relative openness of the Catholic debate at the time.

The Warnock Committee in the United Kingdom

By the time national ethics committees in Europe took up embryo research during the early and mid-1980s technological advances had begun to shift the ethical debate. The rapid spread of proven IVF technology, from Britain and Australia to the United States, Germany, France, and beyond dampened concerns about its safety for mother and child. Continued research would be necessary to improve the efficiency of IVF as an infertility treatment, but with its technical successes and social acceptance, researchers could now turn to other research programs, including the struggle against congenital disease and deeper knowledge about early human development. The prospect of research not directly related to infertility—raised but not addressed by the Ethics Advisory Board in the United States—added a new twist to the bioethical debate and increased its public visibility. The question of how to balance the moral status of the embryo against the promise of biomedical research grew more controversial.

In the United Kingdom, home to the most drawn-out and influential public debate of the 1980s, Edwards's own speculations about the future of embryo research catalyzed the controversy. In January 1982 he appeared to claim in a television documentary that freezing technologies then in development would enable "embryo banks" for experiments.[49] The image of industrialized embryo farming, however unrealistic—and unintended—sparked an outcry in the media and calls within Parliament for an investigative committee. When that September the London *Times* subsequently reported Edwards's claim to have experimented with spare embryos on nonfertility-related projects, the British Medical Association issued a harsh condemnation. Edwards sued for defamation, and the *Times* followed with a remarkable apology that affirmed Edwards's claim that his work was "confined to procedures directly serving currently accepted infertility treatment" and that Edwards had not done "anything concealed from the public eye."[50] The BMA retracted its criticism. Whatever the truth of the matter, public and media attention focused on the ethics of embryo research for the first time.

---

49. "Human Embryo Banks Proposed," *Times* (London), January 28, 1982.

50. "Medical Fears of Live Organ Banks," September 29, 1982; "Dr. Robert Edwards," *Times* (London), October 4, 1982. For Edwards's account, see Robert G. Edwards, *Life before Birth: Reflections on the Embryo Debate* (New York: Basic Books, 1989), 83–87.

In recognition of the importance of the issue secretary of state for social services Norman Fowler announced the formation of the Committee of Inquiry into Human Fertilisation and Embryology in July 1982. Under the leadership of the philosopher Mary Warnock, the Warnock committee (as it came to be known) had sixteen members, mainly doctors and scientists, including one Anglican moral theologian, Anthony Dyson. Over the course of two years the committee grappled with a range of issues raised by IVF, including embryo research, surrogate motherhood, and the regulation of fertility services. It received submissions of evidence from more than two hundred organizations representing scientific, religious, business, and patient-advocacy groups, and sifted through about seven hundred letters from the public. Like the Ethics Advisory Board several years earlier, it heard the testimony of a variety of experts and engaged in heated internal deliberations, many leaked to the press.[51]

The Warnock report, published in June 1984, made two sets of detailed recommendations on the regulation of IVF as an infertility treatment and on embryo research. Its support for an IVF regulatory framework and opposition to surrogate motherhood were relatively uncontroversial. The moral and legal status of the embryo, by contrast, was hotly contested and defied unanimity. As Warnock put it later, "all the other issues we had to consider seemed relatively trivial compared with" embryo research, "concerned as it is with a matter which nobody could deny is of central moral significance, the value of human life." The final report, which Warnock crafted herself, noted "a wide diversity in moral feelings, whether these arise from religious, philosophical or humanist beliefs." Its recommendations were articulated in a pragmatic spirit, reflecting Warnock's own philosophical background and previous experience as head of a government commission grappling with the educational needs of disabled children. While herself relatively unconcerned about the moral status of embryos, she acknowledged a general sense that "there must be *some* barriers that are not to be crossed, *some* limits fixed, beyond which people must not be allowed to go."[52]

In seeking to determine the acceptable range of embryo research, the Warnock committee majority distanced itself from the "strictly utilitarian view," according to which, "as long as the embryo is incapable of feeling pain, it is argued that its treatment does not weigh in the balance." This was the

---

51. On the formation of the committee and its work, see Mary Warnock, *Nature and Mortality: Recollections of a Philosopher in Public Life* (London: Continuum, 2003), chap. 2.

52. United Kingdom, Department of Health and Social Security, *Report of the Committee of Inquiry into Human Fertilisation and Embryology* (London: Her Majesty's Stationery Office, 1984), 2–3.

sentience criterion advanced by Gorovitz in 1978 and later most forcefully articulated by the Australian philosopher and bioethicist Peter Singer. The committee majority also rejected the opposite perspective that the embryo deserved absolute protection as a potential or actual human being or person. It aligned itself with the view that embryos deserved "some added measure of respect beyond that accorded to other animal subjects" but insisted that such respect "cannot be absolute." In seeking to find a middle ground between diametrically opposed pro- and antiresearch positions, Warnock acknowledged that "biologically there is no one single identifiable stage in the development of the embryo beyond which the in vitro embryo should not be kept alive." In keeping with her pragmatism, however, Warnock steered the committee toward a cutoff date beyond which research would be illegal: "Some precise decision must be taken, in order to allay public anxiety."[53]

Without directly referencing the work of the Ethics Advisory Board in the United States, the Warnock committee also settled on the fourteen-day marker as the cutoff for research. The rationale for this juncture was not, as it had been for the EAB, the completion of implantation, but rather the full individuation of the early embryo. Guided by the ideas of Anne McLaren, a leading developmental biologist and committee member, the majority emphasized the point after which the embryo could not split into twins. Häring had suggested the ethical significance of individuation a decade earlier. McLaren now added a new twist: the formation of a fully individual embryo, she argued, coincided with the formation of a "primitive streak," the first outlines of a future nervous system. The existence of an identifiable structural change led McLaren to suggest that the embryo proper only took form at around two weeks. Warnock seized on this argument about the lesser moral status of early embryos to advance a forceful case for experiments with spare embryos from IVF treatments, but also for the creation of embryos expressly for research, "mainly for the alleviation of infertility and the prevention of hereditary disease."[54]

In the end, Warnock mustered majority support behind both positions, but fell well short of unanimity. Thirteen out of sixteen members acknowledged that experiments were essential, "if advances in treatments and medical knowledge are to continue," even as they insisted they did "not want to see a situation in which human embryos are frivolously or unnecessarily used in research." The minority of three, led by a prominent Catholic physician, John Marshall, articulated a secular argument from potential personhood—that it

---

53. Ibid., 62–65.
54. Ibid., 67.

was "wrong to create something with the potential for becoming a human person and then deliberately to destroy it." In her memoir, Warnock relates her frustration at not being able to persuade Marshall, a Catholic supporter of IVF, that research was necessary to improve the safety and reliability of the procedure. The very argument that had persuaded the Jesuit Richard Mc-Cormick to endorse the EAB recommendations for infertility-related research did not prevail five years later, when IVF had shown its safety and effectiveness in practice.[55]

Warnock was even less successful in achieving unanimity for the creation of embryos expressly for research. In her view there was no moral difference between embryos originally created for fertility treatments and those created for research. But only nine out of sixteen members concurred that "to prohibit the generation of embryos specifically for research would severely curtail the range and scientific validity of research." Marshall, now joined by Dyson, the committee's moral theologian, and five other members, rejected this reasoning. "Whatever the handicap to scientific progress," they maintained, "it would be morally wrong to bring human embryos into being solely for the purpose of research."[56] When the Warnock report was published in July 1984, its support for the creation of embryos for research generated the most public and political controversy.

An important contrast with the experience of the EAB five years earlier was the mobilization of the churches around the committee's work and its conclusions. Pope John Paul II's opposition to abortion and insistence on the protection of unborn life from conception, most forcefully articulated from 1982 onward, encouraged Church leaders in the United Kingdom, where Catholics represented about 10 percent of the population, to vehemently oppose all embryo research. While some Catholic moral theologians, including John Mahoney in the United Kingdom (who testified before the Warnock committee), Richard McCormick in the United States, and Norman Ford in Australia, remained open to research necessary to advance IVF therapies for married couples, they now confronted a more vocal antiresearch Church leadership. The Catholic Bishops' Conference of England and Wales, for example, submitted its views to the Warnock committee, insisting that "the human embryo is not a 'potential human being' but a human being with potential." On publication of the committee report, Cardinal Basil Hume, the most senior English Catholic leader, voiced "profound moral objection" to the "destruction of human individuals." The Bishops' Conference called the

---

55. Ibid., 62–90.
56. Ibid., 68, 67.

Warnock committee conclusion that research be allowed for up to fourteen days, to be followed by the destruction of the embryo, "shameful."[57]

The Anglican leadership was more divided. While the Church of England had steadily lost adherents over the postwar decades, it maintained a high visibility in the media and through the representation of bishops in the House of Lords. Running battles over women's ordination, abortion, and other social issues had heightened internal tensions between liberals and social conservatives close to the Church of England's evangelical wing. Such divisions were nothing new, as the Archbishop of Canterbury was traditionally first among equals rather than an authoritative leader. Nevertheless, the Church as a whole did project public positions on critical issues of the day through its Board for Social Responsibility, which was dominated by progressives. In its submission for the Warnock committee, the Church of England sketched out a generally proresearch position, favoring infertility-related projects (as late as forty days after fertilization!) but opposing "the culturing of human embryos for the sole purpose of research."[58]

A key member of the board was the Anglican theologian George Dunstan, who forcefully articulated a Christian case for research, insisting that the idea that truly human life begins at conception was a relatively recent innovation. Before Pius IX's 1869 declaration on protecting life from conception onward, he argued, only killing a "formed" fetus had been equated with murder. "Uterine life has to be protected at some point," Dunstan acknowledged. But "if we put that point too early, forbidding observation and experimental use of pre-implantation embryos in the early stages of cell division, we shall inhibit much useful research of potential human benefit." While the board accepted Dunstan's idea of a forty-day cutoff for research—when "electrical impulses associated with nerves can be detected"—it did not endorse his support for the creation of embryos for research.[59]

Once the Warnock report was published, the board adopted the fourteen-day cutoff point as appropriate for research but maintained its opposition to the deliberate creation of embryos, because "to bring into being embryos purely for research and then to destroy them would be to treat the origins of

---

57. Quoted in Patrick J. O'Mahony, *A Question of Life: Its Beginning and Transmission* (London: Continuum, 1990), 117, 119, 120.

58. Church of England Board for Social Responsibility, "Warnock Evidence," February 24, 1983 (manuscript), 3.

59. Gordon Dunstan, "The Moral Status of the Human Embryo: A Tradition Recalled," *Journal of Medical Ethics* 10, no. 1 (1984): 38–44. Edwards later referred to Dunstan as a "new-found friend" among otherwise hostile religious voices. Robert G. Edwards, "The Bumpy Road to Human In Vitro Fertilisation," *Nature* 7, no. 10 (2001): 1092.

human life with scant respect."[60] The February 1985 General Synod of the Church of England narrowly rejected the board's generally positive stance on Warnock. There followed six months of intense internal debate, during which the board published a fuller explanation of its gradualist understanding of the full humanity of the embryo in a report entitled *Personal Origins*. At the July 1985 synod the majority lined up behind the board's position. A prominent representative of the emergent proresearch majority, the Bishop of York, accepted "with a heavy heart" that if "we are going to relieve the problems of many desperately sad people, we have to go down the road which the Warnock Report spells out for us."[61]

Like the Anglican Church, the rest of Britain's Protestant communities were divided on the moral status of the embryo and the permissibility of research. The Church of Scotland's Board for Social Responsibility, traditionally more conservative than its Anglican counterpart, echoed the official Catholic stance, insisting that the embryo be protected from fertilization onward. Its response to Warnock accused the committee of "utilitarian" thinking and insisted, like the Catholic bishops in England and Wales, that the embryo was not simply "potentially human" but already fully human with the potential to develop further. It was wrong to balance the life of the embryo against the "public good." Other Protestant groups, including the Methodists, were more supportive of research. In its submission to the Warnock committee, the Methodist Division for Social Responsibility agreed that some research on human embryos should be permitted to advance fertility treatments. And in July 1985 a Methodist Church leadership conference recognized "the positive contribution that IVF has made to the life of many childless couples."[62]

The Jewish community in the United Kingdom, like its counterpart in the United States, played a relatively minor role in the developing public ethical controversy. Like Protestantism, Judaism was home to a wide variety of perspectives and lacked any central teaching authority. In his testimony before the EAB, Sid Leiman, an expert on Jewish ethics, had argued that the tradition included resources for both supporters and opponents of embryo research. "Some Jewish authorities rule that during the first 40 days of gestation, the conceptus has little or no moral status, and therefore could be aborted for any

---

60. Church of England Board for Social Responsibility, *Human Fertilisation and Embryology: The Response of the Board of Social Responsibility of the General Synod of the Church of England to the DHSS Report of the Committee of Inquiry* (London: Church of England, 1984), 16.

61. Church of England, *Report of Proceedings: General Synod, February 1985* (London: Church of England, 1985), 326; Board for Social Responsibility, *Personal Origins* (London: Church House Publishing, 1985).

62. Quoted in O'Mahony, *A Question of Life*, 123–24.

constructive medical purpose, such as medical experimentation," he told the board. At the same time, "other, more stringent Jewish authorities accord moral status from the moment of conception on." In the British context, the visibility of Jewish perspectives was raised by the role of Immanuel Jakobovits, who was both chief rabbi and an expert in Jewish medical ethics. In his submission to the Warnock committee, Jakobovits affirmed the value of research in principle, as God calls humankind to heal the world. But he opposed the deliberate creation of embryos for research because it was, as he later put it, "repugnant to generate human life solely for the purpose of destroying it, to produce embryos only to destroy them by experiments."[63]

Germany and the Benda Commission

The first national German bioethics committee took up work in mid-1984, just as the Warnock committee was completing its report. The slower onset of such deliberations in the Federal Republic was, in part, a function of the relative underdevelopment of IVF technology: the first German IVF child was not born until April 1982. But the pace of the technology is not the whole answer. Human embryo research was undertaken in Germany from the mid-1970s onward, particularly in Hamburg and Kiel, without public outcry.[64] Germany would later become known for its strict opposition to all embryo research. But its postwar German political culture was broadly *supportive* of scientific freedom as a break with the legacy of Nazi state control and manipulation of science and medicine.[65] The German Research Foundation (DFG), a federally funded body with a high degree of autonomy, was slow to back any government-led ethical or regulatory oversight of embryo research. A month after the birth of Louise Brown the influential newsweekly *Die Zeit* opined that "in contrast to the Anglo-Saxon countries at least some of our researchers feel left alone by the research organizations of the Federal Republic when it comes to the pressing ethical problems of their work."[66] In February

---

63. Ethics Advisory Board, *Report and Conclusions,* chap. 6, 7. See Immanuel Jakobovits, *Jewish Medical Ethics: A Comparative and Historical Study of the Jewish Religious Attitude to Medicine and Its Practice* (New York: Philosophical Library, 1959). He was quoted in "The Day in Politics: Lords Reject Curbs on Embryo Experiments," *Guardian,* March 7, 1990.

64. In a July 1978 interview Klaus Thomsen related how human eggs had been fertilized in his Hamburg clinic without reaching the implantation stage. "Purer Zufall oder eine echte Hoffnung?" *Der Spiegel,* July 31, 1978.

65. On the importance of scientific freedom in German legal and constitutional thought, see Deutsche Forschungsgemeinshaft, *Forschungsfreiheit: Ein Plädoyer für bessere Rahmenbedingungen der Forschung in Deutschland* (Weinheim, Ger.: VCH, 1996), chaps. 1–3.

66. "Auf dem Weg zum Bio-Babel?" *Die Zeit,* August 14, 1978.

1979, as the Ethics Advisory Board was forging ahead in the United States, a DFG position paper noted that "neither the Science Foundation nor the Medical Association is considering the creation of a central ethics commission at this time."[67]

Outside of scientific and regulatory circles, however, the birth of Louise Brown raised the Nazi legacy in a different and more enduring way—less in support of scientific freedom than in opposition to anything that smacked of eugenics. For example, a leading philosopher, Robert Spaemann, published a February 1979 essay in *Die Zeit* entitled "Concentration Camp Doctors Also Used Biology." Noting science's ambition to push the boundaries of knowledge, he asserted that the "question of utmost importance is how we evaluate the goals for which mankind uses biology." He added: "The concentration camp doctors also used biology, but their goals were appalling." The theme reappeared in the German media over the next decade. In 1988, for example, sociologist Ulrich Beck published an essay in *Der Spiegel* entitled "Eugenics of the Future." Referring to research with embryos and the prospects of genetic engineering, he asserted: "Almost everyone is working, researching, and propagating the new technologies in the conviction that the racial theories and their eugenic insanity disappeared once and for all in the mass graves of the Nazi terror." In its place he raised the specter of a liberal eugenics based on scientific freedom and an ambition to improve, if not perfect, the human race.[68] These arguments, taken up again by the philosopher Jürgen Habermas at the turn of the new millennium, were not foreign to American, British, and French debates. But they resonated particularly strongly in Germany.

The birth of the first German IVF child, Oliver Wimmelbacher, in an Erlangen clinic in April 1982, sparked a first systematic examination of the ethics of IVF and embryo research at the national level. After preliminary consultations with experts in fall 1983, the Federal Ministries of Justice and of Research and Technology appointed a working group in May 1984 to examine the ethical and legal issues raised by IVF, genome research, and gene therapy, and to propose regulatory guidelines. Ernst Benda, a former president of the German Constitutional Court, chaired the group, whose nineteen members included scientists, philosophers, legal scholars, and representatives of the country's major scientific and medical organizations and the Catholic and Lutheran churches. The Benda Commission met nine times between September 1984 and November 1985. Its work was less publicized than that of the EAB

---

67. "Babys im Glas," *Die Zeit,* February 16, 1979.

68. "Auch KZ-Ärzte benutzten Biologie," *Die Zeit,* February 16, 1979; "Eugenik der Zukunft," *Der Spiegel,* November 21, 1988.

or the Warnock committee—with one interesting exception. Benda himself published an essay in January 1985 entitled "The False Path to Bred Humans." He singled out possible interventions in the human genome as an abomination that "violates human dignity and is no different than the well-known human experiments under the Nazis." If science were allowed to set its own limits, he argued, a "scientific totalitarianism would be the result."[69]

The working group report, published in November 1985, reflected the dominant lines of the German debate during the early 1980s—how to weigh concerns about scientific freedom against the dangers of genetic engineering. While acknowledging the centrality of the right to scientific freedom, the report cited the Constitutional Court's view that "the freedom of science does not take absolute precedence over the conflicting values protected by the Constitution," in particular that "human dignity is inviolable" (Article 1). This would have to be borne in mind, the report argued, "in particular when attempts are made to change the genetic material of an egg fertilized in vitro by means of genetic engineering in order to breed an allegedly 'better' human being." Eugenic anxieties underlay the working group's call for a complete ban on cloning, chimeras, or genetic modification and its only cautious support for IVF as a reproductive technology. In setting out these recommendations, the Benda Commission did not explicitly reference the Nazi legacy. But the mention of eugenic concerns in the report, and Benda's own published views, point to the long shadow of the Nazi past.[70]

Despite this historical frame, the Benda Commission majority did not recommend a total ban on embryo research. Its approach to the embryo did emphasize its humanity more than did the reports of the EAB and the Warnock committee. A key passage referred to the embryo as an "individual human (and hence not purely vegetative) life" and as "a human subject in its early form of development" that should "be accorded a status deserving legal protection and which hence must not be made the object of arbitrary manipulation." This language was decidedly deontological, not utilitarian in its thrust; it kept the focus on the status of the embryo itself, and not on different stages of embryonic development. But the careful phrasing here, particularly the reference to *arbitrary* manipulation, did leave the door open to some research. The embryo's moral status was not deemed absolute; its life could "be carefully weighed against the paramount importance of modern genetic research for the health of mankind"—an early, if still vague, reference to the idea of an "ethic of healing." Limits were necessary, but not absolute.

---

69. "Der Irrweg zum gezüchteten Menschen," *Rheinischer Merkur,* January 26, 1985.

70. Benda Commission, *Working Group on In Vitro Fertilisation,* 5–6.

"Respect for human life demands that experiments" be restricted to "cases in which such research can make a decisive contribution to the life of other human beings."[71]

In allowing for research under exceptional circumstances for "medical findings of great value" (*hochrangige Ziele*), the Benda report seemed to allow for a wider range of research goals than had either the EAB or Warnock reports, with their emphasis on combating infertility. The Benda report included favorable mention of experiments that encompassed "the development of techniques for the diagnosis and treatment of cancer as well as of countless diseases of the immunological system and hereditary diseases." In most other respects, however, the German recommendations were more restrictive. In addition to including explicit condemnation of cloning and genetic modification, the commission insisted on limiting the number of embryos produced in an IVF cycle to those to be implanted, so as to reduce the number of surplus embryos potentially available for research. And perhaps most significantly, a "clear majority" of the committee insisted that "as a matter of principle, the procreation of human embryos for research purposes is not justifiable," a sharp contrast with the majority opinion on the Warnock committee.[72]

The Catholic and Protestant representatives on the committee, Franz Böckle and Martin Honecker, did not dissent from the report's recommendations. Böckle, a leading German moral theologian, was a well-known critic of the Church's official teaching on human sexuality. Like Richard McCormick in the United States, he had opposed *Humanae Vitae*'s restrictions on contraception within marriage and had welcomed IVF as a way for couples to deal with childlessness. As early as 1982, two years before he joined the Benda Commission, Böckle had acknowledged that some research with embryos had been necessary to develop IVF as an infertility treatment.[73] As the representative Lutheran on the committee, Honecker did not have to deal with any official teaching office. His Evangelical Church in Germany (EKD), which like the Catholic Church enjoyed state recognition and financial support, was internally divided over embryo research. In November 1985, just as the Benda Commission was completing its work, a group of leading Protestant theologians, including Honecker, published

---

71. Ibid., 6–7, 58.
72. Ibid., 57–58.
73. "Das Maß bleibt Menschlichkeit: Die Technik eilt der sittlichen Bewertung voraus," *Rheinischer Merkur*, June 11, 1982. See also Franz Böckle, ed., *Der Umstrittene Naturbegriff: Person, Natur, Sexualität in der kirchlichen Morallehre* (Düsseldorf: Patmos, 1987).

their reflections on IVF and embryo research under the title, "The Dignity of Early Life." While their statement asserted that "human life is a gift of God and has a special dignity," it articulated a Christian rationale for IVF as a fertility treatment for married couples and did not make the moral status of the embryo absolute. From the moment of conception, a key passage read, a "*future* person is established" (emphasis added). While it critiqued "misuse and experiments with embryos," the statement did not explicitly rule out research designed to improve IVF treatments.[74]

The most striking trend in Germany, in sharp contrast to the United States and the United Kingdom, was the degree of negative *secular* reaction against the Benda Commission's openness to research. The sole dissent to the Benda report's recommendation of embryo research under certain conditions echoed Benda's own ruminations about the shadow of history. Peter Petersen, a committee member and physician concerned about the eugenic applications of the new technologies, cited the zoologist Adolf Portmann, for whom humanity was "on the brink of a dark contemporary era that envisions the biotechnological breeding of human beings." The cautious stance first fully articulated by the postwar bioethics pioneer Hans Jonas—a "heuristics of fear" that insisted on the critical examination of the possible negative future implications of any new technology before its adoption—was echoed in the secular media. In two major stories, *Der Spiegel* charged that Benda had been duped by scientists into backing embryo research with eugenic implications under some circumstances and recounted how protesting students at the University of Tübingen had thrown flour on him, chanting: "We are afraid of genetic technology, but no one is listening to us!"[75] This current of antitechnology anxiety would shape the course of embryo politics in Germany over the next decade.

France's National Consultative Ethics Committee

The French debate, like the German one, developed more slowly than in the United States and the United Kingdom. The country's scientific leadership had greeted news of the first fertilization of a human egg in the laboratory with a certain skepticism. A *Le Monde* editorial had admired the technological prowess of Edwards's work but suggested that it was "for the moment only

74. Evangelische Kirche in Deutschland, *Von der Würde menschlichen Lebens: Eine Handreichung der EKD zur ethischen Urteilsbildung* (Hannover: Evangelische Kirche in Deutschland, 1985).

75. "Gentechnik—der Weg zur Menschenzüchtung?" *Der Spiegel,* December 2, 1985; "Von Menschenzüchtung treibhaft fasziniert," *Der Spiegel,* January 13, 1986.

interesting for researchers." As late as 1977, the renowned French geneticist Jerome Lejeune doubted prospects for IVF children in the foreseeable future. And when Louise Brown did arrive the following year, *Le Monde* showcased experts who emphasized the experimental nature and low success rates of the new technique.[76] A real French debate only started in February 1982, when the embryologist Jacques Testart and the gynecologist René Frydman helped to bring the first French IVF child, Baby Amandine, into the world. While the media echo was generally positive, coverage also highlighted concerns about eugenic abuses of the new technologies and its implications for family and kinship relations.

In response to these concerns, and to a range of other bioethics issues ranging from organ donation to genetic testing, President François Mitterrand announced the formation and duties of a national ethics committee in February 1983. The National Consultative Ethics Committee (CCNE) was the first of its kind in the world—a permanent body that would meet in regular session to analyze issues and advise the government. It was not only more enduring than the Ethics Advisory Board and the Warnock and Benda committees; it also had a larger membership and staff and a clear institutional link to the government through its affiliation with the ministries of health and research. The CCNE initially encompassed some nineteen specialists in ethics and law, fifteen scientists and physicians, and a representative from each of the "principal philosophical and religious families," including a philosopher and a leading Catholic, Jewish, and Protestant thinker, and later a Muslim representative as well.[77] The visibility of the CCNE was heightened by the prestige of the president's office and the prominence of the revolutionary French Enlightenment and human rights tradition. Mitterrand told a bioethics conference in January 1985 that in a new scientific and technological era, France could again assume the leading role "it played at the end of the 18th century, when it was necessary to invent liberty and democracy."[78]

Between 1984 and 1986, under the leadership of the bioethicist and physician Jean Bernard, the CCNE published several recommendations bearing on the problem of embryo research. In its first opinion from May 1984, devoted to work with fetal tissue, the committee called for the "unequivocal recognition

---

76. *Le Monde,* February 16–17, 1969; *Le Monde,* July 27, 1978.

77. For an overview of subsequent adjustments in the composition and precise competences of the CCNE, see http://www.ccne-ethique.fr/founding.php.

78. Quoted in Robert Walgate, "Human Embryology: France Seeks Policy in Haste," *Nature* 313, no. 6005 (1985): 728.

of the human character of the embryo" as a "potential human person." Another opinion that October, on artificial reproductive technologies in general, elaborated: "This potentif human person, whatever one believes about the time when consciousness is awakened, deserves respect, if only because the embryo is a fragment of the human heritage." Both these core ideas—of potential human personhood and of a shared humanity—constituted a deontological approach to the moral status of the embryo. The emphasis was not on sentience or on the first precursors of a nervous system in the "primitive streak" but instead on the embryo as a potential free human being and its relationship with wider human society. More than once the CCNE would distinguish its approach from "utilitarian" alternatives—a veiled reference to the Warnock committee and its pragmatic approach embodied in the fourteen-day marker as a convenient way to distinguish between permissible and impermissible research vistas.[79] French scientists and philosophers who identified more closely with the pragmatic and utilitarian approach that dominated in the United States and the United Kingdom did not shape the work of the CCNE through the 1980s.[80]

The most extensive elaboration of the ethical stakes was the committee's December 1986 opinion on "research and use of in-vitro human embryos." In marked contrast to previous commission reports—EAB, Warnock, and Benda—the committee sought to develop an overarching analytical framework for its analysis. "Without deciding as to the ultimate foundation of the person, but with regard to the diversity of metaphysical or philosophical options," the report read, "the Committee is of the opinion that the foundation of and due respect for the embryo can be based on the rule of reason." Echoing the formulations in its first opinions, the ethical section of the report stated that "from the time it has been conceived the human embryo is a being and not a possession, a person, not a thing nor an animal. It should be considered as a would-be subject, as an 'other' of which we cannot dispose and whose dignity defines limitations for the power or control of others."[81]

The committee had some difficulty in translating this abstract reasoning into concrete recommendations for legislation. A ban on the creation of embryos expressly for research was relatively unproblematic. In such cases,

---

79. Comité Consultatif National d'Ethique (CCNE), "Opinion on Sampling of Dead Human Embryonic and Fetal Tissue for Therapeutic, Diagnostic, and Scientific Purposes," May 22, 1984, http://www.ccne-ethique.fr/docs/en/avis001.pdf; "Opinion on Ethical Problems Arising out of Artificial Reproductive Techniques," October 23, 1984, http://www.ccne-ethique.fr/docs/en/avis003.pdf.

80. For an overview of French schools of bioethics, see Pierre-André Taguieff, "L'espace de la bioéthique: Esquisse d'une problématisation," *Res Publica* 21 (1995): 30–37.

81. CCNE, "Opinion on Research and Use of In-Vitro Human Embryos."

"human embryos would purely and simply be used as tools or objects, and human dignity, which must override scientific research, would not be respected." The issue of surplus IVF embryos was more difficult. The committee expressed the hope that "research will allow fertilisation only of the necessary oocytes for transfer for the birth of a future child." But what about the fate of cryopreserved embryos where they existed? Might one use embryos destined to perish for experiments designed to advance biomedical knowledge? Here, a majority of the CCNE reached a conclusion similar to that of the EAB and Warnock committees: research might be permitted, under restrictive conditions, to battle infertility and support the development of IVF. The majority called its recommendation a "lesser of two evils" and coupled it with the call for a three-year moratorium on the genetic diagnosis of embryos, for fear of its possible eugenic abuses. The CCNE critiqued the fourteen-day marker as arbitrary—without mentioning Warnock by name—and suggested that it would not "be necessary to keep embryos beyond the time of transfer, that is around seven days."[82]

How did the CCNE get from its emphasis on the humanity of the embryo to an allowance of research under some circumstances? It did not make an argument about the stages of embryonic development and the formation of the primitive streak, but began with its relational status. "However embryonic the person may be in the first stages of the human being, our relationship to the embryo is a true reflection of the morality of our relationship to the person as such, to the social community as a whole and even to humanity itself." For the committee majority, the key relationship for the embryo was between it and its would-be parents: "The embryo is not only a human being because it has a specific genome. It is a human being, also, by virtue of parental intention to procreate and the meaning of this project in the family history."[83] This logic culminated in an ethical distinction between the idea of embryos with and without a "parental project." The committee majority suggested that those in the latter category, surplus IVF embryos with no prospect of implantation, had lesser moral status and might be sacrificed in worthy experiments for the greater social good.

Lucien Sève, a leading philosopher and member of the CCNE from its inception in 1983 through 2000, most fully elaborated this relational approach to moral status. He had a strong influence on the December 1986 opinion and authored a 1987 study, published under the auspices of the committee, entitled "Biomedical Research and Respect for the Human Person."

---

82. Ibid.
83. Ibid.

Though himself a Marxist—and a representative of secular philosophy on the committee—he was wedded to the deontological idea of respecting the embryo as a potential person. For Sève, fertilization, and not an arbitrary cutoff point at one or two weeks, was the beginning of an individual human life. To use human life "purely as a means" through "the production of research embryos" was repugnant. It did not follow, however, that all research was taboo. It should only be allowed under limited circumstances, where the "parental project" had been abandoned and where exceptional biomedical promise might be demonstrated.[84]

This emergent approach, with its focus on the importance of human relationships and the presence or absence of a "parental project," was not unanimously shared within the CCNE. Jean Gelamur, the Catholic representative on the committee, refused to endorse the December 1986 report. A leading publisher and member of the Pontifical Commission on Social Communications, he centered his dissent on "the respect due the embryo." In keeping with France's secular political culture, however, he did not invoke the Church's official teaching about treating the embryo as a person from fertilization onward. He referred instead—within the dominant, secular idiom—to the embryo's potential humanity and relationship with society. Because it treats "the embryo as an instrument," research was morally impermissible. Instead of respecting "the autonomy of embryonic life, research creates a relationship of omnipotence over the embryo," he wrote. A leading Catholic layman and friend to Archbishop Jean-Marie Lustiger of Paris, Gelamur nevertheless phrased his objections to embryo research in secular philosophical terms.[85]

The secular cast of the French ethical debate was in part a function of Christianity's institutional weakness. In contrast to Germany, where the Catholic and Protestant churches enjoyed some official recognition and state support, the historically dominant French Catholic community had been stripped of most of its privileges with the 1905 law establishing a strict separation of church and state. The law reduced the Church's property holdings and influence on educational and social policy, strengthening the secularism of the revolutionary tradition. Religious freedom was guaranteed, but religion was largely relegated to the private sphere. The Church had a public

---

84. Lucien Sève, *Pour une critique de la raison bioéthique* (Paris: Jacob, 1994), 100–104. The title was a direct reference to Kant's critiques of pure and practical reason. On related French debates, see François Gros and Gérard Huber, eds., *Vers un anti-destin?: Patrimoine génétique et droits de l'humanité* (Paris: Jacob, 1992).

85. CCNE, "Opinion on Research and Use of In-Vitro Human Embryos." In his dissent Gelamur did not oppose IVF as an infertility treatment for married couples as long as "all procreated embryos can be transferred in satisfactory conditions" and none should remain for research.

voice, represented its views to government, and enjoyed some privileges—for example, the public funding for parochial schools that President Charles de Gaulle had instituted at the dawn of the Fifth Republic in 1958. But Catholics—still a majority of the population, despite steady declines in levels of belief and practice over the postwar decades—were not expected to bring their religious identities or religious arguments into public debate. Gelamur respected this norm, as did the prominent Jesuit bioethics expert Patrick Verspieren, who publicly critiqued the CCNE's core claim that the moral status of an embryo should depend on a "parental project."[86]

French Protestants, much less influential and visible than Catholics, were generally strongly proresearch in their orientation. They were less important numerically than in Germany, the United Kingdom, or the United States and divided into a wide range of different denominations. The Federation of French Protestants (FPF) was a loose amalgam of groups that did, on occasion, articulate shared positions on matters of public policy. In the case of embryo research, this involved a self-reflexive distancing from the position of the Catholic Church. Two years of deliberation by an FPF working group led to the completion of a document offering "elements for reflection" that was endorsed by the larger body in January 1987. The federation was open to research with surplus embryos, as long as it was carefully regulated. It should not proceed "without safeguards" and without the prior demonstration of scientific and medical promise. Olivier Abel, a leading French moral theologian and future Protestant CCNE representative, noted pointedly: "We do not share the Catholic obsession about not losing anything, so that the least embryo is saved."[87]

The legacy of Nazism and eugenics played a significant role in the French debate, though nothing approaching its centrality in the German one. The experience of occupation, collaboration, and resistance had left deep scars in France, reinforcing the traditional emphasis on human rights in its political culture. The preamble to the Fourth Republic's 1946 constitution emphasized the principle of "human dignity." Historical concerns about eugenics informed Mitterrand's decision to form the CCNE in 1983, within a year of the birth of Baby Amandine. And the committee's reports repeatedly warned of the dangers of eugenic abuses. In the mid-1980s, Testart's decision to end his collaboration with Frydman and publish the first of a series of polemics

86. Patrick Verspieren, "Les fécondations artificielles: A propos de l'Instruction romaine sur 'le don de la vie,'" *Etudes* 366, no. 5 (1987): 607–19.

87. "La Fédération protestante de France publie des 'réflexions' sur la procréation artificielle," *Le Monde*, March 21, 1987; Olivier Abel, "Biologie et éthique," *Etudes théologiques et réligieuses*, no. 2 (1987): 208.

against the dangers of a new eugenics sparked a running ethical, philosophical, and historical debate.[88]

The Polarization of Ethical Controversy

By late 1986, national ethics committees on both sides of the Atlantic had taken up the problem of embryo research and come to some broadly similar conclusions. First the Ethics Advisory Board, then the Warnock committee, the Benda Commission, and the CCNE had asserted that the early embryo warranted respect as a developing form of human life but that it might be used up under carefully defined circumstances in research designed to support IVF and, in some cases, other worthy medical goals. There were significant differences across the committees. The greatest divergence was the Warnock committee's endorsement, by a narrow margin, of the creation of embryos expressly for research. Another concerned the rationale for limiting research at around fourteen days—the formation of the "primitive streak" (United Kingdom) or the implantation stage (United States and Germany)—and the particular French connection between the moral status of the embryo and the status of a "parental project." Overall, though, the message of the reports was broadly similar: to assert both the moral status of the embryo and to endorse some research under particular circumstances, especially to advance IVF. During the decade after 1986 it became increasingly difficult to maintain this intermediate stance.

Up through the first phase of work by national ethics committees, controversy surrounding embryo research was heated but not particularly polarized. A great diversity existed within the most influential Christian communities, and the Vatican had not yet reached a definitive position on IVF as an infertility treatment or on embryo research to support it. Catholic moral theologians including McCormick in the United States and Böckle in Germany could sit on ethics committees, endorse research, and not face censure. Leading Protestant groups in the United Kingdom and France tended to favor research, while their counterparts in Germany and the United States, to the extent they grappled with the issue at the time, tended toward skepticism. The Jewish community, a significant voice in the United States and the United Kingdom, was broadly supportive of research, but also marked a plurality of perspectives. Nonreligious actors, too, endorsed a variety of different perspectives on research. Most scientists, doctors, and secular bioethicists

---

88. Jacques Testart, *L'oeuf transparent* (Paris: Flammarion, 1986); and, as editor, *Le magasin des enfants* (Paris: Editions François Bourin, 1990).

tended to acknowledge the question of the moral status of the embryo but place more emphasis on the promise of research. Very few endorsed the view that the embryo, because it could not feel pain, had no moral status at all—a perspective put forward memorably by Peter Singer with his 1982 claim that the early embryo was "far inferior to a tadpole in respect of all characteristics that could be regarded as morally relevant."[89]

From the mid-1980s onward, as media coverage increased and legislatures took up the issue of regulation, this fluid religious-secular constellation began to harden and greater polarization set in. Two simultaneous developments during the late 1980s played a role. The first, and most important, was a growing Catholic and evangelical tendency to link the embryo research issue to a broader pro-life agenda. With the publication of the Vatican instruction *Donum Vitae* in February 1987, John Paul II created a direct link between embryo research and abortion, closing off the lively intra-Catholic debate that Karl Rahner had first sparked two decades earlier. A second development, partly a reaction to the first, was a stronger effort of scientists and some secular bioethicists to downplay the moral status of the embryo and tout the healing potential of research. A key to this strategy was the ultimately unsuccessful effort to introduce the term "pre-embryo" to refer to the preimplantation embryo, suggesting its inferior moral status. On both sides of the Atlantic, many participants in the sharpening controversy adhered neither to the absolute Catholic/evangelical position nor to the strong proresearch alternative. But as policy debate heated up, the sharply opposed positions drew greater public and media attention.

The Church's Restrictive Turn

After years of preparation, the Vatican published *Donum Vitae* ("The Gift of Life") in February 1987, with the full title "Instruction on Respect for Human Life in Its Origin and on the Dignity of Procreation." Authored by the Congregation for the Doctrine of the Faith, which was then led by Cardinal Joseph Ratzinger, the future Benedict XVI, the document reiterated traditional positions on procreation and human dignity in light of technological developments. Its complete rejection of IVF as a fertility treatment reprised the argument of *Humanae Vitae* (1968) against technological interventions in the procreative process. It was the explicit prohibition of IVF for married couples that drew the most media attention. The *New York Times,* for example, printed the instruction verbatim across four

---

89. Peter Singer and Helga Kuhse, *Unsanctifying Human Life: Essays on Ethics* (Oxford: Blackwell, 2002), 185.

pages, and *Le Monde* covered it and the criticisms it unleashed in depth over several days.[90]

Less remarked on at the time, but decisive for embryo politics, was *Donum Vitae*'s extended argument about the full humanity of the embryo and categorical condemnation of all embryo research. Part of its reasoning was theological: human life was sacred from its beginning because it involved the "creative action of God." But the instruction also asserted the existence of "recent findings of human biological science which recognize that in the zygote resulting from fertilization the biological identity of a new human individual is already constituted." Like the Vatican's 1974 instruction on abortion, *Donum Vitae* stopped short of declaring that the personhood of the embryo was a scientific fact: "Certainly no experimental datum can be in itself sufficient to bring us to the recognition of a spiritual soul." Pointing to the existence of a genetic program from fertilization onward, however, it saw science providing "a valuable indication for discerning by the use of reason a personal presence at the moment of this first appearance of a human life." The instruction finished this key passage with a rhetorical question: "How could a human individual not be a human person?"[91]

If the Vatican did not declare that the embryo *was* a person—a common misconstrual of its position—it did insist that it be *treated* as one. Human life was a gift of God to be nurtured from its beginnings and never willfully destroyed: "The human being is to be respected and treated as a person from the moment of conception; and therefore from that same moment his rights as a person must be recognized, among which in the first place is the inviolable right of every innocent human being to life." What of surplus IVF embryos, destined to die in any case without any potential future as children? Here, too, the Church took a restrictive stance, referring to any freezing of embryos as an attack on their human dignity. Those "called 'spare' are exposed to an absurd fate, with no possibility of their being offered safe means of survival which can be licitly pursued." However tragic the existence of surplus embryos, the Vatican argued, their lack of a future did not justify killing them in experiments. Letting them die was the best alternative.[92]

---

90. "Text of Vatican's Doctrinal Statement on Human Reproduction," *New York Times,* March 11, 1987; "Un document du Vatican Jean-Paul II s'oppose à la procréation artificielle: La tentation néopaienne," *Le Monde,* March 10, 1987.

91. Congregation for the Doctrine of the Faith, *Instruction on Respect for Human Life in Its Origin and on the Dignity of Procreation: Replies to Certain Questions of the Day,* February 22, 1987, http://www.vatican.va/roman_curia/congregations/cfaith/documents/rc_con_cfaith_doc_19870222_respect-for-human-life_en.html.

92. Ibid.

From one point of view, *Donum Vitae* was not a new departure. It was in line with *Humanae Vitae's* rejection of artificial reproductive technologies, even for married couples. And it reiterated the view, first fully formulated in the 1974 "Instruction on Procured Abortion," that the embryo should be treated as a person from conception. What was new was the incorporation of the embryo research issue into a pro-life agenda. A first major step in this direction, four years into John Paul II's papacy, had been a 1982 address to the Pontifical Academy of Sciences that critiqued, "in the most explicit and formal way, experimental manipulations of the human embryo," because "a human being from conception to death cannot be exploited for any purpose whatsoever."[93] *Donum Vitae* was a key part of the pope's developing campaign against the "culture of death," which would reach its fullest expression in his 1995 encyclical *Evangelium Vitae* ("The Gospel of Life"). The strong link between the embryo research and abortion issues, once picked up by the Catholic hierarchy and their pro-life allies, contributed to a polarization of controversy, particularly in the United States.

The pope was only partially successful in drawing the Catholic debate about IVF and embryo research to a close. In France, for example, some Catholic hospitals offering IVF as an infertility treatment to married couples protested *Donum Vitae* and continued to offer services. Claude Sureau, a prominent Catholic physician, was more blunt; he called the Vatican instruction both a surprise and a "source of great sadness for Catholics."[94] There was similar protest in Catholic circles in the United States, the United Kingdom, and Germany. On the issue of embryo research, there was less open protest. Priest-scholars who had indicated support for embryo research under some conditions, such as John Mahoney in the United Kingdom and Norman Ford in Australia, now assented to the new teaching. Mahoney, a British Jesuit, had testified before the Warnock committee in support of a gradualist approach to personhood. Ford had published a comprehensive analysis of the scientific and ethical issues that marshaled the available evidence in favor of the fourteen-day stage as a significant developmental marker. They now endorsed the pope's view that, even if personhood cannot be established as a scientific fact, the embryo should always be treated as a person.[95] In the

---

93. John Paul II, "Address of John Paul II to Members of the Pontifical Academy of Sciences," October 23, 1982, http://www.vatican.va/holy_father/john_paul_ii/speeches/1982/october/documents/hf_jp-ii_spe_19821023_pont-accademia-scienze_en.html.

94. Claude Sureau, quoted in Michel Chartier et al., *Aux débuts de la vie: Des catholiques prennent position* (Paris: Editions La Découverte, 1990). Along similar lines, see Böckle, *Der Umstrittene Naturbegriff*, 63–66.

95. Mahoney's 1984 book lost the Church imprimatur originally bestowed on it. See John Mahoney, *Bio-ethics and Belief: Religion and Medicine in Dialogue* (London: Sheed and Ward, 1984);

United States, McCormick was less compliant. Recalling that the Ethics Advisory Board and the Warnock report had sought to cut a middle path between absolute protection of the embryo and support for valuable research, he lamented that "the Holy See has not shown that kind of restraint."[96]

During the late 1980s and early 1990s—an era of what McCormick called the "chill factor" in moral theology—a new generation of Catholic thinkers centered in the United States, including Carol Tauer, Lisa Sowle Cahill, and Margaret Farley, continued to support embryo research under some conditions.[97] In a series of publications these and other scholars echoed Dunstan's argument that the Church had abandoned an earlier, more adequate understanding of the gradual development of the full humanity of the fetus. They insisted that the embryo be treated with respect but were open to worthy experiments with surplus IVF embryos destined to die in any case. Most rejected the creation of embryos for research as an illicit instrumentalization of human life, but some refused to make sharp distinctions between them and surplus IVF embryos and supported research in both cases, under carefully restricted circumstances.[98]

The Catholic Church's turn in a more restrictive direction was followed by powerful Protestant groups in the United States and Germany, but not in France or Britain. In May 1982 the largest evangelical denomination, the Southern Baptist Convention, extended its pro-life position beyond an insistence on the "sanctity of life" to the claim that "both medical science and biblical references indicate that human life begins at conception."[99] Like the Vatican, the Southern Baptist Convention gradually folded embryo research into its antiabortion stance. The Evangelical Church in Germany, which had articulated support for research to advance IVF at the time of the Benda report in 1985, took a restrictive turn in the years that followed. A major statement endorsed by a synod in November 1987, "On Respect for Life," urgently warned "against 'destructive' research on so-called surplus

Norman M. Ford, *When Did I Begin?: Conception of the Human Individual in History, Philosophy, and Science* (Cambridge: Cambridge University Press, 1988).

96. Richard A. McCormick, "The Ethical and Religious Challenges of Reproductive Technology," *Cambridge Quarterly of Healthcare Ethics* 8 (1999): 550.

97. See, for example, Carol A. Tauer, "The Tradition of Probabilism and the Moral Status of the Early Embryo," *Theological Studies* 45, no. 1 (1984): 3–33; Lisa Sowle Cahill, "The Embryo and the Fetus: New Moral Contexts," *Theological Studies* 54, no. 1 (1993): 124–42; and Lisa Sowle Cahill and Margaret A. Farley, *Embodiment, Morality, and Medicine* (New York: Springer, 1995).

98. Carol A. Tauer, "Embryo Research and Public Policy: A Philosopher's Appraisal," *Journal of Medicine and Philosophy* 22, no. 5 (1997): 437–38.

99. Southern Baptist Convention, "Resolution on Abortion and Infanticide," May 1982, http://www.sbc.net/resolutions/amResolution.asp?ID=20.

IVF embryos and the creation of embryos for research," even in pursuit of "medical findings of great value"—a deliberate attack on a key formulation of the Benda Commission. "Even in the stage of a first cell division," the report claimed, "the embryo possesses the same ethical quality as a fetus in early pregnancy."[100] The evolution of the Protestant position enabled the formation of an ecumenical antiresearch alliance for the legislative battles that lay ahead.

In the United Kingdom and France, by contrast, most Protestants followed mainline U.S. denominations in carving out a proresearch position at odds with the Catholic Church. In the United States, Episcopalians, Methodists, and the United Church of Christ had endorsed IVF and some embryo research by the late 1980s. As early as 1971, for example, the UCC had insisted that the embryo be treated with respect, but not as a person. The National Council of Churches issued a policy statement in 1986 along these lines, which expressed concern about any "careless treatment of embryos" but was open to research to combat infertility.[101] While internally divided, the Church of England remained mainly aligned with the proresearch stance carved out by its Board for Social Responsibility in the 1980s. French Protestant leaders, the most openly scornful of *Donum Vitae,* insisted on greater room for scientific freedom in opposition to Rome's top-down efforts to impose its restrictive position within the Church and society.

The Secular Case against Strictures on Research

If many Catholics and evangelicals dissented from the compromise recommendations of various national ethics committees—to allow embryo research, but under restricted circumstances—many scientists and their allies in the secular bioethics community were skeptical as well, for very different reasons. All four national committees had suggested some support for research, but had done so cautiously, according the embryo some respect as a developing form of human life. For researchers and bioethicists more concerned about biomedical progress than about the moral status of the embryo this was a painful compromise. As the Catholic Church hardened its position, the media picked up on the debate, and as politicians prepared to

100. Evangelische Kirche in Deutschland, "Zur Achtung vor dem Leben—Maßstäbe für Gentechnik und Fortpflanzungsmedizin," November 6, 1987, http://www.ekd.de/EKD-Texte/achtungvordemleben_1987.html.

101. National Council of Churches, *Genetic Science for Human Benefit* (New York: NCCCUSA, 1986).

take up legislative controversy, research proponents sought to lay out a more forceful case against strictures on research.

Part of the effort to shift the debate in a more research-friendly direction was the introduction of the new term "pre-embryo" to describe the embryo before fourteen days. This was, in part, a shift in scientific terminology. There were, as research advocates pointed out, good scientific reasons to distinguish among different phases of early embryonic development—movement from the zygote to the morula to the blastocyst. Clifford Grobstein, writing in 1979, had been the first to characterize the embryo during these preimplantation phases as a "preembryo."[102] As ethical and political controversy surrounding human embryo research picked up during the mid- and late 1980s, research advocates seized on the term "pre-embryo" as a way to support moral distinctions between different stages of embryonic development. If the early embryo was not an embryo after all, harming it raised fewer ethical concerns.

The term popped up on both sides of the Atlantic around the same time. In June 1985 the United Kingdom's Voluntary Licensing Authority (VLA), set up to oversee IVF clinics and embryo experiments in the absence of central government legislation, adopted the term.[103] Its most influential proponent was Anne McLaren, a research scientist, a member of the Warnock committee, and a close adviser to Mary Warnock herself. Around the same time, the American Fertility Society, the major U.S. association for IVF professionals, endorsed the term. In guidelines published in 1986 by a committee that included McCormick and Grobstein, the AFS defined the "pre-embryo" as "a living, genetically unique entity with a statistical potential to implant." The embryo, by contrast, was a "far more complex" precursor to "the rapidly growing and maturing fetus." Another leading professional association, the American College of Obstetricians and Gynecologists (ACOG), took up the term, and a joint committee of both organizations set up in January 1991 adopted it as well.[104]

The debate about the appropriateness of the term "pre-embryo" was most heated in the pages of the prestigious British journal *Nature*. Daniel Davies, a former editor, was a critic. "If research on embryos were an uncontentious matter, and if scientists were generally of the opinion that the new terminology

102. Clifford Grobstein, "External Human Fertilization," *Scientific American* 240, no. 6 (1979): 66.

103. On the origins of the term "pre-embryo" in the U.K. context, see Gregory Bock and Maeve O'Connor, *Human Embryo Research—Yes or No?* (London: Tavistock, 1986), 141–51.

104. Excerpts from the 1986 AFS report of the Ethics Committee of the American Fertility Society, "Ethical Considerations of the New Reproductive Technologies," in *Source Book in Bioethics: A Documentary History*, ed. Albert R. Jonsen, Robert M. Veatch, and LeRoy Walters (Washington, DC: Georgetown University Press, 1998), 358–68. For McCormick's views, see his "Who or What Is the Preembryo?" *Kennedy Institute of Ethics Journal* 1, no. 1 (1991): 1–15.

helped their understanding, nobody would have many qualms at the name change," he wrote in 1986. "But those who are introducing 'pre-embryo' into the vocabulary know full well that the research is indeed contentious and that fundamental issues have yet to be resolved." McLaren countered that the reasons for the terminology were scientific, not political, and insisted on the "confusing ambiguity of 'embryo'" to denote sharply different stages of early development. In 1987 a *Nature* editorial sided with Davies and called for an end to use of the term "pre-embryo." It was a "cop-out, a way of pretending that the public conflict about IVF and other innovations in human embryology can be made to go away by means of an appropriate nomenclature." Even research supporters should admit that "on the issue of nomenclature the Vatican is philosophically the more consistent."[105]

In the United States, too, the term "pre-embryo" faced sharp criticism. George Annas commented on the joint AFS-ACOG committee's adoption of it in 1991, charging that "redefining the preimplantation embryo as a nonembryo permitted the committee to advise its members that anything goes with these now nonembryos."[106] The flagship journal in the United States, *Science,* did not integrate "pre-embryo" into its style sheet. In Germany, *Der Spiegel* referred to the concept as "deceptive advertising." As early as its December 1986 report, the CCNE had dismissed the idea as "utilitarian" and dangerous: "The use of a new word (seldom used in scientific publications) 'pre-embryo' may create the feeling that, for some time, the embryo could be treated differently, with less respect."[107] While the term persisted within the bioethics literature, it failed to find wide acceptance within the scientific community and in leading textbooks, not to mention among research opponents.

The fate of proresearch arguments did not hang on any success of the term "pre-embryo." Given the potential of embryo research to help those suffering from infertility and other ailments, thinkers including Peter Singer, based in Australia at the time, John Harris in the United Kingdom, and John Robertson and Bonnie Steinbock in the United States, insisted that embryos, because they were unable to feel pain, did not have any significant moral status. The capacity to suffer and to exercise reason and autonomy were the

---

105. David Davies, "Embryo Research," *Nature* 320, no. 6059 (1986): 208; Anne McLaren, "Embryo Research," *Nature* 320, no. 6063 (1986): 570; "IVF Remains in Legal Limbo," *Nature* 327, no. 6118 (1987): 87.

106. George J. Annas, "Ethics Committees: From Ethical Comfort to Ethical Cover," *Hastings Center Report* 21, no. 3 (1991): 18. For defenses of the term in the moral theology literature, see Thomas Shannon and Allan Wolter, "Reflections on the Moral Status of the Pre-Embryo," *Theological Studies* 51, no. 4 (1990): 603–26.

107. For a critical discussion of the term "pre-embryo" in the French context, see "Les embryons au service de l'homme," *Le Monde,* November 16, 1988.

threshold to personhood and rights. Before that stage—and certainly before the formation of the primitive streak—there was no meaningful moral distinction between surplus IVF embryos and those created expressly for research. As Harris argued it, "I cannot but think that if it is right to use embryos for research then it is right to produce them for research."[108]

Most of these scholars did acknowledge some basis for respect for the human embryo. It was not to be created and used wantonly, for example in the testing of cosmetics. In keeping with utilitarian logic, the reason for restraint and respect lay not with the intrinsic moral status of the embryo but with the sensitivities of fellow citizens for whom it represented human life. Because they lack sentience, Steinbock argued, "embryos do not have interests of their own, and therefore cannot be harmed or benefited." But because others *believe* embryos to be human beings worthy of protection, they have symbolic interests, and deserve some respect. Not surprisingly, for these thinkers the benefits of research easily outweighed any affront to ethical sensibilities, especially when those benefits were calculated not just in terms of knowledge but in terms of alleviating suffering. "Research embryos are not created solely for the purpose of destroying them in experiments," Steinbock argued. "The purpose of the experiments is to gain knowledge that will enable to save lives and prevent misery."[109]

The rise of Catholic/evangelical opposition to all embryo research and the growing impact of utilitarianism, particularly within the Anglo-Saxon bioethics community, polarized the debate from the late 1980s onward. During a first phase marked by the work of national ethics committees, between 1979 and 1986, there was some convergence around the necessity of both granting the embryo some moral status and permitting research with spare IVF embryos, mainly in support of infertility medicine. But just as legislatures began to take up the question of regulation, the polarization of the ethical debate was reinforced by political polarization, particularly in the United States, where the tension between religious antiresearch and secular proresearch arguments mapped most neatly onto the left-right "culture wars" that encompassed abortion and other "family values" issues.

---

108. Anthony Oakley Dyson and John Harris, *Experiments on Embryos* (New York: Routledge, 1990), 62. See also John Harris, "In Vitro Fertilization: The Ethical Issues," *Philosophical Quarterly* 33, no. 132 (1983): 217–37; and Bonnie Steinbock, *Life before Birth: The Moral and Legal Status of Embryos and Fetuses* (New York: Oxford University Press, 1992). Some of Singer's early contributions to the debate are in Peter Singer and Deane Wells, *Making Babies: The New Science and Ethics of Conception* (New York: C. Scribner's Sons, 1985).

109. Bonnie Steinbock, "Ethical Issues in Human Embryo Research," in *Papers Commissioned for the NIH Human Embryo Research Panel* (Bethesda, MD: National Institutes of Health, 1994), 43. On the symbolic angle, see John A. Robertson, "Symbolic Issues in Embryo Research," *Hastings Center Report* 25, no. 1 (1995): 37–38.

The Human Embryo Research Panel, 1993–94

A perfect illustration of increasing polarization was the fate of the last major national bioethics committee before the cloning and stem cell breakthroughs of the late 1990s—the 1993–94 U.S. Human Embryo Research Panel. A decade and a half after the 1979 recommendations of the Ethics Advisory Board, which presidents Jimmy Carter, Ronald Reagan, and George H. W. Bush had effectively ignored, Bill Clinton took office in January 1993 promising a new departure. He charged the National Institutes of Health to take a new look at embryo research and to make recommendations on whether and how the federal government might support it. Under the leadership of NIH director Harold Varmus, a committee of nineteen was assembled, including cochairs Steven Muller, former president of Johns Hopkins University and a political scientist, and Patricia King, a professor at Georgetown Law Center. The committee included scientists, doctors, lawyers, and two bioethicists, Carol Tauer of the University of Minnesota and Ronald Green of Dartmouth. Like the EAB fifteen years earlier, the HERP consulted experts, held public hearings, and published its recommendations in a report, this one dated August 1994.[110]

The parallel with the EAB extended to the substance of its 1994 recommendations, which called for research with embryos during the first two weeks after fertilization under strict guidelines designed to advance biomedical goals. Specific rationales for these conclusions differed somewhat. The EAB had settled on two weeks as the end of the implantation stage, while the HERP borrowed from the Warnock report and focused on the formation of the "primitive streak" that marked the end to any possibility of twinning. The EAB had focused almost solely on gains for infertility medicine, while the HERP pointed to the fight against congenital disease and presciently included the possibility of "research involving the development of embryonic stem cells." Finally, the EAB had not clearly distinguished between such surplus IVF embryos—the latter had only emerged with the introduction of freezing technologies in the mid-1980s—and the creation of embryos expressly for research. The HERP followed the Warnock committee in allowing for the latter possibility; all but two of its members endorsed the creation of embryos for research "to answer crucial questions in reproductive medicine."[111]

---

110. On the work of the HERP, see Harold Varmus, *The Art and Politics of Science* (New York: Norton, 2009), 176–96; Ronald Michael Green, *The Human Embryo Research Debates: Bioethics in the Vortex of Controversy* (New York: Oxford University Press, 2001); R. Alta Charo, "The Hunting of the Snark: The Moral Status of Embryos, Right-to-Lifers, and Third World Women," *Stanford Law and Policy Review* 6, no. 2 (1995): 11–37; and Tauer, "Embryo Research and Public Policy," 423–39.

111. National Institutes of Health, *Report of the Human Embryo Research Panel,* vol. 1 (Bethesda, MD: National Institutes of Health, 1994), xi, xvii.

If the recommendations of the EAB and the HERP were similar in key respects, so too were the ethical rationales they articulated. Both committees took the moral status of the embryo seriously but maintained that research in some cases be allowed. While the EAB had insisted on "profound respect" but that "this respect does not necessarily encompass the full legal and moral rights attributed to persons," the HERP argued that "although the preimplantation embryo warrants serious moral consideration as a developing form of human life, it does not have the same moral status as an infant or child."[112] In both cases, the status of the embryo was weighed against the promise of biomedical research. The EAB report had focused on the benefits for infertility medicine while mentioning, in passing, "potentially valuable information about reproductive biology, the etiology of birth defects, and other subjects." The HERP placed more emphasis on biomedical payoffs. Its report led with the claim that research carried "great potential benefit to infertile couples, families with genetic conditions, and individuals and families in need of effective therapies for a variety of diseases."[113]

The greatest difference between 1978–79 and 1993–94 was the level of media attention and public controversy that accompanied the panel's deliberations. Polarization emerged through a series of public panel hearings magnified by the *Washington Post* and picked up by other media outlets. The 1978–79 hearings had taken place before embryo research was folded into the pro-life agenda. The Catholic Church, more worried about IVF as a reproductive technology than about the moral status of embryos, did not take a strong public stance. Fifteen years later, the National Conference of Catholic Bishops (NCCB) and its spokesman on life issues, Richard Doerflinger, were actively engaged. Doerflinger testified twice to the panel, in front of television lights, laying out the Church's absolute opposition to all embryo research. "I am here to express the Catholic bishops' concern that government decisions on human experimentation be guided by a clear commitment to the dignity of human life at every stage of existence," he told the panel in February 1994 testimony. "At every stage after fertilization, the human embryo is a living, thriving, developing member of the human species, deserving human respect."[114] Doerflinger did not sway the panel. Nonetheless, his relentless attacks raised the public visibility of its deliberations.

---

112. Ethics Advisory Board, *Report and Conclusions,* 101; National Institutes of Health, *Report of the Human Embryo Research Panel,* vol. 1, x.

113. Ethics Advisory Board, *Report and Conclusions,* 111; National Institutes of Health, *Report of the Human Embryo Research Panel,* vol. 1, x.

114. Richard M. Doerflinger, "Public Comment: NIH Human Embryo Research Panel," February 22, 1994, http://www.usccb.org/prolife/issues/bioethic/embryo/rd20294.shtml.

The HERP members were not themselves polarized on the issues; the panel did not include a single principled opponent of embryo research. Green, Tauer, and the only other member of the panel who had written extensively on bioethical questions, Alta Charo, were sympathetic to the creation of embryos for research and the pursuit of research related not just to infertility but to wider biomedical goals. Given the strong proresearch makeup of the panel, it is hard to take at face value the claim in its report that in assembling the group, no attention had been given to members' "positions on the acceptability of embryo research."[115] It is true that two members, King and Tauer, dissented from the panel's recommendations concerning the creation of embryos for research. On a close reading, however, neither was opposed to deliberate embryo creation in principle; they only thought the practice should be more sharply restricted. For King, the panel's support for embryo creation for projects of "potentially outstanding scientific and therapeutic value" was too expansive. Tauer dissented from embryo creation to create stem cells, arguing that the technique was still unproven. Like Mc-Cormick on the EAB fifteen years earlier, she insisted that her openness to work with embryos was compatible with Catholic moral tradition, even as it differed sharply from the Vatican's post-1987 stance.[116]

The panel's support for the creation of embryos for research, leaked to the media in advance of the final report, caused the greatest public furor. It allowed Doerflinger and other opponents of all research, including powerful members of Congress, to mobilize effectively against any and all federally funded embryo research. The story of that mobilization and of Bill Clinton's eventual rejection of his own committee's recommendations is covered in the next chapter. But the roots of its political failure are to be found in the strong association between the embryo research and abortion issues—a peculiarity of the U.S. debate. One of the HERP members, Duke president Nannerl Keohane, asked later whether a different name, such as "Preembryo Research Panel" would have changed the outcome of the controversy. That is unlikely, given the fusion of the embryo research and abortion issues in the United States and the political mobilization of the Catholic Church and its allies.[117] "If this narrative has a villain," Ronald Green wrote in his retrospective account of the HERP's fate, "it is Richard

---

115. National Institutes of Health, *Report of the Human Embryo Research Panel,* 3.

116. According to Tauer, "many types of research that need to be done, such as contraceptive research, couldn't possibly be done unless you create *embryos* in the lab." See "U.S. Panel May OK Human Embryo Study," *New York Times,* August 19, 1994.

117. Keohane, quoted in Ira H. Carmen, *Politics in the Laboratory: The Constitution of Human Genomics* (Madison: University of Wisconsin Press, 2004), 96. According to Tauer, "scientists on the committee had rejected the term 'pre-embryo.'" See Tauer, "Embryo Research and Public Policy," 425.

Doerflinger."[118] Outside the United States, the religious–secular polarization was not as sharp. It was more common in the German and French debates to call for embryo protections on a purely secular or philosophical basis. The principle of human dignity, anchored in both countries' constitutions in the wake of the Nazi catastrophe, was invoked against the creation of embryos expressly for research. And in the United Kingdom, religious arguments in *support* of research were much more prominent than in the United States. The Church of England leadership opposed the deliberate creation of embryos for research but backed work with surplus IVF embryos. Its rationale for an ethic of healing was explicitly theological—that Christians were called to advance biomedical knowledge to alleviate suffering.

Among those who criticized the more polarized U.S. debate was Daniel Callahan, a leading bioethicist. The founder of the Hastings Center, Callahan had left the Catholic Church and did not support its absolute prohibition on embryo research. At the same time, he was critical of the HERP reluctance to recognize the difficult tradeoffs at the core of the embryo research issue. While the HERP insisted on "respect" for embryos, he noted, those "that stand in the way of research are to be sacrificed—as nice a case of the ends justifying the means as can be found." From Callahan's perspective, justifying deliberate embryo creation was "better and more honestly done by simply stripping preimplantation embryos of any value at all." Research "within moral limits is worthy of respect," he argued. "Research that restlessly seeks to find a way around them, holding out some supposedly higher goods, is not."[119] Callahan's own compromise position, support for research with spare embryos destined to perish in any case in order to advance IVF, held limited appeal for pro- and antiresearch forces now arrayed against each other.

Conclusion

One can distinguish three phases in the development of ethical controversy surrounding embryo research from 1968 through the early 1990s. The first phase, roughly the decade following on the first fertilization of an egg outside the womb in Cambridge, England, in 1968, centered on concerns about eugenics, safety, and human sexuality. The focus was on the development of IVF

---

118. Green, *Human Embryo Research Debates,* 7.

119. Daniel Callahan, "The Puzzle of Profound Respect," *Hastings Center Report* 25, no. 1 (1995): 39–40. For a differing perspective on the question, see Michael J. Meyer and Lawrence J. Nelson, "Respecting What We Destroy: Reflections on Human Embryo Research," *Hastings Center Report* 31, no. 1 (2001): 16–23.

as an infertility treatment and the race to produce the first "test-tube" baby. The moral status of the embryo was a subordinate issue. During a second phase, as IVF was gradually established as an infertility treatment, from 1978 to 1986, national ethics committees took up the problem of the respect due to the embryo, on the one hand, and the imperative of biomedical research, on the other. During a third phase, from 1987 to 1994, which coincided with the onset of political and policy struggles, the ethical debate became more polarized. The Catholic Church and its pro-life allies fused the embryo research and abortion issues, and scientists and their allies in the bioethics community increasingly emphasized the healing power of research for infertility and other conditions.

The transition from the middle to the later period proved critical for embryo politics. The mid-1980s saw four sets of recommendations from national ethics committees that sought to combine respect for the embryo with support for promising biomedical research. There was considerable consensus across the committees, which included leading secular and religious thinkers. The embryo was a developing form of human life but did not have the rights of a person. It might be used for very specific purposes, mainly to advance IVF as an infertility treatment. Edwards himself noted the considerable common ground. "Some religions would balance the respective benefits of making a decision on embryo research and whether the embryo should be sacrificed for this purpose," he noted at a November 1985 symposium. "This is not alien to our thought either."[120]

By the late 1980s, however, fronts had begun to harden. As Catholic leaders and their evangelical allies linked the embryo research and abortion issues, scientists and their allies in the bioethics community emphasized more fully the healing potential of research. Both sides in the debate recognized the problem of the moral status of the embryo and the imperative of biomedical progress. But the far-reaching consensus evident during the middle of the decade began to fray. Polarization was most pronounced in the United States and the United Kingdom. In Germany, where the legacy of Nazi eugenics formed a backdrop for controversy, skepticism of embryo research cut across religious and secular communities. The French debate, dominated by a secular political culture and a Kantian approach to human dignity, most resembled the German one. In the context of the political struggle recounted in the next chapter, these national differences took on sharper contours and contributed to very different policy outcomes.

---

120. J. W. Bowker, "Religions and the Status of the Embryo," in *Human Embryo Research—Yes or No?*, ed. Gregory Bock and Maeve O'Connor (London: Tavistock, 1986), 181.

✺ CHAPTER 2

First Embryo Research Regimes

The embryo did not become the object of open political struggle in Atlantic democracies until the second half of the 1980s. Ethical debates that began in the 1970s, centered among scientists, doctors, philosophers, and theologians, gained wider public attention through the work of national ethics committees convened first in the United States and then in the United Kingdom, Germany, and France, over the period 1978 to 1986. Only when governments began take up those committee recommendations and explore appropriate regulatory action did IVF and embryo research gain broader political salience. Parties and interest groups coalesced around different ethical stances and policy proposals, some more supportive of research than others. As ethical controversy morphed into policy struggle, the contours of the debate shifted from one country to the next. In the United Kingdom, and with particular ferocity in the United States, the abortion issue came to frame the debate, pitting Christian conservatives against their mainly liberal and secular opponents. In Germany, and to a lesser degree in France, a deeper historical legacy provided the frame. Anxiety about the abuse of science and the violation of human dignity, informed by the Nazi experience, encouraged a more restrictive approach to research. In all four countries, contrasting national terms of debate combined with electoral shifts and new patterns of interest group politics to generate very different embryo research regimes over the period 1990 to 1995.

In the United States, periodic flashes of political interest in embryo research only slowly gave rise to an open political clash. By never acting on the Ethics Advisory Board's 1979 recommendations, the administrations of Jimmy Carter, Ronald Reagan, and George H. W. Bush—cautious about offending antiabortion forces—upheld a de facto ban on federally funded embryo research, while leaving it unregulated in the private sector. President Bill Clinton's efforts to enable federal funding, through the mechanism of the Human Embryo Research Panel (1993–94), sparked a conservative reaction that culminated in a 1995 congressional funding ban via the Dickey Amendment. In the United Kingdom, the Warnock committee's proresearch recommendations energized the pro-life movement and its parliamentary supporters, who almost succeeded in passing legislation outlawing all embryo research in 1985. After several more years of struggle, however, a broad proresearch coalition, supported by a conservative prime minister, Margaret Thatcher, passed the Human Fertilisation and Embryology Act in 1990, instituting the major Warnock committee recommendations.

German and French political dynamics were very different. In the Federal Republic, the Christian Democrat–led government of Chancellor Helmut Kohl, originally open to research under some circumstances, gravitated toward the total ban favored both by the churches and by Social Democrats and Green activists. The 1990 Embryo Protection Law criminalizing any and all destructive embryo research was more restrictive than the recommendations of the Benda Commission five years earlier, with its support for research for "medical findings of great value." In France, a long drawn-out struggle, marked by a shifting balance of electoral power between Right and Left and periods of cohabitation between Socialist president François Mitterrand and conservative prime ministers, culminated in the national Bioethics Laws of 1994. The legislation included a total ban on destructive embryo research and broke with the recommendation of the National Consultative Ethics Committee, which had supported experiments under some circumstances.

In the United Kingdom, Germany, and France, detailed parliamentary debates preceded the passage of this groundbreaking legislation. Leaders from both major parties wrestled with how best to combine respect for the embryo with an ethic of healing. While the exchanges were pointed, they were marked by a high level of civility; given the ethical stakes, party discipline was relaxed in all three countries, allowing for a more open and full exchange of views. In the United States, by contrast, legislation bearing on embryo research never got past the committee stage for full consideration on the House and Senate floors. This had to do with the decentralized structure of the American state, but also with the passions surrounding embryo politics due to its close association with the country's running controversy over abortion.

The United States: Embryo Research and Abortion Politics

Embryo politics almost got off to an early start in the United States. Even before the first fertilization of a human egg in a laboratory in 1968, Congress had begun to consider the possibility of a national bioethics committee to advise on a range of new technologies, including organ transplantation and artificial life support.[1] In March 1971, just weeks after DNA pioneer James Watson addressed Congress on the topic "Potential Consequences of Experimentation with Human Eggs," the Democratic senator from Minnesota Walter Mondale introduced legislation to create a National Advisory Commission on Health Science and Society. His bill, to address "growing awareness and concern throughout the country about the implications of biomedical advances," passed the Senate but died in the House in 1972.[2] Scientists adamant about freedom of research joined with politicians opposed to government regulation to defeat the measure. Mondale was particularly "disappointed and appalled" by scientific opposition to the commission idea. Public concerns about new technologies that enabled organ transplantations, extended life artificially, and created embryos in the laboratory had not proved salient enough to generate a national policy debate or legislative response.[3]

During the first half of the 1970s, several science-related issues did command public attention, but embryo research was not among them. Breakthroughs with recombinant DNA generated some concern in Congress and the states about genetic engineering and the risks posed by laboratory accidents. In 1975 scientific leaders in the field meeting in Asilomar, California, adopted a voluntary moratorium on gene-splicing research, effectively forestalling federal regulation. The previous year, revelations about postwar syphilis experiments with black Americans in Tuskegee, Alabama, had spurred Congress to set up the first national bioethics body, the National Commission for the Protection of Human Subjects of Biomedical and Behavioral Research. During its 1974–78 life span the commission tackled a variety

1. Office of Technology Assessment, *Biomedical Ethics in U.S. Public Policy* (Washington, DC: U.S. Government Printing Office, 1993), 7.

2. On the hearings that led to the proposed legislation, see Albert R. Jonsen, *The Birth of Bioethics* (New York: Oxford University Press, 1998), 90–94; Amitai Etzioni, *Genetic Fix* (New York: Macmillan, 1973), 55–56.

3. Mondale quoted in "Ethics Debate Set Off by Life Science Gains," *New York Times,* March 28, 1971.

of controversial issues, including research involving prisoners, children, and fetal tissue. But it did not address IVF research or experiments with early embryos. In August 1975, outside of public view, the National Institutes of Health made federal research funding contingent on the approval of an in-house Ethics Advisory Board. The EAB was only formed in early 1978, once a first research proposal had passed the NIH's scientific review and awaited final approval.

As noted in the last chapter, the formation of the EAB and its first deliberations took place out of the public eye. The birth of the first IVF child, Louise Brown, in the United Kingdom in July 1978 represented a political turning point. HEW secretary Joseph Califano then broadened the board's remit to include a full consideration of new reproductive technologies and their ethical implications. Through a series of hearings held around the country, and through the testimony of a variety of stakeholders including scientists and religious leaders, the EAB sought to engage a wider public debate. In certain respects it was successful. The board received 13,000 pieces of mail and, thanks to leaks to the media of its internal deliberations, drew some media attention in early 1979, as its work was drawing to a close. But its main conclusions—recommending research with embryos up to the fourteen-day stage to improve the safety and efficiency of IVF—did not occasion a national debate. The United States was going into a recession and faced an oil shortage. The Iranian hostage crisis was in full swing. With President Carter facing an uphill reelection bid, the question of IVF and embryo research had little public resonance—not least because the Catholic Church and its allies in the pro-life movement had not yet linked it effectively to the abortion issue.

The Carter administration's response—or more accurately, nonresponse—to the EAB recommendations also explains the lack of political controversy. Califano approached the EAB findings cautiously, calling for two months of public discussion before making any decisions about their implementation. He may have feared offending the growing pro-life movement; a Catholic, Califano later related in his memoirs how Carter's support for federal funding of abortion for poor women had provoked the ire of the Church hierarchy. As it happened, Califano left the government in August 1979 as part of a cabinet reshuffle in the run-up to the 1980 election. His successor, Patricia Harris, not only did not act on the EAB recommendations, she also supported a move in Congress that ended up dissolving the body by channeling its funding into the creation of a more comprehensive body, the President's Commission for the Study of Ethical Problems in Medicine and Biomedical and Behavioral Research. At its first meeting in January 1980, the commission decided to take up a range of topics, including genetics and gene therapy and the definition of death—but not embryo research, which the EAB had recently addressed. Embryo experimentation was in limbo. Although the EAB had ceased to exist, HEW regulations requiring EAB approval for federal research funding addressing IVF and embryo research remained in place.[4]

After Ronald Reagan defeated Jimmy Carter in a landslide in November 1980, there was nothing to prevent the new administration from reconstituting the EAB, accepting or rejecting its recommendations, or issuing its own regulations by executive order. But by early 1981, when President Reagan took office, abortion politics had begun to emerge as a public frame for embryo controversy, with far-reaching consequences for the development of policy.[5]

The emergence of the abortion issue as a frame for the U.S. embryo research debate was part of the legacy of the January 1973 *Roe v. Wade* Supreme Court decision that legalized abortion through the second trimester. The Court majority, led by Chief Justice Warren Burger, had built its argument around a woman's right to privacy and a common law tradition that protected the fetus from the time of viability. The majority 7–2 opinion bracketed the question of the moral status of the embryo. "We need not resolve the difficult question of when life begins," it noted. "When those trained in the respective disciplines of medicine, philosophy, and theology are unable to arrive at any consensus, the judiciary, at this point in the development of man's knowledge, is not in a position to speculate as to the answer."[6] Writing for the majority, Harry Blackmun did note that protecting life "from conception" was now, "of course, the official belief of the Catholic Church" and one "strongly held by many non-Catholics as well." But in a rambling aside he also underscored "substantial problems" with this view posed "by new embryological data that purport to indicate that conception is a 'process' over time, rather than an event, and by new medical techniques such as menstrual extraction, the 'morning-after' pill, implantation of embryos, artificial insemination, and even artificial wombs."[7] While the majority opinion here made only passing and inaccurate (artificial wombs as a new medical

4. On the demise of the EAB and the failure to replace it, see Clifford Grobstein, Michael Flower, and John Mendeloff, "External Human Fertilization: An Evaluation of Policy," *Science* 222, no. 4620 (1983): 127–33.

5. On the politics of abortion in the United States, see Kristin Luker, *Abortion and the Politics of Motherhood* (Berkeley: University of California Press, 1985).

6. *Roe v. Wade*, 410 U.S. 113, 93 S.Ct. 705, 35 L.Ed.2nd 147 (1973).

7. Ibid., 60–61.

technique!) references to the moral status of the embryo, the two dissenting justices addressed the issue even less. William Rehnquist, who crafted the minority opinion, centered his argument on the absence of a right to privacy in the Constitution and insisted that abortion was basically an issue for the states to decide. The moral status of the fetus, not to mention the embryo, was not the critical issue.[8]

The Court's decision shocked Catholics and evangelicals opposed to abortion and spurred the formation of a broad, grassroots pro-life movement with strong links to churches. The National Right to Life Committee formed in June 1973 and spearheaded an annual March for Life in Washington, D.C., every subsequent January. Beginning in 1973, congressional Republicans introduced and reintroduced human life amendments designed to overturn the Court's decision by changing the Constitution. While they never came close to the two-thirds majority needed in both houses of Congress, these efforts kept the abortion issue in the media and on the national agenda. During the late 1970s, the increasing political engagement of evangelicals, typified by Jerry Falwell's Moral Majority, strengthened the pro-life movement as a political force within the Republican Party. While the party's 1976 platform endorsed a human life amendment in principle, it maintained that abortion "is undoubtedly a moral and personal issue but it also involves complex questions relating to medical science and criminal justice." In the 1980 platform it was much stronger in its support for "a constitutional amendment to restore protection of the right to life for unborn children."[9] Ronald Reagan's defeat of Jimmy Carter in November 1980 proved a milestone. While the election was fought mainly on economic and foreign policy issues, Reagan's pro-life position—including a pledge to appoint Supreme Court judges who might overturn *Roe v. Wade*—helped to forge a powerful electoral coalition and capture a majority of the Catholic vote.

The Emergence of the Abortion Parallel

Over this entire period, the pro-life movement did not explicitly take up the question of embryo research. Versions of a human life amendment referenced conception as the beginning of life, but conservatives did not seize on its relevance to embryo research. The Vatican's 1974 "Instruction on Procured

8. Ibid., 171–78.

9. Republican Party, "Republican Party Platform of 1976," August 18, 1976, http://www.presidency.ucsb.edu/ws/index.php?pid=25843; "Republican Party Platform of 1980," July 15, 1980, http://www.presidency.ucsb.edu/ws/index.php?pid=25844.

Abortion" had upheld the view that the embryo should be treated as a person from conception but had not mentioned the research issue directly. The parallel between embryo research and abortion did start to emerge as a theme among the thirteen thousand or so letters sent to the EAB as part of its public consultations in 1978–79, but there was no mobilization comparable to what the Human Embryo Research Panel would face in 1994. Ironically, a *New York Times* masthead editorial was among the first high-level mentions of the abortion parallel. In February 1979 the editors suggested that the EAB's anticipated proresearch findings, by allowing for embryo destruction, would adhere "to the standards that were established by the Supreme Court six years ago for assessing the legality of abortion."[10]

Research supporters did not subsequently pick up the idea that a right to abortion might imply a right to conduct embryo research. It was research opponents who would seize on the abortion parallel.[11] A first controversy along these lines took place in late 1979 and early 1980 surrounding the approval of the first IVF clinic in the United States, in Norfolk, Virginia, to be led by Edwards's partners and rivals during his early efforts to fertilize human eggs, Howard and Georgeanna Jones. Failed opposition to the clinic was led by local pro-life forces now concerned less about artificial reproductive technologies—the Church's main concern with IVF to that point—than about the destruction of embryos. "The last thing Virginia needs," the *Washington Post* quoted an "irate antiabortionist," is "a laboratory where scientists will be playing God with babies' lives."[12]

The parallel between abortion and embryo research briefly spilled over into national politics in the spring of 1981. Persuaded that a human life amendment lacked the necessary two-thirds support in Congress, conservatives Jesse Helms in the Senate and Henry Hyde in the House proposed a human life bill that would have deemed the unborn "legal persons." In order "not to deprive persons of life without due process of law," the proposed legislation asserted, "human life shall be deemed to exist from conception."[13] Reagan, who backed the idea of a human life amendment, announced his support

---

10. "Experimenting with Test Tube Babies," *New York Times*, February 17, 1979.

11. On early links between embryo research and the abortion issue in U.S. politics, see Andrea L. Bonnicksen, *In Vitro Fertilization: Building Policy from Laboratories to Legislatures* (New York: Columbia University Press, 1989), 80–82.

12. "Test-Tube Baby Clinic: Approval of Norfolk Hospital Lab Stirs Anger of Abortion Foes, Others," *Washington Post*, January 9, 1980. See also "U.S. Clinic for Conception Outside Body Approved," *New York Times*, January 9, 1980.

13. On the controversy, see "Opposing Sides Step Up Efforts on Abortion Measure," *New York Times*, February 15, 1981; "Determining When Life Begins and Abortion Stops," *New York Times*, April 23, 1981.

for the legislation in a March 1981 news conference, telling reporters that Congress was poised to decide "when and what is a human being."[14] Leading scientists, alarmed at the bill's negative implications for embryo research, launched a public counterattack. The National Academy of Sciences passed a resolution in May maintaining that the bill's claim that "present day scientific evidence indicates a significant likelihood that actual human life exists from conception" could not "stand up to the scrutiny of science." Because the issue of when life begins "must remain a matter of moral or religious values," Congress should not legislate on the matter.[15] The resolution—the first of its kind since an academy statement against creationism in 1972—expressed both anxiety about the prospect of government restrictions and alarm at the rise of abortion as a political frame for embryo research.

As it happened, the human life bill, like its sister amendment, did not secure the necessary votes in Congress. Nor did Reagan make appointments to the Supreme Court that overturned *Roe v. Wade*. Over the course of his two-term presidency, growing frustration within the pro-life movement made Reagan and his domestic advisers wary of doing anything that might further provoke the ire of a core constituency, including federal support for embryo research. A pattern developed: top officials within the NIH pressed for the reestablishment of the Ethics Advisory Board but were rebuffed or ignored by the White House. In 1982, for example, the assistant secretary for health, responding to discontent from scientists and administrators, tried but failed to secure administration support for the reestablishment of the board. A top NIH infertility specialist, frustrated by the blanket research ban, left to join the Norfolk clinic in early 1984.[16] In the meantime, the March 1983 expiration of the presidential ethics commission set up under Jimmy Carter spurred an effort to set up a replacement. After a series of hearings organized by then Tennessee senator Al Gore in 1984, Congress voted in May 1985 to create the Biomedical Ethics Advisory Committee (BEAC) to address controversial questions, including IVF, fetal-tissue research, and genetic engineering.[17]

The fate of the BEAC during Reagan's second term underscored the impact of the abortion issue on the governance of science. The board was to be appointed by a group of six senators and six congressmen. Wrangling over

14. "Reagan Says Ban on Abortion May Not Be Needed," *New York Times,* March 7, 1981.

15. Quoted in "Onset of Human Life: Answer on Crucial Moment Elusive," *New York Times,* May 4, 1981.

16. "Baby Researcher to Join Va. Institute," *Washington Post,* January 18, 1984.

17. Office of Technology Assessment, *Biomedical Ethics in U.S. Public Policy,* 12–13.

the abortion question delayed its composition for almost a year. The senators' group then took more than two more years to agree on the fourteen-member composition of the BEAC itself, and continued deadlock on the abortion issue further delayed the selection of chairman. The BEAC only met twice, in September 1988 and February 1989, before its funding ran out.[18] In the meantime, efforts to reconstitute the EAB continued. In May 1986 an American Academy for the Advancement of Science resolution called for a new EAB to take up research proposals in reproductive biology and other controversial areas. Officials within the Department of Health and Human Services (HHS)—the successor to HEW—appeared more responsive than earlier in the decade. In July 1988, HHS secretary Otis Bowen announced the formation of a board. As the bioethicist Arthur Caplan put it, the EAB appeared poised to begin "rising from the dead."[19]

The move to reconstitute the EAB again ran aground on abortion politics. George H. W. Bush, who succeeded Reagan as president in early 1989, was less committed to an antiabortion agenda but equally reticent about antagonizing the pro-life movement. In keeping his electoral coalition together he had to contend with evangelicals now organized in the Christian Coalition and the Family Leadership Council. He also faced a more conservative Catholic hierarchy, which, in the wake of the strong Vatican linkage of embryo research with abortion in the February 1987 instruction *Donum Vitae* and John Paul's reiteration of the theme during his U.S. visit later in the year, became more politically engaged on the issue.[20] Against this backdrop, the Bush administration's refusal to resurrect the EAB or to authorize federal funding for embryo research—like its rejection of NIH recommendations in support of research with fetal tissue from aborted fetuses—is hardly surprising. Congressional Democrats and their allies among scientific and medical groups were in a weak position. They passed an NIH reauthorization bill in 1992 that called for the reestablishment of an ethics advisory board but could not override Bush's veto.[21]

---

18. For an account of the BEAC's development and demise, see Robert M. Cook-Deegan, *The Gene Wars: Science, Politics, and the Human Genome* (New York: Norton, 1994), 256–82.

19. Colin Norman, "IVF Research Moratorium to End?" *Science* 241, no. 4864 (1988): 405–6. Caplan quoted in "Ethics and Fetal Research: Government Begins to Move," *New York Times,* July 31, 1988.

20. The pope had told Catholic health-care workers in Phoenix that "the Church cannot fail to emphasize the need to safeguard the life and integrity of the human embryo and foetus." See John Paul II, "Address of His Holiness John Paul II to the Leaders in Catholic Health Care," September 14, 1987, http://www.vatican.va/holy_father/john_paul_ii/speeches/1987/september/documents/hf_jp-ii_spe_19870914_organiz-sanitarie-cattoliche_en.html.

21. Joseph Palca, "New Watchdogs in Washington," *Hastings Center Report* 23, no. 2 (1994): 5.

Through the 1980s the development of IVF continued quietly in the private sector and in the states, even without federal research funding, and more and more Americans took advantage of the technology to combat infertility problems. When IVF did make national headlines in the late 1980s, safety and consumer protection issues were the driver—not concern about the status of embryos destroyed or frozen in laboratories and clinics. In March 1989, a House subcommittee released a report on the state of IVF clinics that decried overreporting of success rates and a lack of safety oversight. Congressman Ron Wyden, who noted the lack of "even cursory inspections required at other medical laboratories," introduced a legislative remedy.[22] The Fertility Clinic Success Rate and Certification Act, which easily passed Congress and was signed by Bush in October 1992, directed HHS to set safety standards and collect information about embryo laboratories and IVF practices. The program, conducted through the Centers for Disease Control and Prevention, did not impose regulations on the states and the private sector or restrict IVF and embryo work conducted without federal funds. But it was the first time IVF emerged as a national political and policy issue.

From Clinton's New Departure to the Dickey Amendment

Only with the election of Bill Clinton in November 1992 did embryo research become the object of a drawn-out political struggle. While economic issues had dominated the campaign against Bush, Clinton had run on a prochoice agenda and began to implement it on taking office. By executive order in January 1993 he reversed Bush's opposition to research with fetal tissue from abortions and lifted federal bans on foreign aid to NGOs that offered family planning services in the developing world. An unintended consequence of these measures was to energize the pro-life movement, which had flagged during the Bush years, disheartened by the Supreme Court's reaffirmation of the substance of *Roe v. Wade* in two landmark cases in 1989 and 1992. The annual March for Life in Washington, D.C., which usually drew about 75,000 participants, attracted about a quarter million in late January 1993. New York's Cardinal John J. O'Connor told the crowd: "Your presence here makes very clear that we will not be intimidated" and that "we have only just begun."[23] Embryo research would gradually emerge as a political battleground for antiabortion forces.

---

22. "Test-Tube Babies: What Are the Odds?" *Washington Post*, March 28, 1989.
23. "Clinton Cancels Abortion Restrictions of Reagan-Bush Era," *Washington Post*, January 23, 1993.

In early 1993, with little public fanfare, and with the encouragement of NIH scientists and the American Fertility Society, research backers in Congress moved not to resurrect the EAB but to eliminate the requirement of board approval for embryo research. Democratic senators Ted Kennedy and Henry Waxman quietly inserted language into the February 1993 NIH reauthorization bill to that effect. The technical language in the bill—"The provisions of section 204(d) of part 46 of title 45 of the Code of Federal Regulations (45 CFR 46.204(d)) shall not have any legal effect"—deflected media attention, and research opponents took little notice at the time.[24] Harold Varmus, the new head of the NIH, was legally free to begin funding embryo research projects upon the passage of the legislation. But sensitivity to ethical and political concerns led him to first convene the Human Embryo Research Panel, whose deliberations were recounted in chapter 1. Unlike the EAB, the HERP was conceived as a temporary body to make recommendations to Varmus, who might then, with White House approval, issue regulations to cover federal support for embryo research.[25]

The panel was quietly formed in January 1994, and its nineteen members— mainly medical, legal, and ethics experts, including no principled opponents of embryo research—held its first public hearings the following month. That is when political controversy began. Richard Doerflinger of the National Conference of Catholic Bishops not only shared the Church's strong opposition to research with the panel; he and key allies in the pro-life movement reached out to the media and sought to mobilize constituents and members of Congress against the panel's anticipated proresearch recommendations. Varmus and the panel members received "thousands of nearly identical postcard messages, telling us not to encourage research on early embryos, because they were innocent human beings."[26] Congressman Richard Dornan, a longtime supporter of a human life amendment, proved a key ally. He and some thirty colleagues wrote a letter to Varmus attacking embryo research as "Frankensteinesque" and at odds with "the protection and preservation of human life." The letter contained a veiled threat of legislative action: "Congress has not examined these initiatives, and the American people are largely unaware that the NIH is even contemplating using their tax dollars to fund such bizarre experiments on living human embryos."[27]

---

24. Joseph Palca, "A Word to the Wise," *Hastings Center Report* 22, no. 4 (1994), 5.

25. A useful overview of the panel and its fate is Stephen S. Hall, *Merchants of Immortality: Chasing the Dream of Human Life Extension* (New York: Houghton Mifflin, 2003), 105–22.

26. Varmus, *Art and Politics of Science,* 203.

27. Eliot Marshall, "Rules on Embryo Research Due Out," *Science* 265, no. 5175 (1994): 1024–26.

In an effort to shield the HERP's deliberations from political controversy, Varmus responded to Dornan with a letter of his own. He suggested that embryo research might assist the NIH's ongoing efforts to combat "infertility, pregnancy loss, genetic disease, and cancer." Anticipating arguments that would become more influential after the successful isolation of embryonic stem cells in 1998, Varmus further insisted that research and applications "could spare enormous human suffering and help countless Americans."[28] Not surprisingly, pro-life activists and their supporters in Congress were not reassured. When the thrust of the HERP findings was leaked to the media in August 1994, Catholic, evangelical, and pro-life organizations flooded the White House and Congress with letters and phone calls. Dornan warned Varmus in a second letter that "the American people will be justifiably outraged and appalled if their tax dollars are used to create human life in a laboratory dish only to have it thrown out with the trash."[29]

The release of the actual HERP report, in September 1994, was a political turning point. Its two major recommendations—to allow research with surplus IVF embryos up to the fourteen-day stage and to permit the creation of embryos expressly for research under some circumstances—now drew the concentrated fire of pro-life forces and their supporters in Congress. In the *New York Times,* for example, Judie Brown, president of the American Life League, denounced embryo research as equivalent to "killing little boys and girls."[30] Such opposition from religious conservatives and antiabortion activists was, of course, not unexpected. What put the White House on edge in a mid-term election year was the emergence of broader opposition to the idea of creating embryos expressly for research. Particularly notable was a critical *Washington Post* masthead editorial. "It is not necessary to be against abortion rights, or to believe human life literally begins at conception," the editors argued, "to be deeply alarmed by the notion of scientists' purposely causing conceptions in a context entirely divorced from even the potential of reproduction." William Galston, then deputy assistant to Clinton for domestic policy, later noted that the editorial helped to bring the issue "out of the inner workings of the bureaucracy into the public arena." Just weeks before

---

28. Letter quoted in "U.S. Panel May OK Human Embryo Study," *Boston Globe,* August 19, 1994.

29. Quoted in Andreas Frew, "Congressional Murder Most Foul: Report from the Heady Heights of Capitol Hill," *New Scientist* 144, no. 1949 (1994): 67–78.

30. "Federal Panel Urges U.S. to Drop Its Ban on Financing of Human Embryo Research," *New York Times,* September 28, 1994.

the November elections, the White House formed an ad hoc working group to deliberate on how to respond to the HERP recommendations.[31]

No decisions were made before the November elections. But their outcome—new Republican majorities in both houses of Congress—changed the political situation. Under the leadership of Newt Gingrich, Republicans had swept to victory with the help of an election pledge, the Contract with America, that included a strong antiabortion plank. "If we accepted the Panel's full recommendation," Galston worried at the time, "adverse congressional and public reaction might well lead to the continued cutoff of all funding for embryo research."[32] The White House working group recommended that Clinton reject federal support for embryo creation, and Clinton, already shifting to the political center so as to position himself for his 1996 reelection bid, agreed. "I understand that advances in in vitro fertilization research and other areas could derive from such work," Clinton asserted in a press release in early December. But he continued: "I do not believe that federal funds should be used to support the creation of human embryos for research purposes, and I have directed that NIH not allocate any resources for such research." Clinton announced his decision just hours after Varmus and the NIH leadership had endorsed all of the panel's recommendations.[33]

Clinton's statement was a humiliating surprise for Varmus and HERP members. But it did not rule out all federal funding for embryo experiments— just the creation of embryos expressly for research. NIH officials quietly began to fashion internal mechanisms for the assessment and approval of embryo research grant applications. But politics would overtake these efforts as well. Fulfilling Dornan's threat from early 1994, pro-life forces and their allies in Congress moved to effect a total ban on federal research funding. Chris Smith, cochair of the House Pro-Life Caucus, trumpeted Clinton's reversal on the embryo creation issue as "the biggest victory in the history of the movement," and Dornan threatened to use "every available legislative tool" to fight all forms of federal support for embryo research, insisting that "the Clinton statement did not go far enough." In this new climate, HERP member Alta Charo referred to its recommendations as "a dead duck."[34]

---

31. William A. Galston, *Public Matters: Essays on Politics, Policy and Religion* (Lanham, MD: Rowman and Littlefield, 2005), 78–80.

32. Ibid., 85.

33. Varmus reportedly saw the text of Clinton's statement only half an hour before it became public. Eliot Marshall, "Human Embryo Research: Clinton Rules Out Some Studies," *Science* 266, no. 5191 (1994): 1634. For Varmus's own account, see *Art and Politics of Science*, 206–8.

34. Joseph Palca, "Doing Things with Embryos," *Hastings Center Report* 25, no. 1 (1995): 5; Kurt Kleiner, "Clinton U-Turn on Embryo Research," *New Scientist* 144, no. 1957 (1994): 6–7.

The Republican congressional majority that took up work in January 1995 pressed ahead. That July, by a vote of 30 to 23, the House Appropriations Committee amended the 1995 NIH appropriation bill to bar any federal funding for embryo research. The Dickey Amendment, named for its main sponsor, Republican Jay Dickey of Arkansas, included language outlawing federal funding for any research in which a human embryo or embryos are created or "destroyed, discarded, or knowingly subjected to risk of injury or death." The amendment, which first went into effect in 1996, was attached to subsequent appropriation bills into the next century, implementing a legislative ban in place of the de facto ban in place since 1975. In the future, any federal support for embryo research would require not only executive orders but also new legislative action.

It is worth noting that the Republican majority did not move to outlaw all embryo research in the country, just its federal funding. And it was only barely able to defeat a measure that would have only prohibited embryo creation but allowed for experiments with IVF spares; such an effort failed in committee by a 26–26 tie vote. The Dickey Amendment's cosponsor, Republican Roger Wicker of Mississippi, had argued that once you prohibit the deliberate creation of embryos for research, "you have to conclude that it's unethical to use federal funds to experiment on any human embryo."[35] This political opposition to ethical distinctions between the creation of embryos for research and the use of surplus IVF embryos which were destined to die in any case would have far-reaching policy consequences.

The Dickey Amendment and other legislative measures in 1995, including restrictions on federal funding for family planning, marked important, if rare, victories for the pro-life movement. The American Life League thanked Congress for standing up for "the moral dignity and respect that is due to all human beings, including the tiniest boys and girls." Democratic Congresswoman Nancy Pelosi of California mused: "The Christian Coalition is here to collect."[36]

Over the following years, up through the announcement of the first successful isolation of human embryonic stem cells in November 1998, Democratic leaders close to the scientific and medical communities sought, unsuccessfully,

---

35. The amendment, sometimes also referred to as the "Dickey-Wicker Amendment," was approved by the full House in August 1995 and officially enacted in January 1996. Jim Zook, "House Panel Votes to Bar U.S. Funds for Human-Embryo Research," *Chronicle of Higher Education* 41, no. 6 (July 28, 1995): A33; Irene Stith-Coleman, *Human Embryo Research* (Washington, DC: Congressional Research Service, 1998).

36. Pelosi quoted in "Abortion Foes Prevail In House Panel Votes; Appropriations Committee Rejects Family Planning, Embryo Research," *Washington Post,* July 21, 1995.

to draw public attention to the cause of embryo research. In January 1996, for example, Democrat Barbara Boxer of California told her colleagues on the Senate floor that "all this prohibition does is close out venues for medical research that could save people's lives." Anticipating the stem cell breakthrough that would follow some two years later, she suggested that "human embryo research could help enable hospitals to create tissue banks which would store tissue that could be used for bone marrow transplants, spinal cord injuries, and skin replacement for burn victims." Boxer laid the blame for restrictive policies on antiabortion forces. "Prohibiting federal funding of human embryo research," she lamented, "will hold the health of millions of Americans hostage to antichoice politics."[37]

In the two decades between the 1975 NIH moratorium on embryo research and the 1995 passage of the Dickey Amendment, the abortion issue emerged as the frame for embryo politics in the United States. The moral status of the embryo, overshadowed by IVF safety issues through the 1970s, gained some public salience through the work of the 1978–79 Ethics Advisory Board. During the 1980s, as Catholics and evangelicals incorporated embryo protection into their existing antiabortion agenda, Presidents Reagan and Bush refused to resurrect the EAB or act on its recommendations. Only in the early 1990s did the political and policy struggle break out into the open. Clinton administration efforts to allow research sparked a conservative reaction that, in conjunction with the 1994 Republican sweep in Congress, culminated in a restrictive research regime. The historical legacy of the abortion struggle, and unfavorable electoral trends, had dealt research supporters a series of setbacks.

In an important 1996 article, the bioethicist George Annas lamented the prominence of the abortion frame for the political struggle over embryo research in the United States. "Even though the abortion debate in the United States is not likely to be resolved by ethical argument," he argued, "it should not be permitted to hold every related issue of medical ethics hostage, as it now does." Annas criticized the work of the HERP for not tackling the question of the moral status of the embryo head-on. "Ethics panels debating an abortion-related issue," he insisted, "must persuasively distinguish their subject from abortion itself and provide a strong ethical reason for the

---

37. *Congressional Record*, 104th Cong., 2nd sess., vol. 142, no. 102 (July 11, 1996): H7340. Efforts to lift the ban on funding for research with spare embryos while maintaining it for those created deliberately failed again in 1996—and would in subsequent years as well. Stephen Burd, "House Unit Votes to Bar Federal Funds for Research on Embryos," *Chronicle of Higher Education* 42, no. 43 (July 5, 1996): A24.

research and its need for public funding." In some sense, Annas was lamenting the inevitable simplification of complex intellectual and ethical questions in the political mix. Politicians assimilate new issues to old ones; they draw on and adapt existing frames with a proven capacity to reduce complexity and rally constituents around a point of view. The divisive and passionate abortion issue served that function in U.S. embryo politics.[38]

Annas's lament raises a further, interesting question: Is it possible to have a political and policy argument about the moral status of the embryo and the promise of biomedical research that is not framed mainly by the abortion question? The European experience suggests the answer is yes.

The United Kingdom: Toward a Liberal Research Regime

Embryo politics in the United Kingdom were similar to those in the United States in some respects. A pro-life movement that emerged in response to the liberalization of abortion laws in the late 1960s seized on the embryo research issue in the mid-1980s. In contrast to the United States, however, it did not have enough political clout to shape the national research regime. The Catholic Church was less than half as large as its U.S. counterpart—about a tenth as opposed to just under a quarter of the population—and evangelicals remained overshadowed by the leaders of the establishment Church of England, which was less stridently opposed to abortion and more supportive of embryo research. The government of Prime Minister Margaret Thatcher (1979–90), while generally conservative in outlook, was unabashedly proresearch and less deferential toward social conservatives than Republican administrations in the United States. It welcomed the recommendations of the Warnock committee (1982–84)—to allow research on embryos up to fourteen days old and to permit their creation for research under certain circumstances—and turned back the efforts of pro-life forces to rally antiresearch majorities in Parliament in 1985–86. Supported by a coalition of scientific and patient-advocacy groups, the government secured passage of the Human Fertilisation and Embryology Act in late 1990.[39]

---

38. George Annas, "The Politics of Human-Embryo Research—Avoiding Ethical Gridlock," *New England Journal of Medicine* 334, no. 20 (1996): 1329–32.

39. The most comprehensive account of the British case is Michael Mulkay, *The Embryo Research Debate: Science and the Politics of Reproduction* (Cambridge: Cambridge University Press, 1997). See also Jennifer Gunning and Veronica English, *Human In Vitro Fertilization: A Case Study in the Regulation of Medical Innovation* (Aldershot, UK: Darmouth, 1993); and Lynda Birke, Susan Himmelweit, and Gail Vines, *Tomorrow's Child: Reproductive Technologies in the '90s* (London: Virago Press, 1990).

It is striking how little political interest was roused by embryo research in the United Kingdom before 1982. The efforts of Robert Edwards and Patrick Steptoe to produce the first IVF child during the 1970s occasioned periodic media attention. But while the Medical Research Council, the government's main mechanism for funding science, refused to support their work for safety reasons, no larger debate emerged at the level of society and politics. Not a single parliamentary debate during the Labour-led governments of Harold Wilson (1967–74) and James Callahan (1974–79) directly addressed IVF or embryo research. And, in contrast to the United States, no concerted efforts to create national bioethics committees to oversee new scientific and technological developments took place. A young Liberal Party leader and later founder of the Social Democrats, Shirley Williams, was among the few who called for greater democratic oversight. In a 1971 essay she quoted Edwards's admission that "this work presents challenges to a number of established social and ethical concepts" and asked why scientists should operate in a political vacuum. "Failure to create the institutions in which such notions can be discussed and such guidance can be evolved," she wrote presciently, "may lead to bitter mutual recriminations between scientists and politicians."[40]

Even the birth of Louise Brown in July 1978 did not precipitate a political debate. A flurry of stories in the media appeared about possible extensions of IVF to cloning, genetic manipulation, and the creation of a "brave new world." But most of the coverage of the Browns and of Edwards and Steptoe's feat was positive and congratulatory. Calls for government regulation were muted. The day after the announcement, a leading Welsh member of Parliament, Leo Abse, asked the secretary of state for education and science whether a low-level advisory committee on genetic research might not also examine "what control is required over research involving human fertilisation in vitro and embryo transplants" and be expanded "to enable the ethical and social aspects to be reviewed." Margaret Jackson, the Secretary at the time, responded negatively. The advisory committee was not the right body, and the MRC had already determined "some time ago that it would not support research in these fields until there was satisfactory evidence from work with animals of the safety of the techniques." There would be no immediate government action. And there was not any clamoring for such action within the media or within Parliament.[41]

---

40. "The Responsibility of Science," *Times* (London), February 27, 1971.
41. United Kingdom (UK), *Parliamentary Debates, Commons,* 5th ser., vol. 954 (July 25, 1978), col. 669.

As in the United States, the pro-life movement would eventually help to place embryo research on the national political agenda. The United Kingdom's 1967 Abortion Act had not recognized a right to abortion on the model of *Roe v. Wade,* but it had lifted the threat of criminal prosecution from physicians who performed an abortion, as long as it was determined that "the continuance of the pregnancy would involve serious risk to the life or of grave injury to health, whether physical or mental, of the pregnant woman" or that her "capacity as a mother will be severely overstrained by the care of a child or of another child." For abortion opponents, this inclusive language was tantamount to abortion on demand during the first twenty-eight weeks of pregnancy. As in the United States, a protest movement took shape. The Society for the Protection of Unborn Children (SPUC) was formed in 1966, amid the parliamentary debates over the Abortion Act, and an even more conservative organization, LIFE, followed in 1970. While they lacked any official Catholic Church affiliation and sought to make the case against abortion in human rights terms, both organizations drew mainly on support from Catholics and evangelicals. Their base of support was much narrower than that of the U.S. movement.[42]

Often disparaged in the media and the public sphere as fanatics and "prolifers," the antiabortion movement never seriously threatened to overturn the 1967 Abortion Act. During the 1970s and into the 1980s, the small All-Party Parliamentary Pro-Life Group, with predominantly Catholic membership, periodically sought to amend the law by tightening the conditions for abortion or reducing the timeframe to twenty-four or twenty weeks into pregnancy. Their campaign gained momentum in 1975, when Parliament almost passed legislation that would have narrowed the provisions of the Abortion Act. As it happened, the mobilization of women's groups, who insisted on abortion as a right, played a role in the defeat of the effort, as did lukewarm support for abortion restrictions within the Anglican hierarchy. While generally opposed to abortion and eager to reduce its practice, Church of England leaders were wary of a recriminalization strategy. In response to a strong statement of the Catholic hierarchy against abortion in 1980, for example, the Anglican Board for Social Responsibility affirmed opposition to abortion as a general matter, but was also attentive to its tragic aspects. "We as Christians are aware that it is quite inadequate to limit ourselves to expressions of moral disapproval," they insisted. "Our moral concern for the

---

42. For a historical and political overview of abortion in the United Kingdom through the mid-1970s, see Malcolm Potts, Peter Diggory, and John Peel, *Abortion* (Cambridge: Cambridge University Press, 1977), 277–376.

protection of human life will only have or be seen to have integrity if it also finds expression in an equal concern for whatever enhances human life."[43]

Given this political constellation, and her own passion for economic and foreign policy, Thatcher downplayed the abortion issue, which had the potential to divide her Conservative Party. In June 1979, for example, only several months after she took office, a law that would have restricted abortion to twenty weeks passed a first parliamentary hurdle but went no further—in part because she did not throw her full support behind it. Initially, Thatcher's proresearch orientation, not any concern about the divisive abortion issue, probably best explains her government's lukewarm reception of the idea of a national committee to examine IVF and embryo research when it was first raised in early 1982. It was media reports about Edwards's embryo research agenda that had aroused a handful of MPs and sparked a call for ethical review of IVF and embryo research. In a March 1982 debate in Parliament—the first ever devoted to the topic—a government spokesman acknowledged that "once the possibility of manipulation of the act of conception exists, a whole area of possible scientific inquiry opens up" and that "there are many paths down which some of us, at least, would be most unhappy to see scientists wander." But he also insisted that the creation of any ethics oversight body should await recommendations being discussed within the MRC, the British Medical Association, and the Royal College of Obstetricians and Gynaecologists.[44]

The Political Backlash against the Warnock Committee

Continued media coverage of the statements made by Edwards and agitation by Leo Abse and some of his colleagues in the Labour Party eventually led the government to change course. In July 1982, without awaiting recommendations from other bodies, Secretary of Health Norman Fowler announced the formation of the Warnock committee, acknowledging the need for a "wider examination of the social, ethical and legal aspects of these developments."[45] The professional bodies, when they did weigh in during late 1982 and 1983, remained skeptical of the need for government regulation. In November 1982 the Medical Research Council insisted that

---

43. Church of England Board for Social Responsibility, *Abortion and the Church: What Are the Issues?* (London: Church House Publishing, 1993), 27.

44. Under-Secretary of State for Health and Social Security Geoffrey Finsberg in UK, *Parliamentary Debates,* Commons, 6th ser., vol. 21 (March 30, 1982), cols. 283–84.

45. Quoted in "Inquiry into Test-Tube Baby Births," *Times* (London), July 24, 1982.

research must be "scientifically sound" but preferred to leave the initiative to scientists, provided fertilized embryos were not cultured in vitro "beyond the implantation stage." In April 1983 the Royal College of Obstetricians and Gynaecologists dismissed the view that "the question of research on experimentation with early human embryonic material is a matter for the law" and insisted instead that "the problem is a strictly ethical one." The prestigious Royal Society admonished that local ethics committees, not legislators, should provide oversight.[46]

In setting up the committee, whose deliberations were recounted in chapter 1, the government acknowledged embryo research as a political and not just expert policy issue. The media attention given to the formation of the Warnock committee and its subsequent work dashed hopes of professional self-governance. In the run-up to the publication of the committee's report and proresearch recommendations in July 1984, the pro-life movement's seizure of the parallel between abortion and embryo research also transformed the political constellation. A key juncture was the flurry of negative media attention in September 1982 surrounding Edwards's reputed statements about cultivating embryos for research. LIFE denounced Edwards, accusing him of pursuing "laboratory-reared unborn children" to be "cannibalized for the benefit of others."[47] International developments also reinforced the abortion parallel in British politics. The U.S. pro-life movement, a model for many British activists, had taken up parallel efforts in early 1981 with a renewed drive for a human life amendment under Reagan's presidency. And, in an October 1982 Rome address to doctors, Pope John Paul II made a first strong public connection between Catholic opposition to abortion and to any "experimental manipulations of the human embryo."[48]

While the abortion parallel emerged as a theme of the written testimony supplied by SPUC, LIFE, and the Catholic bishops to the Warnock committee, it played little role in the deliberations of the committee itself. By most accounts, the committee members were surprised by the criticisms they faced from opposite directions. Concerned about undue restrictions on research, the editors of *Nature* argued that "the time limit should be dropped"—a position

46. The BMA and MRC reports were published in "Appendix VI: Interim Report on Human In Vitro Fertilisation and Embryo Replacement and Transfer," *British Medical Journal* 286, no. 6377 (1983): 1594; and Medical Research Council, "Research Related to Human Fertilisation and Embryology: Statement by the Medical Research Council," *British Medical Journal,* vol. 285, no. 6353 (1982): 1480. See also Royal College of Obstetricians and Gynaecologists, *Report of the RCOG Ethics Committee on In Vitro Fertilization and Embryo Replacement or Transfer* (London: Chamelion Press, 1983).

47. "Medical Fears of Live Organ Banks," *Times* (London), September 29, 1982.

48. John Paul II, "Address of John Paul II to Members of the Pontifical Academy of Sciences."

that Edwards, Steptoe, and the MRC would endorse as well. Antiabortion MPs and their allies concerned about possible eugenic abuses of the new technology demanded legislative action along stricter lines than the committee's recommendations.[49] Speaking for the government in July 1984, Fowler acknowledged that "the issues raised by the report arouse strong and widely differing opinions." In keeping with the government's cautious approach, he invited responses to the report and promised to hold a parliamentary debate by year's end, but called any formal legislation premature.[50]

Initial debates about the report in the House of Commons in November 1984 revealed a high degree of skepticism among MPs drawn from all three main parties: Conservatives, Labourites, and Liberals. Members of the Pro-Life Group were particularly outspoken in their criticism of the recommendations, but other MPs, more concerned about potential eugenic abuses and the instrumentalization of human life in the laboratory, weighed in as well. Fowler was generally cautious about promising biomedical breakthroughs beyond infertility medicine and distanced himself from any purely "utilitarian" approach, while still insisting that "desirable outcomes from research are possible." He quoted the Anglican Board for Social Responsibility's majority conclusion that "until the embryo has reached the first 14 days of its existence, it is not yet entitled to the same respect and protection as an embryo implanted in the human womb and in which individuation has begun." Without directly revealing his preferences, Fowler indicated his overall sympathy with the majority proresearch perspective within the board and on the Warnock committee.[51]

Bernard Braine, a prominent Catholic who would play a role in subsequent parliamentary debates as well, grounded his pro-life argumentation in religious language unusual in British politics. "Practising Christians and Jews will recall the message that the Lord God delivered to the prophet Jeremiah," he declared. "Before I formed thee in the belly I knew thee; and before thou cameth forth out of the womb I sanctified thee." He also placed emphasis on slippery slope arguments about potential eugenic abuses of the new technology. The Warnock report had revealed "developments in embryology that are already under way that will have dire legal, social, ethical and eugenic

---

49. "Confused Comment on Warnock," *Nature* 312, no. 5993 (1984): 389; "Pioneers Defend Embryos Research," *Times* (London), December 19, 1984.

50. UK, *Parliamentary Debates,* Commons, 6th ser., vol. 64 (July 18, 1984), cols. 203–4.

51. An MP from the floor remarked: "It is important to have on record the fact that many members of the Church of England think that the bishops would be far better sticking to the virgin birth than to the test tube birth." UK, *Parliamentary Debates,* Commons, 6th ser., vol. 68 (November 23, 1984), cols. 531–32.

consequences for our nation and perhaps for all mankind." Braine countered MPs who held up embryo experiments as a potential means to combat diseases, including genetic disorders, by citing a prominent French geneticist opposed to research, Jerome Lejeune, who had submitted testimony to the Warnock committee. "The use of the embryo for experimentation is an affront to humanity," Braine insisted, "and there is no room whatever for compromise on the matter."[52]

The scientific community observed the debate and developments around it with alarm. By the end of the year, more than one hundred organizations had responded to the government's request for comment on Warnock, the majority negative. While reassured by the government's proresearch stance and its desire not to rush into legislation, *Nature*'s editors had presciently warned that a member of Parliament might seek to introduce legislation directly, without government approval.[53] This is precisely what happened. In February 1985, Enoch Powell, a one-time mentor to Thatcher and former rival for Conservative party leadership, introduced the Unborn Children (Protection) Bill, which would "render it unlawful for a human embryo created by in vitro fertilisation to be used as a subject of experimentation or, indeed, in any other way or for any other purpose except to enable a woman to bear a child." LIFE and the SPUC helped to assemble more than one million signatures on a petition in support of the bill. The leader of England's Catholics, Cardinal Basil Hume, wrote to every MP asking for their support. The combination of eugenic concerns and the abortion frame appeared to be generating momentum for the restrictive legislation.[54]

Interestingly, Powell himself was not a member of the pro-life movement. He was mainly concerned about the instrumentalization of human life and possible eugenic abuses. As he put it in the February 1985 Commons debate: "When I first read the Warnock report I had a sense of revulsion and repugnance, deep and instinctive, towards the proposition that a thing, however it may be defined, of which the sole purpose or object is that it may be a human life, should be subjected to experiment to its destruction for the purpose of the acquisition of knowledge." While he had aligned himself with pro-life forces, allowing them to put their imprint on the name of his bill, Powell insisted—somewhat disingenuously—that abortion was not the issue. As he put it, "the Bill does not concern itself in any way with questions such

---

52. Ibid., cols. 542.
53. "Confused Comment on Warnock," 389.
54. For an overview of the controversy surrounding the Powell bill, see Mulkay, *Embryo Research Debate,* chap. 2.

as those of surrogacy, abortion, or the source of the gametes of a fertilised ovum." He was aware that many of his supporters believed that his bill "was authorised by and in accordance with their religious beliefs," but his approach was broader. "The repugnance with which those of many religious persuasions or none view the actions that the Bill would forbid," he argued, was "an instinct implanted in a human society."[55]

While clearly on the defensive in the debate, Warnock supporters led by Jo Richardson of the Labour Party developed three arguments that would be honed over subsequent years. The first was a head-on attack on the abortion parallel. Richardson related that many of her constituents equated research, wrongly, with "doctors and technicians chopping away at perfectly formed miniatures the size of tadpoles." When she explained to them that a fertilized embryo was "at day one smaller than the point of a pin and invisible to the naked eye, they were nonplussed." The second was an argument about consistency—that one could not support IVF, as did Powell, and oppose embryo research designed to assure its safety and effectiveness. The third argument was that embryo research could bring biomedical benefits, particularly but not exclusively in the area of infertility medicine. "To rush into legislation, as we are doing, that will close the door entirely on the beneficial effects of the years of patient research," was premature, Richardson warned, especially regarding research that had "resulted not in a generation of Frankensteins but in a movement towards eliminating the pain and suffering of children and their parents." Minister of Health Kenneth Clarke warned in a similar vein that "those who support the Bill must face the fact that they are probably stopping beneficial research."[56]

These arguments did not carry the day. Buoyed by an impressive public petition-and-letter-writing campaign—and by a lack of interest on the part of many MPs, who did not show up for the debate and vote—the Commons gave its initial approved to the Powell bill by a vote of 238 to 66. The vast majority of Conservative MPs broke with Clarke and Fowler in supporting the bill, as did a majority of Labour representatives.[57] The scientific community now raised the alarm. "Probably the worst consequence imaginable to scientists working in a political democracy," Edwards had written as early as 1971, "would be the pre-emption by the state of a branch of science such as human embryology."[58] He, Anne McLaren (the leading scientist on the

---

55. UK, *Parliamentary Debates,* Commons, 6th ser., vol. 73 (February 15, 1985), cols. 640–41.

56. Ibid., cols. 642–45, 683.

57. "Big Majority for Embryo Bill," *Times* (London), February 16, 1985.

58. Robert G. Edwards and David J. Sharpe, "Social Values and Research in Human Embryology," *Nature* 231, no. 5298 (1971).

Warnock committee), and other scientists now spoke out against scientific skeptics of embryo research and emphasized its capacity to alleviate suffering. Responding directly to Lejeune's claims, the head of the Royal Society, Andrew Huxley, wrote the *Times* that a ban on research might mean "the infliction of misery on numerous children and on the families into which they will be born."[59]

In the run-up to the highly anticipated final parliamentary debate on the bill in June 1985, Warnock engaged in a direct exchange with Cardinal Hume in the *Times*. Not one to mince words, she wrote an editorial that laid out her committee's careful efforts to navigate a pragmatic path on both regulating and permitting research and warned that "the law should beware of following the ideals of extremists." Referring to the Powell bill's equation of embryo research with the destruction of children, she decried "the great tide of moral fundamentalism, sweeping across from America" that "cannot be wholly distinguished from dogmatism, intolerance, and fanaticism."[60] Hume published a response a week later headlined "Why Warnock Is Wrong." It was not fanatical, he insisted, to maintain that life begins at fertilization: "The intellect is readily able to grasp what recent scientific knowledge has illustrated, the continuum that stretches from the moment of fertilization up to birth and beyond." Hume insisted that no democracy could survive without a common morality. And what other tradition besides Christianity, he asked, "is a realistic alternative for providing the nucleus of the moral community?"[61]

As it turned out, the anticipated showdown over the Powell bill did not take place. The government used its control over the legislative timetable to prevent its consideration before the end of the parliamentary session. Pro-research forces now had breathing room to mobilize, should another bill like Powell's be introduced the following year. The British Medical Association, the Royal Society, and the Medical Research Council now aligned themselves more fully with the Warnock report's recommendations. Warnock and McLaren began to crisscross the country making the scientific and ethical case for carefully regulated embryo research. A critical juncture was the formation of the Progress Campaign in November 1985, an umbrella organization aligned with influential patient-advocacy groups, including the

---

59. "Embryo Research," April 6, 1985. Lejeune had written a letter of his own to the *Times* attacking scientific critics of his claims and expressing satisfaction that his name had been invoked no fewer than six times in the Commons debate; "Embryo Research," *Times* (London), March 26, 1985.

60. "Absolutely Wrong," *Times* (London), May 30, 1985.

61. "Why Warnock Is Wrong," *Times* (London), June 6, 1985.

Genetic Interest Group and the Parkinson's Disease Society.[62] An emerging coalition of scientific, medical, and advocacy organizations gradually turned the political tide against Powell and his supporters in the pro-life movement, who did not muster enough support to reintroduce their bill for parliamentary consideration in 1986.

The Human Fertilisation and Embryology Bill

In the meantime, the government went ahead on two tracks: putting regulatory structures in place and gradually preparing its own legislation. In June 1985 the MRC set up the Voluntary Licensing Authority to govern IVF and embryo research along the lines advocated by the Warnock committee. With Powell's defeat, the government was not in a rush to reintroduce the issue in Parliament. The pro-life movement, much weaker than in the United States, could not mount a political challenge without the support of a broader coalition of research opponents like Powell, who were concerned about its possible eugenic implications. In a country where Catholics represented only about 10 percent of the population, the critical reception of the Vatican's February 1987 blanket condemnation of all embryo research and IVF, the instruction *Donum Vitae,* did not help matters. Confident that arguments about the biomedical potential of embryo research would carry the day, the government published a white paper in December 1987 outlining its legislative strategy: an open vote of conscience within Parliament on two opposing measures, one supportive of the Warnock recommendations, the other opposed to all embryo research.[63]

By fall 1989, when the Human Fertilisation and Embryology Bill was finally put on the parliamentary agenda, the abortion issue had not faded completely as a frame for the issue. The government agreed to consider an amendment to the legislation that would reduce the timeframe for legal abortion from twenty-eight to twenty-four weeks. This initially made some research advocates anxious. The Royal Society insisted that "the abortion issue should be kept separate from the discussion of embryo research" and called for a "reasoned debate based on the facts of embryological research rather than one dominated by the emotions evoked by the issue of abortion."[64] As it

---

62. See Birke, Himmelweit, and Vines, *Tomorrow's Child,* 271–72.

63. Simon Hadlington, "British Government Hedges Bets on Embryo Research," *Nature* 330, no. 6147 (1987): 409.

64. Quoted in "The Queen's Speech: Analysis—A Straight Choice and a Free Vote," *Financial Times,* November 22, 1989.

turned out, these fears were unfounded. The incremental adjustment of the Abortion Act passed by a large majority. If anything, its linkage to the embryo issue probably hurt the antiresearch cause, allowing research supporters to dismiss opponents as narrow-minded "pro-lifers" and to align themselves, by contrast, with the biomedical promise of the research.

This dynamic was evident in the parliamentary contest itself. In the first debate in the House of Lords in December 1989, Warnock struck a combative tone. A no to embryo research, she argued, would "put ourselves back into the seventeenth century," an explicit reference to Galileo's persecution at the hands of the Catholic Church. "We cannot undo the Enlightenment," she argued, "and it would be morally wrong to place obstacles, derived from beliefs not very widely shared, in the path of science."[65] A leading Anglican bishop in the House of Lords, John Habgood, made a proresearch argument in a less polemical vein, casting doubt on "the tremendous significance attached by some people to the moment of fertilisation." The Duke of Norfolk, a leading Catholic layman in the United Kingdom, countered that embryo research of any kind "inevitably results in mutilation and destruction of human life at its earliest stage" and that "another better way has to be found to relieve human suffering." Chief Rabbi Immanuel Jakobovits, an expert in Jewish medical ethics, staked out a middle position, supporting research with surplus IVF embryos for worthy goals but insisting that "no embryo should ever be generated for the purpose of experimentation." He lauded the high quality of the debate in which "both sides are clearly equally sincere in wishing to promote the protection and the sanctity of human life."[66]

The political isolation of the pro-life position was evident in the outcome of the Lords vote; the government's proposed legislation passed in February 1990 by a margin of 234 to 80. As the debate moved to the House of Commons, the antiabortion lobby stepped up its campaign, at one point sending every member of Commons a life-size model of a fetus at twenty weeks. Progress and the Genetic Interest Group intensified their lobbying efforts as well, organizing scientific briefings for MPs. By all accounts, public opinion had now swung decisively in favor of research with surplus IVF embryos that were destined to die in any case. The idea of an ethic of healing articulated in a Christian idiom emerged as a key component of the proresearch cause. As Habgood put it in a widely referenced editorial the day of the Commons debate, "under suitable safeguards" embryo research opened the way "to a reverential sharing in the mystery of God's creativity, as well as the relief of

---

65. UK, *Parliamentary Debates,* Lords, 6th ser., vol. 513 (December 7, 1989), col. 1036.
66. Ibid., cols. 1020, 1032, 1072–73.

human suffering." Support for human life and dignity was compatible with an emphasis on biomedical progress. As he put it, the "belief that human beings are made in the image of God points both to reverence for human life as actually given, and also to our human possibilities for creative change."[67]

This ethic of healing featured prominently in the decisive April 1990 Commons debate. "In this House we all share a moral duty to respect and protect the sanctity of human life," Minister of Health Clarke told his colleagues, adding that "we also all share a moral duty to alleviate suffering and to fight against disease." A vote for life-saving research, he insisted, was "compatible with both those moral duties."[68] Bernard Braine, head of the Commons Pro-Life Committee, led the attack on the legislation, emphasizing the moral status of the embryo and dismissing the term "pre-embryo" as a cynical ploy to advance research. He lamented the growth of frozen IVF embryos as material for experiments and insisted that the Archbishop of York, a research supporter, "does not speak for the majority of Christians." Braine pointed with approval to the more complete prohibition on embryo research being debated simultaneously in Germany, where recollection of "what was done by perverted science remains stronger." (Not everyone took kindly to the parallel. One leading research supporter did "not see why we should take lessons in morality from the Germans.")[69]

The pivotal April 1990 vote was an overwhelming victory for proresearch forces: 364 to 193 in favor, with Thatcher and a majority of her cabinet supporting the measure by a 3 to 1 margin. In May and June, research opponents placed their hopes in an amendment that would have prohibited the creation of embryos expressly for research, focusing their appeals on MPs who may have backed research with surplus IVF embryos but viewed their deliberate creation and destruction as a dangerous instrumentalization of human life. Here, research proponents also prevailed, but by a narrower margin, fighting off the amendment with a 246 to 208 vote. In the final Commons vote, the proresearch legislation passed by a margin of 303 to 65. It set up a new state institution, the Human Fertilisation and Embryology Authority (HFEA), to regulate IVF infertility treatments and to license permissible embryo research to advance knowledge in four main areas: infertility, contraception, congenital disease, and preimplantation genetic diagnosis.[70]

---

67. "When Genesis Is in Conflict," *Times* (London), April 23, 1990.
68. UK, *Parliamentary Debates,* Commons, 6th ser., vol. 171 (April 23, 1990), col. 42.
69. Ibid., cols. 52–53, 64.
70. On the votes and the politics behind them, see Mulkay, *Embryo Research Debate,* chaps. 2–3.

Antiresearch forces, who appeared to have had the upper hand through most of the decade, suffered a stunning setback. In a bitter reaction, Cardinal Hume, the leader of the Catholic Church in England and Wales, warned that "we have dispensed with the traditional Christian vision of the sanctity of human life. We can no longer claim to be a truly Christian society."[71] In contrast to the United States, the linkage with the abortion issue had not played out to the advantage of research opponents. Catholic and evangelical leaders in America had been able to work first through Republican administrations and then, after 1994, through congressional majorities to stymie any federal funding for embryo research. In the United Kingdom, where the pro-life movement was considerably weaker, Catholics were a smaller minority, and most of the Anglican leadership was proresearch, a government supportive of research with control of the legislative agenda was able to carry the day. By 1989–90, a strong parliamentary majority emerged around the imperative of research to advance IVF therapies and other biomedical agendas. The ethical arguments that prevailed in the policy struggle centered less on the moral status of the embryo than on the healing promise of research.

Germany: Eugenic Anxieties and a Research Ban

German political controversy about embryo research was strikingly different than in the United States and the United Kingdom. The abortion issue played a marginal role. An uneasy but stable policy compromise on the issue, achieved by the mid-1970s, prevented its emergence as a central frame for the contestation of embryo research. The leadership of the state-supported Catholic and Protestant churches had converged in opposition to research by the mid-1980s but cast their arguments less in terms of a "right to life" than in terms of the dignity of human life and opposition to its manipulation for scientific and medical ends. Concern about dignity and anxiety about eugenics, reinforced by the long historical shadow cast by Nazism, had informed the conclusions of the Benda Commission's 1985 recommendation for embryo research in exceptional circumstances. But as the issue moved to the Bundestag and onto the political agenda, that negative historical legacy was a rallying point for a broad antiresearch coalition that encompassed not only Christian Democrats but much of the secular political Left, including the Social Democrats and the Greens. Once the parliamentary struggle began in earnest in 1989–90, arguments about the potential of research to alleviate

---

71. "Hume Attacks Embryo Vote," *Guardian,* April 27, 1990.

human suffering, so effective in the British political context, did not gain traction. The Embryo Protection Law that passed in 1990 criminalized all embryo research in the Federal Republic.

The legacy of Nazi eugenics did not predetermine this outcome. As noted in chapter 1, embryos had been created, observed, and discarded in the laboratory in Germany during the late 1970s, without drawing broader media or political attention.[72] Freedom of research was explicitly mentioned in the postwar German constitution, partly in reaction to the state-sponsored scientific abuses of the Nazi era. By the time the first German IVF child was born in April 1982, however, research with embryos had run up against a growing cultural skepticism of science and technology, particularly on the German Left. Among the Greens and Social Democrats, concerns about genetically modified organisms, their potential use in agriculture and medicine, and the eventual genetic engineering of humans reinforced skepticism about IVF-related research and its potential eugenic applications.[73] Scientists, while still jealous of their autonomy, began to acknowledge the importance of democratic oversight for their work. Some regulation began to appear attractive, given the alternative of more drastic government action. "One could do much," German IVF pioneer Liselotte Mettler put it in October 1983. "But one does not know if one is allowed."[74]

Like the Thatcher government in the United Kingdom, the Christian Democratic–Liberal coalition that took office in October 1982 under Chancellor Helmut Kohl adopted a cautious approach. It consulted a range of experts and eventually set up the Benda Commission in May 1984, just as the work of the Warnock committee was winding down in Britain. When it reported, in November 1985, the commission's recommendations—to oppose embryo research in principle but to allow it in pursuit of "medical findings of great value"—drew much less comment and analysis than had Warnock. There was no storm of controversy about embryo research in Germany akin to that in the United Kingdom. Initial discussion in the media centered on the group's recommendations concerning reproductive technologies—its endorsement of IVF as an infertility treatment and opposition to surrogate

---

72. Interview with Klaus Thomsen, "Purer Zufall oder eine echte Hoffnung?" *Der Spiegel,* July 31, 1978.

73. In a response to a 1984 query from Green deputies, the government documented earlier IVF research involving the creation, observation, and discarding of embryos. It distinguished this from the destruction of embryos to obtain scientific knowledge, which the government opposed. See Bundestag, *Antwort der Bundesregierung auf die grossen Anfragen der Abgeordneten Frau Dr. Hickel und der Fraktion Die Grünen, Drucksache 10/1153* (Bonn: Deutscher Bundestag, 1984), 22–23.

74. "Kinder nach Katalo," *Die Zeit,* October 28, 1983.

motherhood. Questions of genetic engineering and gene therapy taken up in the report also received attention, as they coincided with the deliberations of an investigative commission on genetics looking into a bundle of issues ranging from agricultural biotechnology to the use of genetic information.

This initial lack of political controversy surrounding embryo research was partly a function of its relative underdevelopment in Germany. But it was also related to the absence of abortion as a frame for controversy. In 1974–75 the Bundestag had passed and the Federal Constitutional Court had approved a legislative compromise that construed abortion as the taking of innocent human life but suspended prosecution if mandatory counseling revealed evidence of a mother's mental or physical duress. This creative, if controversial, construction offered something to both sides. Abortion supporters could and did claim that the procedure was now allowed de facto in Germany. For their part, opponents lauded state recognition of abortion as the taking of innocent human life, if not as a crime to be prosecuted in practice. With some reservations, the Catholic and Protestant hierarchies accepted this pragmatic compromise, which affirmed the value of human life, acknowledged the tragic nature of the abortion decision, and provided for counseling services.

In upholding this legal compromise, the Constitutional Court was able to affirm the preamble of the Basic Law, with its insistence on the inviolability of human life, while enabling (if not legalizing) abortion in practice. Unlike the U.S. Supreme Court two years earlier, in its *Roe v. Wade* decision, the German court did not sidestep the question of the moral status of the fetus. It did remain almost completely silent on the embryo, however. A key passage in the February 1975 ruling read: "Life in the sense of the historical existence of a human individual, according to reliable biological and physiological knowledge, exists in any case [*jedenfalls*] from day 14 after conception (implantation, individuation)"—a formulation which left open the moral status of the embryo before that juncture.[75] Later, research opponents would argue that the logic of the decision, with its insistence that "where human life exists, it is invested with human dignity," implied that the early embryo, too, deserved constitutional protection. However, the judges had not said so explicitly. With their reference to implantation and individuation as key developmental markers—years before the reports of the Ethics Advisory Board in 1979 and the Warnock committee in 1984—they suggested the possibility of a lesser moral status for the embryo. The Benda Commission,

75. Bundesverfassungsgericht, *BVerfGE 39, 1 (37)—Schwangerschaftsabbruch I*, February 25, 1975, http://www.servat.unibe.ch/dfr/bv039001.html.

in supporting research on early embryos in the service of "medical findings of great value," had exploited that possibility.[76]

From the Benda Commission to the Embryo Protection Law

In March 1986 the Kohl government moved cautiously to legislate along the lines of the Benda report's recommendations. Minister of Justice Hans Engelhardt of the Liberal Free Democratic Party (FDP) put forward a legislative framework for discussion that banned embryo research in principle but would allow state governments and local ethics committees to make exceptions for work on surplus IVF embryos in some cases. The medical and scientific communities, worried about a restrictive interpretation of what constituted "medical findings of great value," nevertheless welcomed the government's response. In May 1985, during the Benda deliberations, a congress of the German Medical Association had declared that "experiments with embryos are to be rejected in principle" unless they should "serve the improvement of the [fertility] method or the well-being of the child." The association rejected the deliberate creation of embryos for research as incompatible with the principle of human dignity but held open the possibility of work with spares given "scientific questions that can only be addressed successfully through experiments with human embryos."[77]

Gradually, however, embryo politics moved in a more restrictive direction—and the scientific and medical communities proved powerless to stop it. In the context of the Federal Republic's federal system of government, a Federal-State Working Group was set up in fall 1986 to propose specific legislation. The working group, made up of legal and medical experts and representatives of different parties at the national and state levels, took up a wide range of issues linked with reproductive medicine, including artificial insemination and surrogate motherhood. On the critical issue of embryo research, it gravitated toward a more restrictive position than either Benda or Engelhardt had envisioned. The working group's initial recommendations, dated November 1987, called for a ban on destructive embryo research—with no exceptions. In February 1988 a Kohl government cabinet report officially adopted this position as its own, with the pragmatic argument that "there are at this point

---

76. As late as 1982, an editorial in the conservative *Frankfurter Allgemeine Zeitung* suggested that embryo research was legal as long as abortion was allowed—a view that later shifted as the issue moved onto the legal and political agenda. *Frankfurter Allgemeine Zeitung,* April 24, 1982.

77. Declaration reprinted in Rolf Keller, Hans-Ludwig Günther, and Peter Kaiser Keller, *Embryonenschutzgesetz: Kommentar zum Embryonenschutzgesetz* (Stuttgart: Kohlhammer, 1992), 265.

still no concrete medical questions that make research on human embryos in the interest of protecting the life of third parties indispensable."[78] While the FDP and the Federal Ministry of Justice under its control resisted, momentum was building for a complete research ban with no exceptions.

What explains this political turn in a more restrictive direction? The mobilization of the churches, a key constituency for Kohl's Christian Democratic Union, played a role. In November 1985, it should be recalled, a prominent Catholic theologian, Franz Böckle, sat on the Benda Commission, endorsed its qualified support for embryo research, and did not face any Church censure. At a 1985 meeting the German bishops had been critical of IVF but did not reject it altogether. After the publication of the Vatican Instruction *Donum Vitae* in February 1987, however, the German Catholic Church's stance on IVF and embryo research hardened considerably.[79] In contrast to the United States and the United Kingdom, German Church leaders rarely linked embryo research with abortion—like their Protestant counterparts, most came to terms with the 1975 abortion compromise. In opposing embryo research church leaders tended not to invoke a "right to life" argument but instead emphasized the constitutional norm of the inviolability of human dignity, which was anchored in the Basic Law.

A similar pattern was evident in the Evangelical Church in Germany. In contrast to mainline churches in the United States and the Anglican Church in the United Kingdom, the EKD, while progressive on a range of social issues, gravitated toward a restrictive position on embryo research, a development complete by the time of its November 1987 synod.[80] The contrast with strong proresearch currents among Anglicans and mainline U.S. Protestants was striking. German Protestants, like their Catholic counterparts, latched on to the human dignity provision of the constitution. In late 1989, on the eve of parliamentary consideration of legislation, Protestant and Catholic leaders issued a joint statement centered not on the abortion parallel but on the constitutional norm. "No matter how great the research goals," they argued, "the dignity of human life forbids that it should be used simply as a means to an end, let alone created for that purpose." The statement called "the idea of sacrifice" totally inappropriate: "Only of his own free will can one human

---

78. Bundestag, *Kabinettbericht zur künstlichen Befruchtung beim Menschen, Drucksache 11/1856* (Bonn: Deutscher Bundestag), 8.

79. On the bishops' stance in the run-up to *Donum Vitae*, see David Seeber, "Die neuen Techniken menschlicher Fortpflanzung," *Herder Korrespondenz* 40, no. 3 (1986): 146–47.

80. Evangelische Kirche in Deutschland, "Zur Achtung vor dem Leben—Maßstäbe für Gentechnik und Fortpflanzungsmedizin," November 6, 1987, http://www.ekd.de/EKD-Texte/achtungvordemleben_1987.html.

being give his life for another." It concluded that "Even the smallest step on the path toward destructive embryo research crosses an important line."[81]

Just as consequential for the restrictive turn in the German debate was the opposition to embryo research among *secular* forces in the Social Democratic (SPD) and Green parties. During the middle of the decade, the strongest opposition to scientific self-governance came from the Social Democrats. A key figure was the party's leading science expert, Wolf-Dieter Catenhusen. In addition to chairing the investigative commission on genetics, Catenhusen pressed hard for restrictive governance of IVF and embryo research. "We have to eliminate the law-free zone that today allows for experiments on fertilized human eggs," he argued in a January 1985 Bundestag debate.[82] The Social Democratic leadership endorsed the idea of a total ban on embryo research in late 1985. The SPD in the state of Baden-Württemberg, in a colorful declaration, denounced the work of "Anglo-Saxon institutes such as the Kennedy Institute of Ethics, the Hastings Center, or the Center for Human Bioethics (in Australia)" as "incompatible with the norms of the Constitution."[83]

In a Bundestag debate called by the SPD in February 1988, Herta Däubler-Gmelin, the party's health spokesperson, welcomed the government's shift in a more restrictive direction but chided it for not moving sooner. She pushed for a comprehensive, restrictive agenda on reproductive medicine that would include detailed strictures on IVF and artificial insemination designed to protect women and prevent eugenic abuses. Invoking the work of scientists on nuclear weapons, she critiqued the "research imperative" and quoted Felix Oppenheimer on the seductions of "sweet science." For Social Democrats and their Green allies in opposition, the moral status of the embryo itself played a subordinate role in the debate, although Däubler-Gmelin did refer to the union of sperm and egg as yielding a "human life on the way to birth." The Greens, in supporting broad-based restrictive legislation, focused almost exclusively on potential eugenic abuses. In the debate Rita Süssmuth, the Christian Democratic minister of health, also placed warnings about Nazi eugenics ahead of concerns about the moral status of the embryo. Invoking Hitler's legacy, she hoped that "we will never again come to the point" at

---

81. Evangelische Kirche in Deutschland, "Gott ist ein Freund des Lebens: Herausforderungen und Aufgaben beim Schutz des Lebens," November 30, 1989, http://www.ekd.de/EKD-Texte/44678.html.

82. Bundestag, *Verhandlungen des deutschen Bundestages. Stenographischer Bericht,* ser. 11 (January 17, 1985), 8513.

83. Quoted in Eric B. Brown, "The Dilemmas of German Bioethics," *New Atlantis,* no. 5 (2004): 46.

which "science and ethics are ripped apart." In a finishing flourish she quoted the bioethicist Hans Jonas: "Don't open the Pandora's box!"[84]

The hostile reception given the Australian bioethicist Peter Singer during a visit to Germany in 1989, where he was invited to speak at a symposium in Marburg on ethical issues linked to disabilities, reflected this focus on eugenics. Singer was on record as being against the idea of the sanctity and inviolable dignity of every human life; he insisted instead on the concrete evaluation of the quality of life in question. When the media publicized his view that parents of severely disabled infants condemned to a life of physical suffering should have the euthanasia option in some cases, the symposium organizers bowed to pressure and disinvited him and eventually canceled the event. A lecture at the University of Dortmund was canceled for the same reason. Singer finally did speak at the University of Saarbrücken during the same trip, where he was harassed and continually interrupted by shouts of "Out with the Fascist!" The media coverage of what came to be called the "Singer affair" pointed to widespread opposition to utilitarian bioethics informed by anxiety about history and its lessons. Singer himself later noted that vocal advocates for the disabled "were strongly supported and encouraged by various coalitions against genetic engineering and reproductive technology."[85]

During the critical 1988–89 years, when political and policy debate was starting in earnest, German research supporters could not count on the support of powerful allies within the government bureaucracy (like the NIH in the United States or the MRC in the United Kingdom) or on a coalition of scientific, medical, and patient-advocacy groups like Progress in the United Kingdom. The Liberals placed more emphasis on scientific freedom and were represented in the governing coalition by the justice minister. But they, too, found themselves swimming against a tide of elite and public opinion concerned about the eugenic potentials of emergent technologies—a stark contrast with the simultaneous growing emphasis on an ethic of healing in the British debate. Some scientific groups were more supportive of regulation than others. The prestigious Max Planck Society, a government-financed network of laboratories, declared itself open to a moratorium on embryo research in 1989. By contrast, the German Research Foundation maintained the view that a ban on all research would end work in a critical field.[86]

84. Bundestag, *Verhandlungen des deutschen Bundestages*, ser. 11 (February 25, 1988), 4290–91, 4302–3.

85. Peter Singer, "On Being Silenced in Germany," *New York Review of Books* 38, no. 14 (1991): 36–42; "Euthanasie: Bizarre Verquickung," *Der Spiegel*, August 21, 1989.

86. "Leicht zu beseitigendes Opfer," *Die Zeit*, September 22, 1989.

The struggle over the shape of the legislation turned on whether a ban would be complete or allow research aimed at "medical findings of great value." In June 1989, Minister of Justice Engelhard, who still supported some exceptions, struck a deal with the minister for family affairs, Ursula Lehr, who favored a total ban. The legislation called for a comprehensive ban but justified it not with respect to the moral status of the embryo, but through reference to the dearth of worthy research projects. The prohibition should only last as long as there were no prospects for successful research. According to press reports, some justice ministry officials expected such prospects to materialize before the parliamentary vote on the law; they even mentioned areas such as AIDS and cancer.[87] But, by the fall of 1989, on the eve of the first Bundestag debate devoted expressly to the government's legislative proposals, a strong coalition across the parties, the churches, and legal scholars had emerged in favor of a total ban. State governments represented in Germany's upper house, the Bundesrat, also signaled their support for such an approach.

The decisive parliamentary debate took place in early December 1989, two weeks after the fall of the Berlin Wall. Not surprisingly, it did not get much media attention. A high degree of consensus across the parties was in evidence, with the principle of human dignity serving as common ground. Engelhard opened with the comment that "new methods in reproductive medicine open not only opportunities but especially potentials for abuse." Referring to the early embryo, he insisted that "life and human dignity require comprehensive protection." Däubler-Gmelin and Schmidt of the Greens chided the government for not doing enough by leaving IVF infertility procedures out of the law. For Schmidt, the proposed legislation left enough "loopholes for scientific drive, eugenics and genetic selection." To prevent such practices and to protect women from exploitation, she argued, one should abandon artificial reproductive technologies altogether.[88] Whatever their differences, the parties, including the more research-friendly FDP, had converged around an embryo research ban in the name of human dignity.

The government's determination to secure as large a majority as possible, and the SPD and Green desire to see even stricter legislation, delayed final approval of the Embryo Protection Law until October 1990, the same month as German reunification and at the start of a national election campaign for the new Germany.[89] Eugenic dangers were a key theme. In one of the final debates before passage, the lead Christian Democratic speaker,

---

87. "Bonner Hintertür," *Der Spiegel,* June 26, 1989.

88. Bundestag, *Verhandlungen des deutschen Bundestages* (December 8, 1989), 14166, 14172.

89. Bundestag, *Verhandlungen des deutschen Bundestages* (October 23, 1990), 18206–20.

Heinz Seesing, led off by celebrating the fact that protecting the embryo would "forbid in advance the application of therapeutic measures that are not yet technically mature but that could change entire future generations." We created our constitution, he argued, "to force the state to protect human dignity in perpetuity." In order to "prevent any possibility of manipulation, that protection must extend from the beginning to the end of life." Work with surplus embryos for worthy goals, he insisted, would lead down a slippery slope; research that might advance medicine could also be exploited for eugenic ends. He welcomed the explicit prohibition of cloning and human genetic modification and extolled the fact that "no other country had instituted a similarly strict protection of human life." Here was a Christian Democratic leader opposing research in all circumstances but not asserting the embryo's right to life or the abortion parallel.[90]

The lead speaker for the SPD, Däubler-Gmelin, was even more outspoken in her emphasis on the eugenic implications of the technology. While acknowledging the popularity of IVF as an infertility treatment, she emphasized its potential abuses. "If we are not careful, new IVF techniques become a gateway for the construction of new people." She added, strangely, that she meant the construction of a "homunculus" akin to the miniature human being created by Goethe's Faust in the epic poem, something now "within the realm of possibility." The SPD deputies, she declared, would oppose the Embryo Protection Law not because it was too strict but because it was not strict enough. She claimed that its provisions against the creation of animal-human hybrid embryos and genetic modification were too weak and she lamented the absence of an explicit prohibition of the freezing of embryos left over from IVF treatments.

The lead Green spokesperson in the debate, Ulla Schmidt, also took a hard line on embryo research, echoing Däubler-Gmelin's view that the ban did not go far enough. As long as there was IVF, she argued, there would be experiments with embryos that might lead to eugenic abuses, such as the negative selection of embryos for certain traits, including the presence or absence of congenital diseases. Schmidt explicitly evoked the parallel of the 1933 Nazi forced sterilization law. She also critiqued the legislation's allowance for freezing of sperm and egg just before fertilization as a de facto way to create surplus embryos either for IVF treatments or for experiments. In contrast to most research opponents, she echoed Däubler-Gmelin's opposition to IVF itself, pointing to its "enormous physical and psychic burdens on women."[91]

---

90. Bundestag, *Verhandlungen des deutschen Bundestages* (October 24, 1990), 18207–9.
91. Ibid., 18209–11, 18213–14.

By this point the cross-party consensus against destructive embryo research was robust and extended even to the leadership of the FDP. In the final October 1990 debate, the party's representative, Rainer Funke noted the importance of scientific freedom but insisted that—in light of the Basic Law's provisions on human life and dignity—embryos should not be "created or used for other purposes."[92] The final vote did not reflect a split between pro- and antiresearch forces. Many SPD and Green deputies voted against the legislation because they felt it did not go far enough. The Embryo Protection Law that went into effect in January 1991 criminalized all research destructive of embryos, outlawed cloning and the creation of chimeras, and bound doctors to only create the exact number of embryos they should implant, as a way to obviate the problem of surplus embryos.

The negative legacy of Nazi eugenics and the Holocaust, and the norm of the inviolability of human dignity connected to it, framed the German political debate and promoted a convergence of secular and religious forces around a restrictive research regime. While the outcome was starkly different from that in the United Kingdom, it reflected a conviction—largely absent in the United States—that rules for embryo research should bind both the public and the private sectors. Where fundamental values were at stake, the German Constitutional Court had declared in its seminal abortion ruling that the democratic state must "not evade such a task by accepting a 'legal vacuum' and refraining from making its own assessment, thus leaving it to the individual's own decision."[93] The drive for clarity in the democratic governance of ethically charged life sciences research was even more pronounced in the case of France.

France: A Comprehensive and Restrictive Approach

Embryo politics in France, like those in Germany, were colored more by concerns about genetic engineering than by the abortion controversy. In both countries, questions of human dignity were widely seen to be at stake. And while the idea of human dignity had biblical roots and was forcefully espoused by the churches and Jewish groups, it found its most powerful political expression in France in a secular register. In Germany, the norm of human dignity was enshrined in the constitution as a conscious, collective response to the horrors of Nazism. In France, too, the World War II era served as a backdrop, heightening sensitivities about the abuse of science. But the

92. Ibid., 18212.
93. Quoted in the report of the Benda Commission, *Working Group on In Vitro Fertilisation*, 7.

centrality of dignity was articulated on a different philosophical and political foundation: the humanistic values of the Enlightenment and their embodiment in the French Revolution and the Republican tradition it inaugurated. Public ideals of freedom, equality, and solidarity, embedded in the legal system and in the broader political culture, favored a comprehensive approach to bioethical questions, especially those with implications for human rights. The question was not whether the state would regulate, but how. It was answered through a decade-long political struggle that led to the Bioethics Laws of 1994, which addressed issues as diverse as organ donation, genetic therapy, and surrogate motherhood. One of their core components was an absolute ban on destructive embryo research—an outcome that paralleled the German one several years earlier.

The French political and policy controversy, like the German one, can be traced back to the birth of the country's first IVF child, Baby Amandine, in February 1982. The media echo was enormously positive, and IVF clinics spread throughout the country over the 1980s. Gradually the absence of government regulation became an object of controversy. Jacques Testart, who had helped to bring Baby Amandine into the world, had worked with French Institute of Health and Medical Research (INSERM) funds and informed its ethics board of his research and clinical work on IVF. His success now drew the attention of politicians. For Minister of Health Jack Ralite the breakthrough showed the need for "an imaginative effort to grapple with the ethical aspect of these questions." As he put it, "the scientists should not be the only ones to reflect on the matter."[94] Minister of Science and Technology Jean-Pierre Chevènement encouraged INSERM to form a broader ethics committee that might supervise embryo and IVF research at other institutions as well. He envisioned the participation of legal experts as well as members of various "spiritual families."[95]

This discussion culminated in the March 1983 announcement of a permanent national ethics committee to advise the government—the first of its kind in the world. It was to include scientists, doctors, philosophers, and one representative each from the Catholic, Protestant, and Jewish communities. In charging the committee in December 1983, President Mitterrand reflected on two decades of rapid advances in the life sciences and the need for a comprehensive democratic regulatory framework. "We believed for some time that rationality would be enough of a guide, but the very success of science is proving us wrong," he argued. Alluding to work on IVF

---

94. "Satisfactions ministérielles," *Le Monde,* February 26, 1982.
95. "Ethique et fécondations artificielles," *Le Monde,* February 28–March 1, 1982.

and human genetics, he insisted that "what is possible or may be soon is not necessarily permissible." While he warned against a blanket skepticism that might bring scientific progress to a halt, he also called for critical reflection and ethical guidance to inform a broader democratic debate.[96] In his charge to the committee, Mitterrand invoked an Enlightenment conception of reason grounded in core beliefs about the dignity of the human person—the "kind of reason that reason alone cannot always achieve." He mixed enthusiasm about science with some anxiety about its impact on humanity's future. Scientists, he argued, must learn to ask: "What risks does my work pose for the human species?"[97]

Mitterrand's intervention was exceptional in two respects. First, in contrast to the United States, United Kingdom, and Germany, a national leader was taking the initiative. As a Socialist, Mitterrand was concerned about technologies of exploitation. As a veteran of the Resistance, he was troubled by the Nazi legacy of eugenics. He articulated these concerns in the secular idiom of the Republic, with its founding ideals of human dignity and equality. His personal convictions and the authority of his office gave bioethical questions considerable salience. Second, Mitterrand called for a comprehensive national debate to be structured within a permanent ethics body. In contrast to the Ethics Advisory Board, the Warnock committee, and the Benda Commission, the National Consultative Ethics Committee had an extensive staff and reported to the Ministry of Health. It was explicitly charged with the development of recommendations that should inform deliberation and decision within the French parliament and the powerful lower house, the National Assembly, in particular. The centralized structure of the French state, backed by the authority of the president, generated a visible space for discussion and debate about embryo research over the next decade—even if French political leaders did not always follow the committee's lead.

While the CCNE produced a stream of opinions bearing on embryo research in the mid-1980s, it initially did not draw much media attention. As in Germany, the absence of an advanced research program—and of a colorful personality like Robert Edwards pointing to new research frontiers—was part of the reason. The committee's early opinions in 1984

---

96. Présidence de la République, "Allocution de M. François Mitterrand, Président de la République, à l'occasion de la mise en place du Comité consultatif national d'éthique pour les sciences de la vie et de la santé," press release, December 2, 1983, http://lesdiscours.vie-publique.fr/pdf/837208100.pdf.

97. Ibid.

setting out the idea that the embryo represented "potential human life" and therefore deserved respect did not occasion a legislative response. Not until December 1986, when the CCNE issued its first in-depth opinion on embryo research did conservative prime minister Jacques Chirac, then in a power-sharing cohabitation arrangement with Mitterrand, take up the issue. He charged the State Council, a legal advisory body, with an examination of the legislative issues at stake. Developments in different fields, Chirac noted, "posed moral questions, the solutions to which seemed to reside, at least in part, in an adaptation of our law, or even in the creation of novel legal norms."[98]

Initially, leading French scientists and medical professionals did not react as negatively to the prospect of regulation as did their counterparts in the United States, the United Kingdom, and Germany. IVF researchers were broadly receptive to the idea that they had a wider responsibility to society grounded in humanist ideals, and the French medical association was a traditionally conservative voice on ethical questions. Testart had called soon after Amandine's birth for a broader societal discussion about the new technology, particularly in light of its potential eugenic applications. He would raise these concerns more vocally in the years that followed. René Frydman, his closest collaborator, also endorsed Chevènement's suggestion for some kind of national ethics body. The spread of IVF and the emergence freezing technologies that enabled surplus IVF embryos, he argued, necessitated a secure regulatory environment for scientists. His main concern was not the moral status of the embryo but instead the imperative of some democratically legitimated oversight of practices with wider implications for society and its values.[99]

Not all French researchers welcomed the prospect of a comprehensive legal framework. Most participants in a major January 1985 colloquium in Paris on "Genetics, Procreation, and Rights" agreed that effective regulation would be possible without blanket national legislation.[100] Two years later, after Chirac had placed the issue on the policy agenda, a leading French scientist, François Gros, claimed that legislation was not necessary, given the work's

---

98. "Un rapport du Conseil d'Etat sur l'éthique médicale, et le droit," *Le Monde,* March 26, 1988; "La loi en souffrance," *Le Monde,* June 13, 1991.

99. "Un bébé venu d'ailleurs," *Le Monde,* February 26, 1982; Jacques Testart, *L'oeuf transparent* (Paris: Flammarion, 1986); René Frydman, *Dieu, la Medecine et l'embryon* (Paris: Éditions Odile Jacob, 1999). See also Robert Walgate, "French Scientist Makes a Stand," *Nature* 323, no. 6087 (1986): 385.

100. Some of the participants later contributed to François Gros and Gérard Huber, eds. *Vers un anti-destin?: Patrimoine génétique et droits de l'humanité* (Paris: Éditions Odile Jacob, 1992).

scientific promise. It was enough to have "frequent meetings among specialists" and consider "the stances of ethics committees," he insisted. French research teams were pressing ahead without much ethical or legal oversight. In the absence of regulations, *Le Monde* reported, embryos were being created expressly for experiments.[101]

As it happened, it took the lumbering French state machine almost two years to develop legislative proposals that addressed embryo research together with a range of other bioethical issues. The research section of the State Council, under the leadership of Guy Braibant, published its report and recommendations under the title "From Ethics to Law" in March 1988.[102] The Braibant report addressed a broad range of bioethical subjects, from human experimentation to organ donation to DNA testing. On the issue of the embryo, the report called for a ban on the creation of embryos for research and a five-year limit on the freezing of embryos. In line with the CCNE's December 1986 recommendations, the Braibant report made allowance for some experiments with surplus IVF embryos less than fourteen days old, but called for a ban on cloning, chimeras, and any modification of the human genome. The report was not, it self-consciously noted, "an effort to take the place of the government or the parliament" but rather "to illuminate the choices at stake" by the light of reason. It sought to translate the "common morality" of the Republic into prescriptions, without special attention to the concerns of the Roman Catholic Church or any other religious body. It was, in the words of one of the Council's vice presidents, Marceau Long, "an approach of great humanism, and perhaps of an atheist humanism."[103]

Electoral Politics and the Bioethics Laws

Chirac did not remain prime minister long enough to act on the Council's recommendations. In the wake of his May 1988 reelection as president, Mitterrand called for legislative elections, which his Socialists won handily, consigning Chirac and the conservatives to the opposition. In September 1988 the new prime minister, the Socialist Michel Rocard, asked Braibant to move from the initial report to a concrete set of legislative recommendations,

---

101. "Un entretien avec le professeur François Gros: 'La France est un pays moteur pour la réflexion sur la bioéthique,'" *Le Monde,* October 26, 1989; "Les embryons au service de l'homme," *Le Monde,* November 16, 1988.

102. Conseil d'Etat, *Sciences de la vie: De l'éthique au droit* (Paris: La Documentation française, 1988).

103. "Un rapport du Conseil d'Etat sur l'éthique médicale Feux verts et garde-fous," *Le Monde,* March 26, 1988.

which were published in March 1989 under the title "The Life Sciences and the Rights of Man"—an appropriate reference to France's revolutionary bicentennial. This second report included more detailed legislative language. It insisted that embryos only be created for procreative purposes but suggested that surplus IVF embryos might eventually be put to three uses: later implantation, donation, or research.[104] Research with surplus embryos would be possible, on condition that such research "not be susceptible to threaten the integrity of the human species or to lead to eugenic practices." A limit of research to seven days after conception was proposed, with exceptions up to fourteen days. Marveling at the breadth and comprehensiveness of the French approach, which encompassed a range of issues beyond embryo research, the U.S. weekly *Science* noted: "Exactly 200 years after a revolution that embodied the newly conceived rights of man, France has announced that it is to become the first Western nation to introduce a wide-ranging law on bioethics."[105]

Hopes of passing the legislation during the symbolic year 1989 were not realized, not least because of the complexity of the proposals and Rocard's express desire to prepare the laws carefully through consultations with ministries and other state institutions. For example, the government also asked the National Consultative Commission on Human Rights to weigh in. In its September 1989 report, the commission was broadly supportive of the proposals. It held up "respect for the dignity of the human person" as a core principle, as well as the "rejection of all eugenic practice."[106] The commission was divided on the question of embryo research, but insistent that it under no circumstances "threaten the integrity of the human species." Braibant seconded the Commission's call for legislation and expressed impatience with the government's cautious approach. Without a clear legal framework, he suggested somewhat cryptically, scientific and technological pressures would lead to "situations of a kind we will no longer be able to master" and to "influences emanating from other cultural conceptions that we will no longer be able to oppose."[107]

Delays into 1990 fueled speculation that President Mitterrand and his advisers were having second thoughts about legislating on IVF and embryo

104. "L'avant-projet de loi sur les sciences de la vie et les droits de l'homme: Le modèle français de l'éthique médicale," *Le Monde,* March 3, 1989.

105. David Dickson, "France Introduces Bioethics Law," *Science* 243, no. 4896 (1989): 1284.

106. Commission nationale consultative des droits de l'homme, "Avis sur les sciences de la vie et Droits de l'Homme," September 21, 1989, http://www.cncdh.fr/article.php3?id_article=276.

107. "Un entretien avec M. Guy Braibant: 'Il y a urgence à légiférer sur la bioéthique,'" *Le Monde,* October 29, 1989.

research, partly out of a concern with burdening French science with too much regulation. Hubert Curien, the research minister, had gone public with some of his concerns in October 1989.[108] To buy more time and head off parliamentary pressures for rapid action, Rocard now commissioned yet another report in October 1990, from a committee under the leadership of Noëlle Lenoir of the State Council. The committee, made up of scientists, philosophers, and religious representatives, published its findings in June 1991, noting that embryo research was "unquestionably the most difficult question" it had faced. In the absence of regulation, the committee report noted, French practices, had "remained relatively opaque." On the model of the U.K.'s new Human Fertilisation and Embryology Authority, the report advocated the creation of a "National Council on Medicine and Research on the Beginnings of Life" to oversee IVF and embryo research. Three core principles should guide its work: nonproduction of embryos solely for research; consent of the donors to use surplus embryos for research; and no implantation of any embryo that has been the object of research. The report warned against any clear legal definition of the rights of the embryo, given that society had "not yet" arrived at a consensus and different political and religious groups were at odds.[109]

The publication of the Lenoir report generated greater interest in bioethical questions in the media and wider society—and among parliamentarians. The Catholic Church, under the leadership of Cardinal Jean-Marie Lustiger, began to mobilize against the proposed legislation. In a public debate with research minister Curien in early 1992, for example, Lustiger argued that science succeeds best where "it rids itself of scientism"—the belief that it is self-sufficient and requires no ethical oversight. Curien, for his part, insisted on the importance of scientific freedom and reasoned debate, noting that even for theologians, "revelation does not obviate the need for rational investigation of scientific knowledge."[110] In the meantime, the issues finally moved onto the parliamentary agenda. Franck Serusclat, a Socialist bioethics expert in the Senate, and Bernard Bioulac, a conservative member of the National Assembly, organized public hearings and expert consultations that culminated in a major report outlining legislative options on the key bioethical issues.[111]

---

108. Ibid.

109. Noëlle Lenoir, *Aux frontières de la vie: Une éthique biomédicale à la française* (Paris: La Documentation française, 1991), 195–203.

110. La Croix, *Science et foi: Colloque, 1er février 1992* (Paris: Centurion, 1992).

111. Frank Sérusclat, *Sciences de la vie et droits de l'Homme: Bouleversement sans contrôleu législation à la française* (Paris: Office parlementaire d'évaluation des choix scientifiques et technologiques, 1992); *Rapport d'information sur la bioéthique* (Paris: Assemblée nationale, 1992).

At long last, the Rocard government's proposed bioethics legislation was approved by the Council of Ministers in March 1992 and taken up by the National Assembly in November 1992. Minister of Health Bernard Kouchner dramatically introduced the bill, suggesting that "many countries are watching how the country of the Rights of Man will speak on biomedical ethics." He spoke of "respect for human dignity" and of the "values that France has defended since the Enlightenment." Kouchner carefully set out the government's position that research with surplus embryos should be allowed for worthy research. While he acknowledged that the CCNE had defined the embryo as "the potentiality of a person," he warned against an absolutist stance against research, given the presence of some twenty thousand frozen IVF embryos, many without hope of a "parental project." While Kouchner evoked "the eternal combat of science and morality, of knowledge and duty which starts in Genesis in the earthly paradise"—an interesting appeal to biblical imagery—he also argued that morality informed by a "humanist conscience" would emerge victorious.[112]

A leading spokesman for the conservative opposition, Christine Boutin, professed herself appalled by this line of argument. Whether or not an embryo was part of a "parental project" did not determine its moral status. She considered the embryo an actual, and not just a potential, person. Although Catholic, Boutin did not dwell on the parallel between abortion and embryo research or invoke religious arguments. She did call the embryo a "miracle" and "the most precious gift." But the only time she mentioned the Church was in defensive mode, lashing out at those who categorized her as a Catholic in order to dismiss her point of view. In keeping with France's secular political culture she instead invoked "our humanist tradition," insisting the embryo should not be a "hostage" to parents or scientists. The "dignity of the human person" necessitated a complete research ban, she argued, praising the German law passed two years earlier. (As in the U.K. debate, this earned a rebuke from a colleague who charged one should not take moral lessons from the Germans.)[113]

The peculiar mix of antiresearch arguments in secular idiom was also evident in the contribution of Jean-François Mattei, a prominent physician and bioethics expert aligned with the conservative opposition and generally

---

112. *Assemblée nationale, Compte rendu intégral, November 19, 1992,* 5726–32. For an overview of the debates, see "L'examen des projets de loi sur la bioéthique: Les députés veulent limiter strictement la procreation médicalement assistée," *Le Monde,* November 26, 1992.

113. *Assemblée nationale, Compte rendu intégral,* November 19, 1992, 5738–51.

opposed to embryo research. Mattei, also a Catholic, nevertheless warned against the imposition of a "moral order"—a reference to the Church's authoritarian role in French politics and society under the ancien régime. He insisted that reason, not authority, should dictate the direction of governance on sensitive bioethical questions. He referred to a "sacred dimension to man"—a phrase that, whatever its religious origins, had been assimilated to France's secular political culture—and insisted on "a society in the service of human values." Mattei acknowledged the ethical quandaries linked to the status of the embryo and the potentials of research. But he came down against any and all destructive embryo research. "Potential or not," he opined, "in my view, we are dealing with a human person."[114]

The Rocard government appeared to have the votes to pass the legislation permitting some embryo research, over the opposition of conservatives. But then a conservative victory in the March 1993 legislative elections transformed the political constellation. Mitterrand spoke out publicly on the need to move the legislation forward. But Mattei, charged by the new majority with adapting the legislation, opted for delay and more consultations and deliberation before any next steps.[115] After several months of work on yet another report laying out the scientific and ethical issues, Mattei noted in a meeting with scientific leaders that the problem of embryo research "crystallizes passions" and was "without a doubt one of the most difficult that has been examined." The report that bore his name repeated Lenoir's strong opposition to the creation of embryos for research but deviated sharply from her allowance for research with surplus embryos. The only research permitted would be the kind that did not harm embryos—practically speaking, none at all. Mattei did reject calls from Boutin and other Catholic conservatives to grant the embryo legal rights.[116] In the end, though, his support for a total ban allied him with conservatives. The French legislative process had now produced a draft law comparable in its restrictions to the German one.

Although France was a majority Catholic country, the Church opposed all embryo research, and Mattei himself was Catholic, he continued to adhere to a secular line of argument. In an extended interview in *Le Monde* in October 1993, he invoked the 1975 abortion law and its call for "respect for

---

114. *Assemblée nationale, Compte rendu intégral,* November 20, 1992, 5781–88.

115. "1988–1993. Regards sur la législature bioéthique: Une pénible valse-hésitation," *Le Monde,* March 19, 1993; "Dans un entretien au journal 'La Vie' François Mitterrand souhaite l'adoption définitive des projets de loi sur la bioéthique," *Le Monde,* April 15, 1993.

116. Jean-François Mattei, *La vie en questions, pour une éthique biomédicale* (Paris: La Documentation française, 1993), chap. 5.

human life from its beginnings." He did not argue that the Constitutional Court had called for the protection of the embryo from conception; like the German Supreme Court, it had not defined when an individual human life worthy of protection began. But he insisted that the principle of respect for human life—even if to be compromised in tragic cases where abortion was permitted—should inform a cautious, restrictive approach to embryo research. When asked whether his Christian faith informed his approach, Mattei responded negatively, citing the Gospel injunction, "render to Caesar what is Caesar's and to God what is God's." France was, he insisted, "a *laïciste* and pluralist republic," and it was "absolutely necessary, when it comes to ethics, to recall the principle of the separation of church and state."[117]

Over the next several months the multiple bills that would become the 1994 Bioethics Laws were readied for parliamentary consideration. The one prepared by the justice ministry centered on eugenics and human rights, gene therapy, and surrogacy. The second, from the health ministry, centered on IVF and included the restrictive provisions on embryo research. The third, developed mainly within the research ministry, centered on protection of information. The proposed ban on embryo research drew the most criticism. Axel Kahn, a leading scientist and CCNE member, called the proposed ban "philosophically incoherent" and argued that one could respect the dignity of the embryo but still do research on it under some circumstances. He warned against the "ideological and religious grounding" of the legislative proposal. In December 1993, Mitterrand signaled his own hesitation about the direction of the legislation, suggesting that he was "unsure that morals could be changed by a law."[118]

In the final April 1994 debate in the National Assembly, Simone Veil, the respected socialist legislator after whom the 1975 abortion law was named, led the opposition. "The progress of knowledge is a challenge for the collective conscience," she argued. While she acknowledged that the idea of making the embryo's status dependent on a "parental project" was questionable, she noted the existence of a range of opinions among Catholic moral theologians on when life truly began.[119] Given the healing potential of research, she suggested, it should be supported for the sake of society. Other socialist deputies were even more direct in attacking a perceived unacceptable case of Church influence on politics. One insisted that bioethics legislation respect

---

117. "Un entretien avec le professeur Jean-François Mattei," *Le Monde,* October 10, 1993.

118. Declan Butler, "Ethics Bill Prompts Second Thoughts among Scientists," *Nature* 367, no. 6460 (1994): 209.

119. *Assemblée Nationale, Compte rendu intégral,* April 7, 1994, 635–37.

the 1905 law on the separation of church and state and the Declaration of the Rights of Man and of the Citizen, while another warned against "Galileo syndrome" and against any "integrist" abuses, a reference to the Church's traditional view that politics and society should be governed in an integral fashion by a binding morality.[120]

In the debate, Mattei continued to insist on the rational, not religious foundation for his position. He acknowledged that up through eight or ten days, the embryo was "not a human being in its reality." But he also insisted that it was a stage in a continuum and therefore deserving of protection. The utilitarian idea that it might be destroyed in pursuit of biomedical knowledge was anathema. The 1990 U.K. law was no model, as the "the pragmatism of our British friends" was at odds with "the French human rights tradition." Mattei reassured his colleagues that he was against "the installation of a moral order" understood as "a political power that authoritatively defines what is good and what is evil." He even quoted Cardinal Joseph Ratzinger, the future Benedict XVI, on the need for "a minimum of consensus on the ethical bases of our social existence," adding that "it would be absurd to want to return to a system of political Christianity." His reasoning, he insisted, was secular—the embryo was a "potential patient" that merited protection."[121] While she disagreed on this key issue, Veil acknowledged that the ethical and policy debate did not amount to a "religious war" and underscored the cross-party consensus against the deliberate creation of embryos for research as incompatible with the country's humanist and human rights tradition.[122]

The legislation bearing on embryo research carried the meandering title: "Law relative to respect for the human body and the donation and use of parts or products of the human body, medical assistance for procreation, and prenatal diagnosis." One of its central provisions was that a human embryo "cannot be conceived except for assisted reproduction" and that "the conception of human embryos in vitro for purposes of study, research, or experimentation is prohibited." While the law allowed for the cryopreservation of embryos within the context of IVF therapies, it did not permit their donation for research. "All experimentation on the embryo is forbidden."[123]

In a July 1994 decision, the Constitutional Court upheld the law. For the first time it explicitly affirmed the "dignity of the human person" as a

---

120. *Assemblée Nationale, Compte rendu intégral,* April 13, 1994, 758; *Assemblée Nationale, Compte rendu intégral,* April 14, 1994, 799.

121. *Assemblée Nationale, Compte rendu intégral,* April 7, 1994, 649–52.

122. *Assemblée Nationale, Compte rendu intégral,* April 14, 1994, 817–20.

123. Jacques Lansac, "French Law Concerning Medically Assisted Reproduction," *Human Reproduction* 11, no. 9 (1996): 1843–47.

constitutional principle, noting its roots in the 1946 Constitution that had endorsed it "after the victory secured by free peoples over the regimes that sought to enslave and degrade the human person."[124] The Court did not incorporate the embryo into the principle of "respect for every human being from the beginning of his life." As with the German Constitutional Court, the issue was left ambiguous. But it also did not rule that restrictions on embryo research violated scientific freedom.

As in Germany, the outcome of the political struggle was a cause for consternation among some scientists—but not for public outcry. The restrictive embryo research regime was embedded within a broad legislative framework designed to express the historic French commitment to human rights and dignity, pillars of the revolutionary tradition, and to prevent the emergence of any eugenic abuses. Even Frydman, who lamented the strictures on embryo research, praised the Bioethics Laws as a whole as an expression of the appropriate democratic governance of science for the greater good of society. The legislation, he wrote, "lets modern science develop its most ambitious projects all the while fixing limits on them" for the benefit of "the individual and, without a doubt as well, of science."[125]

Conclusion

By 1995, on the eve of the cloning and stem cell breakthroughs, national embryo research regimes were in place in the United States, the United Kingdom, Germany, and France. Each had its own peculiar characteristics. In the United States, a ban on federal funds for embryo research went hand in hand with a laissez-faire approach in the private sector. Britain instituted a comprehensive policy that was also the most permissive, allowing embryo research—and the creation of embryos for experiments—under careful regulatory oversight. After extended policy debates about the possibility of allowing some research with surplus IVF embryos, both France and Germany imposed restrictive regimes that criminalized all destructive embryo research within their borders.

On both sides of the Atlantic the scientific challenges were broadly similar, as were the basic ethical arguments. But the policy outcomes diverged sharply. Electoral trends and historical legacies best explain those

---

124. Conseil constitutionnel, "Décision no. 94–343/344 DC du 27 juillet 1994," http://www. conseil-constitutionnel.fr/conseil-constitutionnel/francais/les-decisions/acces-par-date/decisions-depuis-1959/1994/94–343/344-dc/decision-n-94–343-344-dc-du-27-juillet-1994.10566.html.

125. Frydman, *Dieu, la Medecine et l'embryon,* 238.

differences. In the United States, the divisive legacy of abortion informed embryo politics. Three successive presidents, wary of offending pro-life groups who had seized on the abortion-embryo research parallel, neglected to implement the 1979 Ethics Advisory Board recommendations in support of federal funding for some embryo research. And when a Democrat, Bill Clinton, tried to move in that direction, his effort ran aground on the opposition of the Catholic Church and its allies and the 1994 Republican sweep of Congress. In the United Kingdom, abortion controversy overshadowed the first wave of political struggle over embryo research, in 1984–85, but then faded, as a proresearch Conservative-Labour majority was able to steer liberal legislation through Parliament. In Germany, the legacy of Nazism served as glue for a multiparty coalition opposed to research that rejected the recommendations of a national ethics committee to allow research under some circumstances. In France, too, committee recommendations for research under exceptional circumstances were overturned by conservative electoral victories and political mobilization around secular arguments opposed to the exploitation of human life and possible eugenic abuses of new technologies.

These outcomes did not fit a "culture wars" prism that pits religious conservatives against secular liberals and their supporters in the scientific community. In the United States, conservative Catholics and evangelicals supported a federal funding ban; they did not mobilize against research in the private sector, which went forward unregulated. In the United Kingdom, the government of Prime Minister Margaret Thatcher, allied with Conservatives and their Christian base on many social issues, nevertheless supported a liberal research regime—with considerable support from within the Anglican hierarchy. France, with its secular political culture and politically marginal Catholic Church, implemented a restrictive regime. And in Germany, secular parties on the left—the Social Democrats and the environmentalist Greens—were instrumental in securing a total ban on embryo research.

In the national controversies through the mid-1990s, the moral status of the embryo was set against the biomedical promise of scientific research. But debate focused squarely on the former. When the embryo should be considered a human individual, whether at conception or two weeks later, was hotly debated in academic circles, national bioethics commissions, and in legislatures. The potential of biomedical research to reduce suffering received less attention, with the exception of the United Kingdom, where it emerged as a major argument by the late 1980s. But there, too, discussion focused on research designed to improve IVF as an infertility treatment, not its other potential biomedical applications. This was to change dramatically in the late 1990s. The cloning and embryonic stem cell breakthroughs of 1997–98 raised the prospect of a new era of regenerative medicine, generating new ethical controversies and policy struggles that would build on those of previous decades.

✍ CHAPTER 3

The Ethics of Embryonic Stem Cell Research

The successful isolation of human embryonic stem cells in a Wisconsin laboratory in 1998 marked a critical juncture in embryo politics. Over the previous three decades, ethical and political controversy had revolved mainly around the moral status of embryos and whether to use them in experiments to improve the safety and efficacy of infertility treatment. With the exception of the United Kingdom, the future potential of embryo research to address a wider range of medical problems had not figured prominently in policy controversies of the late 1980s and early 1990s. This was now to change. Echoing other major news outlets around the world, the *Washington Post* saw in embryonic stem cells "a self-replenishing supply from which scientists hope to grow replacement tissues for people with various diseases, including bone marrow for cancer patients, neurons for people with Alzheimer's disease, and pancreatic cells for people with diabetes."[1] A future horizon of regenerative medicine burst onto the public imagination. What French prime minister Lionel Jospin later fittingly called "cells of hope" would transform embryo politics.[2]

---

1. Rick Weiss, "A Crucial Human Cell Is Isolated, Multiplied," *Washington Post,* November 6, 1998.

2. "Allocution de Monsieur Lionel Jospin, Premier ministre, devant le Comité consultatif national d'éthique pour les sciences de la vie et de la santé," November 28, 2000, http://infodoc.inserm.fr/inserm/ethique.nsf/937238520af658aec125704b002bded2/dfa9bb7b3ffbafccc12570a500515047.

Few could object to the prospect of regenerative medicine; established research programs involving stem cells from adult and fetal tissues and umbilical cord blood were already in place. But because the derivation of stem cells from embryos involved their destruction, controversy circled back to the well-worn question of the embryo's moral status and when and if it might be destroyed for biomedical ends. As the debate unfolded, the prospect of regenerative medicine shifted the terms of controversy against opponents of research with embryos—in two ways.

A first shift concerned the proper ends of research. The promise of stem cell research pointed beyond infertility, which plagued a small, if significant, portion of the population, to include the struggle against deadly diseases with wider reach, including Parkinson's and Alzheimer's. Now the fate of surplus IVF embryos, destined to perish in any case, could be set against the suffering of actual existing men, women, and children. Opponents of embryo research could and did argue that adult stem cells, in particular, offered alternative and morally unobjectionable means to the same end. But the exceptional promise of embryonic stem cells, given their apparent capacity to multiply in the lab and to grow into every kind of human tissue, made them the greater object of hope. An ethic of healing gained traction—the view that solidarity with the sick overrode concern with the moral status of embryos.

A second shift in the terms of debate concerned the origins of the embryos to be used in research. In the earlier period, many research supporters welcomed work with surplus embryos from IVF treatments but opposed their deliberate creation for research purposes. It was one thing to create an embryo for reproductive purposes and then, if it turned out not to be needed, to eventually use it for valuable research, with the consent of the parents. But many saw the creation of an embryo just for science as an illicit instrumentalization of human life. With the stem cell breakthrough, advocates of embryo creation had a new argument—that the creation of embryos with cloning technology might generate stem cells that would match the DNA of a patient, lessening the chances of immune rejection. The prospect of what came to be known as "therapeutic cloning"—made more real by the announcement of the first cloning of an adult mammal, Dolly the sheep, in February 1997—added a new twist to familiar arguments about the creation of embryos for research.

The decade after 1998 saw a shift not only in the terms of ethical controversy but also in the number and type of participants. As in the preceding decade, a series of national committees served as a locus for ethical contestation and for recommendations to policymakers: the National Bioethics Advisory Commission (NBAC) and the President's Council on Bioethics in the United States; the Chief Medical Officer's Expert Group (Donaldson committee) in the United Kingdom; two bodies in Germany, the Bundestag Investigative Commission on Law and Ethics in Modern Medicine and a new National Ethics Council; and the existing French National Consultative Ethics Committee (CCNE). But these bodies would prove less successful than their predecessors in framing the ethical debate and policy alternatives, in part because the public salience of embryonic stem cell research—a function of the hopes it raised—broadened the range of actors participating beyond scientific and medical associations and churches to include biotech companies and patient-advocacy groups.

A comparison of the four national debates that ensued reveals a degree of convergence combined with persistent differences in the framing of the key issues. The rise of an ethic of healing was evident in the United States and the United Kingdom as well as in Germany and France. In the former two countries, however, a utilitarian approach dominated that cast research and therapies as a way to alleviate suffering, increasingly isolating Catholics, evangelicals, and others who equated embryo destruction with abortion. In Germany and France, by contrast, most embryonic stem cell research supporters remained wedded to an emphasis on human dignity: the embryo should be protected in principle as a potential person, but abandoned IVF embryos might be made available for potentially life-saving research under carefully circumscribed circumstances. This concern about the instrumentalization of human life, articulated in both a religious and a secular register, framed the terms of ethical controversy, stiffening opposition to any deliberate creation of embryos, including therapeutic cloning.

This chapter first tracks the path of stem cell research that culminated in the isolation of human embryonic stem cells in 1998 and the prospect of therapeutic cloning. It then charts the rise of an ethic of healing in the field of bioethics, across religious communities, and among public intellectuals in all four countries, setting out the main arguments that would be seized on by proresearch scientific, medical, biotechnology, and patient-advocacy organizations. A final section looks to the work of national ethics committees in articulating the major arguments and making recommendations that set the stage for new policy and political struggles into the first decade of the twenty-first century.

The Path of Science

Scientific interest in stem cells has a long history. Since the early 1900s researchers have observed the capacity of blood cells embedded in bone marrow to renew themselves by dividing and maintaining the ability to divide again. During the 1960s scientists isolated these hematopoietic stem cells; over subsequent decades bone marrow transplants with adult stem cells were used to treat leukemia, lymphoma, and some other inherited blood diseases. Nerve cells represented another promising research and clinical front. After experiments with rats in the 1960s revealed the existence of brain stem cells, scientists moved to study the reproduction of nerve cells in humans. First transplant therapies were developed, most notably grafts of fetal brain tissue for some victims of Parkinson's disease. Scientists subsequently isolated other stem cells in umbilical cord blood and adult tissues, including skin and liver. But these cells generally proved difficult to culture and grow in the laboratory and did not exhibit the pluripotency necessary to generate diverse cell and tissue types.

Parallel to these developments, advances in embryology over the postwar decades alerted scientists to the importance of stem cells at early developmental stages. Once stem cells matured beyond the five- to seven-day blastocyst stage, they appeared to become committed to reproducing a single cell type. What if stem cells could be isolated during the first few days after fertilization, before they had become specialized, and then induced—in the laboratory—to develop into a range of tissue types? Robert Edwards reported some initial success in deriving rabbit embryonic stem cells in 1963 but was unable to preserve them in culture for any length of time. A first mammalian breakthrough came in 1981, when a team of researchers isolated stem cells from an early mouse blastocyst and got them to begin to multiply in culture. Over the next two decades, success was reported with sheep (1987), cows (1992), and other mammals. In 1995 a University of Wisconsin team under John Thomson reported success with monkeys. By this stage efforts to treat degenerative diseases in mice with stem cell therapies had achieved some initial successes.[3]

By the early 1990s, the race to isolate human embryonic stem cells was well underway. Edwards had initially put human stem cell research on the back burner during the 1970s, as he focused his attention on IVF techniques. After the birth of Louise Brown, he made some efforts to isolate stem cells from surplus IVF embryos. He reports to have had partial success in 1982, although the isolated cells did not survive and multiply in vitro. In 1984, he relates that his "work on stem cells ended with an ethical decision" to "cryopreserve all excess embryos for their parents."[4] Two years later, Peter

---

3. Robert G. Edwards, "Stem Cells Today: Origin and Potential of Embryo Stem Cells," *Reproductive Biomedicine Online* 8, no. 3 (2004): 275–306.

4. Robert G. Edwards, "IVF and the History of Stem Cells," *Nature* 413, no. 6854 (2001): 350.

Hans Hofschneider of the German Max Planck Society made the case for embryonic stem cell research, noting that "in the somewhat distant future differentiated organ tissues could be developed from embryonic cell lines and used as organ replacement."[5] In its 1994 report, the U.S. Human Embryo Research Panel raised the promise of "pluripotential embryonic stem cell lines for eventual differentiation and clinical use in transplantation and tissue repair." And in March 1997, only a year before the Wisconsin breakthrough, the French National Consultative Ethics Committee pointed to the isolation of stem cells from sheep and monkey embryos as possibly heralding the "creation of human embryonic stem cells for which the field of potential applications is vast."[6]

By the mid-1990s two teams were leading the race to the goal: one in Singapore, where Ariff Bongso was collaborating with Australian IVF pioneer Robert Trounson; and the other in Wisconsin, where Thomson and his team were building on their successful work with primates. Bongso succeeded in 1994 in isolating stem cells from human embryos but was unable to get them to form stable in vitro cultures. With the financial support of Geron, a leading biotechnology firm, the Wisconsin team forged ahead. In early 1998 they successfully cultured thirty-six embryos to the blastocyst stage. They isolated the inner-cell mass from fourteen of them, and five of those gave rise to stable stem cell cultures. The cells continued to multiply on a bed of mouse cells. Once scientists figured out how to guide the development of stem cells into specific cell types, Thomson and his coauthors suggested in their landmark November 1998 article in *Science,* there would be a "potentially limitless source of cells for drug discovery and transplantation therapies." They noted that many diseases, including Parkinson's, "result from the death or dysfunction of just one or a few cell types" and that "replacement of those cells could offer lifelong treatment."[7]

The next several years saw a rapid internationalization of the knowledge and technology for deriving and culturing embryonic stem cells. By January 2001, more than two dozen cell lines had been created using the techniques pioneered by Thomson and his team. During the three years that followed, some 128 new cell lines came into being. A global network of researchers took shape spanning the United States, the United Kingdom, Denmark,

---

5. Quoted in "Markenartikel Mensch," *Die Zeit,* September 22, 1989.

6. Comité Consultatif National d'Ethique (CCNE), "Opinion on the Establishment of Collections of Human Embryo Cells and Their Use for Therapeutic or Scientific Purposes," March 11, 1997, http://www.ccne-ethique.fr/docs/en/avis053.pdf.

7. James A. Thomson et al., "Embryonic Stem Cell Lines Derived from Human Blastocysts," *Science* 282, no. 5391 (1998): 1147.

Sweden, Finland, Israel, Japan, South Korea, and other nations. Further technological improvements drove the work forward. One was the capacity to grow the stem cells on a medium composed of human—not mouse—cells, which reduced the potential for tissue abnormalities as the cells multiplied. Another was progress in coaxing stem cells to develop into different kinds of human tissue. By 2008, ten years after the original breakthrough, companies had begun to approach government regulators about permission to start clinical trials for certain replacement therapies. An initial clinical trial was approved in the United States in January 2009.

Parallel to the expansion of embryonic stem cell research was a flurry of work on cloning. The procedure, also known as somatic cell nuclear transfer (SCNT), involves removing the nucleus from an egg, inserting the genetic material from a body cell, and stimulating the growth of an embryonic organism. Scientists had succeeded in cloning frogs in the 1950s, and work with nuclear transfer on mammals pressed ahead slowly over subsequent decades. At this early stage the future link between cloning and stem cells was far from obvious. While scientists, like most everyone else, condemned the prospect of human reproductive cloning, little notice was taken of the potential therapeutic applications of the technology. As late as 1983, DNA pioneer James Watson suggested that, in theory, "cloning could be attempted with human eggs and embryonic cells," but he had added: "for what reason? There is no practical application."[8] The following year, the U.K. Warnock report intimated a link between cloning research and regenerative medicine, noting "that one day it might be possible to produce immunologically identical organs for transplantation." Nonetheless, it did not elaborate on the prospect.[9]

The announcement of the birth of Dolly the sheep in February 1997 placed the issue of therapeutic cloning squarely on the scientific agenda. Working in a lab in Scotland, Ian Wilmut and his team had inserted the genetic material from an adult cell into a hollowed-out egg and stimulated it to begin the process of embryonic development, before transferring it into Dolly's mother. As had been the case in 1978 with the birth of Louise Brown and before that in 1968 with the first in vitro fertilization, a flurry of reports about a "brave new world" and "designer babies" dominated media coverage. "It's unbelievable," the *New York Times* quoted Princeton geneticist Lee Silver marveling on the announcement of Dolly's birth. "It

8. Watson quoted in Jane Maienschein, *Whose View of Life?: Embryos, Cloning, and Stem Cells* (Cambridge: Harvard University Press, 2003), 124.

9. United Kingdom (UK), Department of Health and Social Security, *Report of the Committee of Inquiry into Human Fertilisation and Embryology* (London: Her Majesty's Stationery Office, 1984), 73.

basically means that there are no limits. It means all of science fiction is true." In similar sensationalist fashion the article referenced a fictional "tale about a scientist who obtains a spot of blood from the cross on which Jesus was crucified and then uses it to clone a man."[10]

Almost alone among the major media, the *Financial Times* commented on Dolly's birth by drawing attention to the therapeutic potential of cloning technology. Its editors referred not directly to stem cells, but to the "creation of embryonic cloned cells, which would be induced to develop into specific tissues rather than a complete foetus." The editorial continued: "Such a project may sound like science fiction—and it would certainly take many years to achieve—but it is a legitimate field of research, with great potential for improving human health."[11] In the summer of 1997, the U.S. National Bioethics Advisory Commission made a similar observation: "One could imagine the prospect of nuclear transfer from a somatic cell to generate an early embryo and from it an embryonic stem cell line for each individual human, which would be ideally tissue-matched for later transplant purposes." But the report added: "This might be a rather expensive and far-fetched scenario."[12]

In January 1998—more than half a year before the announcement of the stem cell breakthrough—the U.K.-based Human Genetics Advisory Commission suggested "a distinction between two types of cloning: on the one hand, human reproductive cloning, where the intention is to produce identical fetuses or babies; and, on the other hand, what may broadly be called therapeutic cloning." The latter, while "not coterminous with conventional scientific usage," encompassed "studying cell development or creating stem cell lines with the aim of developing therapeutic applications."[13] With the commission's report the term "therapeutic cloning" was born, in quiet fashion. Interestingly, Thomson's landmark article in *Science,* while it discussed the problem of immune rejection of stem cell tissues, did not raise the cloning issue at all. "Strategies to prevent immune rejection of the transplanted cells need to be developed," he argued. These could include banking cells of

---

10. "Scientist Reports First Cloning Ever of Adult Mammal," *New York Times,* February 23, 1997.

11. "Baaad Baaan," *Financial Times,* March 6, 1997.

12. National Bioethics Advisory Commission, *Cloning Human Beings: Report and Recommendations of the National Bioethics Advisory Commission* (Rockville, MD: National Bioethics Advisory Commission, 1997), 30–31.

13. Human Genetics Advisory Commission and Human Fertilisation and Embryology Authority, *"Cloning Issues in Reproduction, Science and Medicine,"* Human Genetics Advisory Commission (January 1998): 2–3. http://www.dh.gov.uk/prod_consum_dh/groups/dh_digitalassets/@dh/@ab/documents/digitalasset/dh_104394.pdf.

certain types or manipulating them genetically to combat immune rejection. Nuclear transfer was not mentioned.

What brought the possibility of therapeutic cloning to wider public attention was a November 1998 announcement by Advanced Cell Technology, a biotechnology firm and Geron rival. ACT claimed that its scientists had created genetically matched stem cells by fusing adult human cells and a cow embryo. The purported breakthrough, said to have taken place two years earlier but not documented in an authoritative scientific publication, drew media attention to the link between stem cells and cloning. The *New York Times* noted ACT's claims that "the method could eventually be used to grow replacement body tissues of any kind from a patient's cells, sidestepping the increasing scarcity of organs available for transplant and the problems of immune rejection." But most of the coverage focused on the ethical issues raised by the combination of human genetic material with cow eggs—and on whether ACT had timed the release of the undocumented study to benefit from the wave of media attention surrounding the embryonic stem cell breakthrough the same month.[14]

Over the next decade, several international teams worked to clone human embryos with an eye to developing genetically matched stem cells. In addition to ACT, Bongso was involved in the race, as were several Chinese teams working in relative international obscurity. The most advanced team, it appeared at the time, was led by Hwang Woo Suk of South Korea. In February 2004 he and his coauthors claimed to have successfully cloned a human embryo and to have derived stem cells. The results, published in *Science* and announced at a press conference at the Seattle meeting of the American Association for the Advancement of Science before a battery of some twenty television cameras, created an international sensation. A year later the Korean team published even bolder claims—cloning experiments with a success rate ten times greater than the year before.[15] For one of Hwang's collaborators, Gerald Schatten, it was "a breakthrough that I didn't think would happen for decades."[16]

---

14. ACT announced in November 1998, just days after the announcement of Thomson's breakthrough, that one of its scientists had cloned an embryo. Nicholas Wade, "Researchers Claim Embryonic Cell Mix of Human and Cow," *New York Times,* November 12, 1998.

15. Hwang Woo Suk et al., "Evidence of a Pluripotent Human Embryonic Stem Cell Line Derived from a Cloned Blastocyst," *Science* 303, no. 5664 (2004): 1669–74; Hwang Woo Suk et al., "Patient-Specific Embryonic Stem Cells Derived from Human SCNT Blastocysts," *Science* 308, no. 5729 (2005): 1777–83.

16. Quoted in Gretchen Vogel, "Korean Team Speeds Up Creation of Cloned Human Stem Cells," *Science* 308, no. 5725 (2005): 1096.

In fact it was a breakthrough that had not happened. Hwang and his team had fabricated key data and fooled the scientific community. The revelations of the scandal in late 2005 had tremendous scientific fallout; Hwang resigned from his laboratory and faced criminal charges in South Korea, and *Science* published a retraction and apology. But the race to clone human embryos continued apace, with more investments and more scientific teams. Harvard's new Stem Cell Institute, the source of some of the best new stem cell lines, pressed forward with cloning research. In the United Kingdom, the International Centre for Life, located in Newcastle, received the first license to clone human embryonic cells for research in August 2004. The following May the Newcastle lab announced success in cloning a human embryo from an embryonic—not an adult—skin cell. A key breakthrough came in January 2008, when researchers at the California-based biotechnology firm Stemagen succeeded in cloning a somatic cell and published their results in a major journal. They claimed to show "for the first time" that "SCNT can produce human blastocyst-stage embryos using nuclei obtained from differentiated adult cells." They did not, however, manage to culture stem cells from them.[17]

Parallel to these developments in embryonic stem cell and cloning research, work with adult stem cells proceeded rapidly. A series of publications in 1999–2000 pointed to the potential for adult stem cells in blood and brain tissue, in some circumstances, to revert back to a pluripotent state and to develop into different cell types. Proven bone marrow transplant technology was further refined, and replacement tissues had some success against diabetes and advanced kidney cancer. This and other work with adult and fetal stem cells held out the possibility of a reservoir of genetically compatible stem cells for therapies without any destruction of embryos. But it also faced impressive technical hurdles. Evidence of the reprogramming of mature stem cells to an undifferentiated state remained fragmentary, and adult stem cells often proved difficult to preserve and multiply in culture. If adult stem cells promised a simpler and ethically unproblematic path to regenerative medicine, its scientific and clinical potential—like that of embryonic stem cells—still remained unproven.

At the end of the first decade of the new century, a rash of new discoveries pointed to potential ways to secure more versatile stem cells without destroying embryos. Articles published in 2004 and 2005 suggested how, through the genetic manipulation of sperm and egg, scientists could create embryolike

17. Andrew French et al., "Development of Human Cloned Blastocysts Following Somatic Cell Nuclear Transfer with Adult Fibroblasts," *Stem Cells* 26, no. 2 (2008): 485–93; Gretchen Vogel and Constance Holden, "Nuclear Transfer: Still on the Table," *Science* 319, no. 5863 (2008): 563.

organisms, incapable of growing into children, that might serve as a source of stem cells. Another research program centered on techniques to isolate stem cells from embryos without destroying the embryo itself. In August 2006 a team at Advanced Cell Technology claimed success in removing a single stem cell from a two-day-old embryo without damaging the latter. A further line of research involved deriving stem cells from sperm-producing cells. A German breakthrough in March 2006 achieved the removal of sperm-producing cells from mice and their transformation into stem cells with many of the properties of embryonic stem cells. And, in early 2007, a U.S.-based team announced the isolation of embryonic stem cells in amniotic fluid. All of these alternative techniques were in early developmental stages, but each suggested a possible alternative to more controversial embryonic stem cell research.[18]

The most revolutionary development, with the potential to thoroughly transform the landscape of stem cell research, was success in reprogramming adult body cells to act like embryonic stem cells. Announced in August 2006 by a team led by Shinya Yamanaka at the University of Kyoto, induced pluripotent stem cell (IPS) technology involved genetic manipulation of adult cells to allow for their controlled differentiation into different kinds of body tissue. First established with mouse cells, the technique was successfully extended to human skin cells in 2007. Rapid breakthroughs in 2008–9 suggested that IPS cells could be created and cultured without genetic manipulation, increasing the prospects for their eventual safe use in tissue replacement therapy. Like adult stem cells, the rapidly developing IPS research program held out the prospect of regenerative medicine without the destruction of embryos.[19] But the breakthrough did not put an end to ethical controversy. As long as the future clinical potential of all three research programs remained unproven, embryonic stem cell research remained a contentious issue—a potential path to regenerative medicine for some and an illicit exploitation of early human life for others.

The Rise of an Ethic of Healing

Late twentieth-century scientific advances cast ethical controversy over embryo research in a new light. The central question of the preceding two

---

18. For an overview of some of these alternatives, see *Alternative Sources of Pluripotent Stem Cells: A White Paper* (Washington, DC: President's Council on Bioethics, 2005). See also Helen Pearson, "Early Embryos Can Yield Stem Cells…and Survive," *Nature* 442, no. 7105 (2006): 858.

19. The seminal article documenting the original IPS breakthrough with mice was Kazutoshi Takahashi and Shinya Yamanaka's, "Induction of Pluripotent Stem Cells from Mouse Embryonic and Adult Fibroblast Cultures by Defined Factors," *Cell* 126, no. 4 (2006): 663–76.

decades remained: whether and under what circumstances embryos might be destroyed in laboratory experiments. Respect for the human embryo was still to be weighed against hoped-for biomedical progress. But the future vista of that progress had changed dramatically. Through the mid-1990s the focus had been improved IVF technologies and greater knowledge about genetics and congenital disease. From now on progress would also encompass a wide range of stem cell therapies for a host of degenerative diseases. An appeal to solidarity with the sick heightened the pressure on research opponents opposed even to the use of frozen embryos slated for destruction anyway. It also cast the efforts to create embryos for research—in cloning experiments designed to derive genetically matched stem cells for therapies—in a more positive light. As Claude Sureau, president of the French National Academy of Sciences, put it in July 2000: "From a problem of human procreation that did not interest many people, we have moved to a therapeutic issue for the whole society that interests everyone."[20]

As the debate about stem cell and cloning research spread in the media and civil society, it raised a number of controversial issues beyond the moral status of the embryo and an ethic of healing. One growing concern was the exploitation of women as a source of eggs. The number of embryos utilized in research increased with the stem cell breakthrough, and the importance of egg donation increased in the context of cloning research. Reports that Hwang Woo Suk, the disgraced South Korean researcher, had pressured women who worked in his laboratory to donate eggs drove new concerns about exploitation and the importance of consent procedures.[21] Another line of argument, more prominent in public debates, focused on national scientific competitiveness amid globalization. Research supporters argued that ethical restrictions might lead to a mass exodus of scientific talent and that it was immoral to ban research and later import its therapeutic benefits. Because science and technology had economic and social consequences for the health of a society, this strategic argument for research had a moral undertone of its own. It was more prominent at the turn of the century than at any previous juncture.[22]

---

20. Quoted in Bernard Charles and Alain Claeys, *Rapport d'information déposé par la mission d'information commune préparatoire au projet de loi de révision des lois "bioéthiques" de juillet 1994, vol 2. Auditions* (Paris: Office parlementaire d'évaluation des choix scientifiques et technologiques, 2001): 212.

21. On the international debate about the ethics of egg donation and selling, see Françoise Baylis and Carolyn McLodd, "The Stem Cell Debate Continues: The Buying and Selling of Eggs for Research," *Journal of Medical Ethics* 33, no. 12 (2007): 726–31.

22. See, for example, then German chancellor Gerhard Schröder, "Der Neue Mensch," *Die Woche,* December 20, 2000. Schröder's insistence that the economic competitiveness argument was an ethical one never found its way to the mainstream of debate in Atlantic democracies.

Still, as it had in the 1980s and 1990s, the moral status of the embryo and the biomedical potential of research remained the central object of public controversy and established a basic continuity with the earlier era. What had changed with the isolation of human embryonic stem cells was not the central issue but its contours. The tremendous potential of the embryonic stem cell to address a broad range of illnesses placed principled opponents of all embryo research on the defensive on both sides of the Atlantic and cast the issue of deliberate embryo creation in a new light.

In early 1999 two American bioethicists, Glenn McGee and Arthur Caplan, were among the first to make a comprehensive case for an ethic of healing. In an essay in the *Kennedy Institute of Ethics Journal,* they hailed the Wisconsin breakthrough as a way to move beyond the familiar embryo research debate. "The plan to sacrifice embryos for a revolutionary new kind of research," they argued, had "reawakened a long-dormant academic debate about the morality of destroying developing human life." In their view, given that "128 million Americans suffer from diseases that might respond to pluripotent stem cell therapies," stem cell research was "a moral imperative akin to national self-defense. Not even the most insidious dictator could dream up a chemical war campaign as horrific as the devastation wrought by Parkinson's disease, which destroys our grandparents, parents, and finally many of us." Supporters of life-giving research, Caplan and McGee argued, were in good company: "The desire to ameliorate the suffering of the ill motivated Hippocrates, St. Francis of Assisi, Cicero, and Florence Nightingale."[23]

McGee and Caplan did not sidestep the problem of the moral status of the embryo. As proresearch voices in the debates of the 1980s and 1990s, they had acknowledged the idea that the embryo should be treated with some respect. To square the idea of respect for embryos with their destruction, they now emphasized the idea of sacrifice—that is, the worthy death of embryos abandoned and therefore destined to die in any case. "What need is so great that it rises to the level where every member of the human family, even the smallest of humans might sacrifice?" they asked. "Already it is clear that we believe that no need is more obvious or compelling than the suffering of half the world at the hand of miserable disease." McGee and Caplan anticipated the counterargument that no end, however noble, could justify the sacrifice of a human being. They acknowledged the early embryo as a member of the human family in its earliest stage of development but insisted it did not deserve the same protection as a fully developed human individual:

23. Glenn McGee and Arthur A. Caplan, "The Ethics and Politics of Small Sacrifices in Stem Cell Research," *Kennedy Institute of Ethics Journal* 9, no. 2 (1999): 152–54.

the "sacrifice of an early embryo, whether it involves a human person or not, is not the same as the sacrifice of an adult because the life of a 100-cell embryo is contained in its cells' nuclear material."[24]

The argument that healing potential necessitated research—and that research that destroyed embryos was compatible with respect for them—extended positions articulated in the American context over the previous two decades. The Ethics Advisory Board (1978–79) had insisted on "profound respect" for the embryo but allowed for research to ensure "the safety and efficacy of embryo transfer."[25] The Human Embryo Research Panel (1994) had granted the embryo "serious moral consideration as a developing form of human life" but supported research on a wider set of goals, with infertility medicine still the main concern.[26] Five years later, McGee, Caplan, and other research supporters shifted their emphasis. It was now the alleviation of suffering more than infertility-related issues that was critical. One could respect embryos while also sacrificing them for a new set of noble and compelling ends.

In the United Kingdom, an early utilitarian case for embryonic stem cell research from an ethic-of-healing perspective was made within the Nuffield Council on Bioethics, a leading national body. Founded in 1991 as a public-private partnership with support from the state-funded Medical Research Council and a private organization, the Wellcome Trust, the Nuffield Council held a 1999 roundtable on stem cell research dominated by scientists, physicians, and ethics professionals generally sympathetic to embryo research. The biologist Anne McLaren, who had played an instrumental role in the work of the Warnock committee (1982–84), was among the participants. The roundtable culminated in an April 2000 paper that articulated a healing rationale for stem cell research. The paper acknowledged that embryo research "involves using the embryo as a means to an end" but asserted matter-of-factly that support for stem cell research was a natural extension of an earlier readiness to use embryos for research on infertility and congenital diseases: "Since we accept the morality of doing so in relation to currently authorised embryo research, there seems to be no good reason to disallow research on the embryo where the aim is to develop therapies for others." The argument for healing, already established in the case of infertility-related research and applied to genetics and congenital disease in the British policy

24. Ibid., 155.

25. Ethics Advisory Board, *Report and Conclusions: HEW Support of Research Involving Human In Vitro Fertilization and Embryo Transfer* (Washington, DC: Department of Health, Education, and Welfare, 1979), 111.

26. Ibid., 101; National Institutes of Health, *Report of the Human Embryo Research Panel,* vol. 1 (Bethesda, MD: National Institutes of Health, 1994), x.

debates of the late 1980s and early 1990s, could now be trumpeted more broadly. As with McGee and Caplan, the roundtable argued that noble ends of research proffered respect for the embryo, even in its destruction: "The removal and destruction of cells from a donated embryo does not indicate lack of respect."[27]

The idea of respect coupled with destruction—however problematic— distinguished the most common articulation of an ethic of healing from its most radical variants.[28] The Australian bioethicist Peter Singer, who moved to Princeton University in 1993, had insisted on reducing the suffering of all sentient beings, including animals, since the 1980s. He had long argued in a consistent utilitarian vein that consciousness and the ability to feel pain were critical markers in biological development and that no living crea- ture, human or otherwise, had a fundamental claim on the respect of others until that stage. After the stem cell breakthrough, with its healing potential, he reiterated his view that limitations on embryo research in the name of human dignity were an ethical obfuscation. As Singer put it in August 1999: "Other things being equal, there is less reason for objecting to the use of an early human embryo, a being that has no brain, no consciousness and no preferences of any kind, than there is for objecting to research on rats, who are sentient beings."[29]

Secular bioethicists who shared Singer's utilitarian premises nevertheless often resisted his conclusions. In a 2003 article, the prominent British bio- ethicist John Harris echoed Singer's premise as a point of departure, rejecting the concept of human dignity as "platitudinous but also totally incoherent."[30] More than Singer, however, Harris acknowledged the importance of respect for the embryo—not in itself, but as a symbolic recognition of "strongly held beliefs regarding the moral status of the embryo and fears of instrumentaliza- tion against the promise of remarkable advances in the treatment of disease."[31] In this perspective, respect was not compelled by the humanity of the embryo

---

27. Nuffield Council on Bioethics, "Stem Cell Therapies: The Ethical Issues" (April 2000). The council also gave conditional support to therapeutic cloning.

28. Daniel Callahan questioned the "obligation to carry out a war against disease" and insisted that "respect for embryos in any meaningful sense is, at the least, incompatible with destroying them solely for our medical benefit. They obviously gain nothing but death." Daniel Callahan, "Promises, Promises: Is Embryonic Stem-Cell Research Sound Public Policy," Commonweal, January 14, 2005, 12–14.

29. Peter Singer, "Sense and Sentience," Guardian, August 21, 1999.

30. John Harris, "Stem Cells, Sex, and Procreation," Cambridge Quarterly of Healthcare Ethics 12, no. 4 (2003): 369, n. 2.

31. John Harris, "The Ethical Use of Human Embryonic Stem Cells in Research and Therapy," in A Companion to Genethics, ed. Justine Burley and John Harris (Malden, MA: Blackwell, 2002).

but rather by the emotional sensitivities of those who considered it a human being worthy of protection. With embryonic stem cells, "what level of costs in lost research are acceptable to maintain a symbolic commitment to human life" had shifted.[32] Not surprisingly, those who viewed the moral status of the embryo as a symbolic issue now gave it even less consideration than previously, in light of embryonic stem cells' potential to alleviate the suffering of men, women, and children afflicted by degenerative diseases.

The inflection of the debates in Germany and France was somewhat different, both in terms of participants and main lines of argument. Both countries lacked a well-developed cadre of professional bioethicists; a more diverse group of scientists, physicians, philosophers, and other experts articulated the core arguments in specialist literature and in the media. In both countries, the idea of the fundamental human dignity of the embryo, developed during the policy debates of the late 1980s and early 1990s, remained a more widely shared point of departure. In Germany the Nazi legacy and the postwar constitutional guarantee of the "inviolability of human dignity" was a frame of reference, while in France a humanist emphasis on the embryo as a potential human individual—as long as it was part of a "parental project"—was a starting point for the debate. In both countries, the idea of the humanity of the embryo had led national ethics committees only to envision research under exceptional circumstances, with IVF embryos destined to perish in any case. Legislators had gone even further, imposing total bans. The healing potential of embryonic stem cells opened up the German and French debates, but a sense of caution and an almost universal determination to draw a line at the creation of embryos for research remained.

In Germany, some of the most prominent public intellectuals urged caution in the wake of the cloning and stem cell breakthroughs of 1997–98. The country's leading philosopher, Jürgen Habermas, took up bioethical questions systematically for the first time in his career. In a series of talks, interviews, and publications he articulated an anxiety about technological progress akin to that first articulated by Hans Jonas, the giant of postwar German bioethics. Some of his concern was for the moral status of early human life. In a December 2001 interview, for example, Habermas argued that cloning and stem cell research demanded striking the right balance between the "collective good of health and freedom of research" and "the protection of the life of the embryo in vitro." However, his main concern was

---

32. John A. Robertson, "Symbolic Issues in Embryo Research." *Hastings Center Report* 25, no. 1 (1995): 38. Robertson tackled the stem cell issue in a utilitarian vein in "Ethics and Policy in Embryonic Stem Cell Research," *Kennedy Institute of Ethics Journal* 9, no. 2 (1999): 109–36.

not the embryo but the possibility of future genetic manipulation and what he called a liberal eugenics driven by parents' wishes, not state coercion. The "instrumentalization of pre-personal human life" through embryo research, he argued, "has put us on a slippery slope."[33]

Habermas's concerns were in part a response to a controversy unleashed by a rival philosopher, Peter Sloterdijk, in 1999. In July of that year, Sloterdijk had given a wide-ranging lecture provocatively entitled "Rules for the Human Zoo," which described a new "evolutionary horizon" enabled by breakthroughs in the life sciences. An atheist in the Nietzschean tradition, Sloterdijk suggested that in the absence of God, humankind must assume the responsibility for its own evolutionary future. He discerned a "long-term development towards the genetic reform of species characteristics" and the transition from "birth fatalism" to "prenatal selection."[34] Not surprisingly, given the Nazi legacy, Sloterdijk's use of the term "selection" occasioned outrage. In September 1999 a number of leading thinkers, closer to Habermas's Enlightenment rationalism, condemned Sloterdijk's vision as a eugenic project reminiscent of Nazism. The influential weekly *Der Spiegel* devoted a cover story to the controversy, under the subheading: "Hitler, Nietzsche, Dolly, and the New Philosophers' Debate."[35]

Other influential secular voices rejected both Sloterdijk's Nietzschean vision and Habermas's more deontological concern about a liberal eugenics. A prominent philosopher based in Berlin, Volker Gerhardt, placed greater emphasis than Habermas on the healing potential of the stem cells. "Through embryo research we can gain knowledge that promises far-reaching therapeutic perspectives," he argued, cautioning against research restrictions that would isolate Germany from future biomedical applications.[36] Gerhardt, who served as chair of the German Science Foundation's Bioethics Commission and, after 2000, as a member of the National Ethics Council, downplayed the importance of dignity and respect as points of reference in the debate but distinguished his approach from utilitarianism. Echoing the symbolic argument put forward by Harris, he saw the embryo representing

33. "Auf schiefer Ebene: Ein Gespräch mit Jürgen Habermas über Gefahren der Gentechnik und neue Menschenbilder," *Die Zeit*, January 24, 2002. Many of Habermas's contributions on the theme were later published in English as Jürgen Habermas, *The Future of Human Nature* (Cambridge: Polity, 2003).

34. "Regeln für den Menschenpark," *Die Zeit*, September 16, 1999. Sloterdijk's address was later translated into English as "Rules for the Human Zoo: A Response to the Letter on Humanism," *Environment and Planning D: Society and Space* 27, no. 1 (2009): 12–28.

35. *Der Spiegel*, September 29, 1999. Among the many interventions was an open letter by the philosopher Manfred Franck, "Geschweife und Geschwefel," *Die Zeit*, September 23, 1999.

36. Volker Gerhardt, "Die Frucht der Freiheit," *Die Zeit*, November 27, 2003.

"human life in the process of becoming" that deserved some consideration, not "because the mass of cells is already a human being," but because a person cannot accept that "one treats that out of which one emerges in an abject or indifferent way." Research, Gerhardt insisted, should only be allowed "under strict medical controls."[37]

In contrast to the 1980s, the public debate saw a range of prominent public voices in Germany with even fewer moral qualms about destructive embryo research. Julian Nida-Rümelin, holder of the first German chair in bioethics and an adviser to Chancellor Gerhard Schröder on cultural questions, articulated a straightforward utilitarian stance. While he acknowledged that "every single embryo has the full genetic complement of a human individual that under favorable circumstances will grow into a human individual," he refused to apply the concept of human dignity to the embryo in an "inflationary manner," given its inability to feel pain.[38] Another prominent thinker and legal theorist, Reinhard Merkel, concurred that the concept of human dignity should not be extended to the embryo. He agreed that the goals of battling Alzheimer's, Parkinson's, and other degenerative diseases could not "justify destructive research on embryos" if they were "legal subjects with basic rights to life and human dignity." But he argued that embryos did not have that moral and legal status, noting that the 1975 constitutional court ruling on abortion had not explicitly extended the concept of human dignity to preimplantation embryos. For Merkel, embryo research for worthy goals was clearly "morally acceptable."[39]

The proresearch views of Merkel and Nida-Rümelin provoked sharp reactions. In a heated exchange in the influential newsweekly *Die Zeit,* the philosopher Robert Spaemann accused Nida-Rümelin of breaking with the ethical principle of universal human dignity. Spaemann also insisted, against Merkel, that most German constitutional scholars extended the principle of the inviolability of human dignity to life in all its stages as a conscious reaction against the horrors of Nazism. In the same extended exchange, the philosopher Hans Joas agreed that the "only acceptable criterion for drawing a line around those to whom the term 'human dignity' applies is biological belonging to the human family." But he was careful not to go as far as Spaemann in insisting that the constitution and the court's rulings necessitated

37. Volker Gerhardt, "Vom Zellhaufen zur Selbstachtung: Warum Nida-Rümelins Definition des Menschen richtig ist," *Focus,* January 22, 2001.

38. Julian Nida-Rümelin, "Wo die Menschenwürde beginnt," *Der Tagesspiegel,* January 3, 2001. Given its early developmental stage, he argued, "the embryo's self-esteem [*Selbstachtung*] cannot be damaged."

39. Reinhard Merkel, "Rechte für Embryonen?" *Die Zeit,* January 25, 2001.

absolute protection for the embryo from the moment of conception. The concept of human dignity that informed the restrictive legislation of 1990 remained a point of departure for the German debate. But its constitutional and legal implications were now more contested.[40]

The French ethical debate, too, grew more diverse and contested during the decade after the isolation of human embryonic stem cells. A focus on the moral status of the embryo as a "potential person" or the "potentiality of a person," remained, as did the idea that only embryos created for procreation that were no longer part of a "parental project" could be utilized in research. Within this general framework, however, there was a change in tone. Several key figures who had treated research as a necessary evil to maintain the effectiveness and safety of IVF as a fertility treatment now cast it as a positive good in the struggle against degenerative disease. Axel Kahn, for example, who chaired the National Consultative Ethics Committee from 1992 to 2004, backed research with surplus embryos in June 2001 "in the name of the sacredness of life" and in the service of a "humanitarian vocation." Experimentation to further regenerative medicine, he insisted, would give a "surplus embryo, destined to never become a child, more dignity than to disappear by thawing in a test tube."[41] In 2007 he further developed this key idea—that research in the service of healing was compatible with the dignity and respect owed the embryo. "Medicine progresses thanks to research on all ages of human life," he insisted, "and the embryo's nature of potential humanity would not be an argument against performing research upon it."[42] Anne Fagot-Largeault, a leading biologist and former CCNE member, linked the case for research back to the ideal of solidarity so anchored in French political culture. Work with embryonic stem cells expressed "a morality of solidarity with those who suffer and who one must help with all the means at one's disposal."[43]

As in Germany, some prominent thinkers went even further, rejecting the argument from potential personhood and human dignity altogether. In an influential 1999 edited volume that addressed cloning and embryo research, CCNE member Henri Atlan characterized "the sacred character of life as

---

40. Hans Joas, "Grenzen der Verfügbarkeit," *Die Zeit,* February 15, 2001.

41. Axel Kahn, "La Science n'est pas diabolique," *Le Monde,* June 21, 2001.

42. Kahn at a National Assembly hearing, *Compte rendu de l'audition publique ouverte a la presse,* November 29, 2007, http://www.assemblee-nationale.fr/13/rap-off/i1325-tII.asp.

43. Her lecture upon her election to the Collège de France is reported in National Assembly hearings in November 2001, *Rapport fait au nom de la commission spéciale sur le projet de loi relatif à la bioéthique* (Paris: Assemblée nationale, 2002), 141.

an empty notion"—a theme echoed by other contributors.[44] Like utilitarian thinkers in the United States and the United Kingdom, and Nida-Rümelin and Merkel in Germany, these thinkers refused to extend the idea of human rights to human life that could not feel pain. In France this secular antipathy to the argument about the moral status of the embryo was magnified by its association with the Catholic Church. For the philosopher Roger-Pol Droit, for example, the very term "human dignity" implied "a concealed theology" and a "trace of transcendence." Another prominent supporter of research, Bernard Debré, argued in a 2001 article that "by prohibiting research and prohibiting knowledge, you certainly are not going to protect human ideals."[45]

The more aggressive proresearch argumentation was partly a reaction against the restrictive Bioethics Laws of 1994, through which conservatives had overturned the cautious proresearch recommendations of the CCNE. But it was also a response to the promise of stem cell research. Not all secular voices went along. In early 2001, Lucien Sève, a Communist philosopher and CCNE member who had been instrumental in the development of the ethics council's cautious proresearch stance during the 1980s, wrote that the "embryo incontestably represents the potentiality of a human being."[46] Didier Sicard, the physician who succeeded Kahn atop the CCNE in 2004, continued to espouse the view that research should be embarked on carefully, under exceptional circumstances. "A human embryo, whatever its ontological status, remains a possibility of a human being and not of a rabbit or a mouse," he told a conference that year. "To make of it a bank of stem cells," for Sicard, was "a considerable step toward its instrumentalization."[47] Sève, Sicard, and other prominent figures continued to back work only with surplus IVF embryos and only under exceptional circumstances—but most were willing to broaden those circumstances to include the struggle against degenerative disease. The philosopher Sylvain Reboul, for example, remained skeptical of any manipulation of the embryo in principle but favored it on a case-by-case basis, in order to address "illnesses suffered here and now by individuals."[48]

---

44. Henri Atlan et al., *Le clonage humain* (Paris: Editions du Seuil, 1999).

45. Bernard Debré, "Pour la recherche," *Libération,* July 4, 2001. Debré, a physician and former minister of (international) cooperation, joined the CCNE in 2008.

46. Lucien Sève, "L'humain n'est pas une marchandise," *L'Humanité,* February 9, 2001.

47. Didier Sicard, "Réflexions sur le progrès en médecine," *Contrepoint Philosophique,* October 2004, http://www.contrepointphilosophique.ch/Ethique/Sommaire/ProgresEnMedecine.html?Article=ProgresEnMedecine.htm.

48. Sylvain Reboul, "L'embryon malade de la loi," *Libération,* February 26, 2000.

Religious Communities and an Ethic of Healing

The emergence of embryonic stem cell research and the horizon of regenerative medicine also sparked a reformulation of ethical controversy within religious communities in the United States, the United Kingdom, Germany, and France. The official stance of the Roman Catholic Church did *not* change. As stem cell debates picked up on both sides of the Atlantic, the Vatican issued a statement in August 2000 reiterating the view that any destruction of embryos was "a *gravely immoral* act and consequently *gravely illicit.*" The statement addressed the rise of an ethic of healing head-on. *"No end believed to be good,* such as the use of stem cells for the preparation of other differentiated cells to be used in what look to be promising therapeutic procedures, *can justify an intervention of this kind."* Its conclusion: "A good end does not make right an action which in itself is wrong."[49] U.S. and European bishops reiterated this argument in different forums. In a June 2001 statement, the French bishops recalled that "some practices honor humanity, others injure it." The embryo, the "weak link in the human chain," should therefore be treated with respect.[50] A month later, Richard Doerflinger, spokesman for the U.S. Conference of Catholic Bishops, told a congressional hearing that embryonic stem cell research "violates a central tenet of all civilized codes on human experimentation beginning with the Nuremberg Code: It approves doing deadly harm to a member of the human species solely for the sake of potential benefit to others."[51] Greek Orthodox bishops in the United States represented a similar position.[52]

There were dissenting voices within the Catholic Church. A Catholic moral theologian at Yale University, Margaret Farley, insisted that "a growing number" of her peers did "not consider the human embryo in its earliest stages (prior to the development of the primitive streak or to implantation) to

---

49. Pontifical Academy for Life, "Declaration on the Production and the Scientific and Therapeutic Use of Human Embryonic Stem Cells," August 25, 2000, http://www.vatican.va/roman_curia/pontifical_academies/acdlife/documents/rc_pa_acdlife_doc_20000824_cellule-staminali_en.html.

50. Conférence des évêques de France, "L'embryon humain n'est pas une chose," June 21, 2001, http://www.cef.fr/catho/espacepresse/communiques/2001/commu20010625embryon.php.

51. "Testimony of Richard M. Doerflinger on Behalf of the Committee for Pro-Life Activities, United States Conference of Catholic Bishops before the Subcommittee on Labor, Health and Human Services, and Education Senate Appropriations Committee Hearing on Stem Cell Research," July 18, 2001, http://www.usccb.org/prolife/issues/bioethic/stemcelltest71801.htm.

52. In October 2001, a synod of the Greek Orthodox Church in the United States reiterated the view that "human life is sacred from its very beginning, since from conception it is ensouled existence. As such, it is 'personal' existence, created in the image of God and endowed with a sanctity that destines it for eternal life." See The Holy Synod of the Orthodox Church in America, "Embryonic Stem Cell Research in the Perspective of Orthodox Christianity," October 17, 2001, http://www.oca.org/Docs.asp?ID=50&SID=12.

constitute an individualized human entity with the settled inherent potential to become a human person." Farley's arguments harkened back to those of Richard McCormick, the Jesuit who served on the Ethics Advisory Board in 1978–79, and Franz Böckle, the German moral theologian who had served on the Benda Commission. They had been willing to countenance some embryo research to improve the safety and effectiveness of IVF. Now, Farley and certain other Catholic thinkers, including Carol Tauer and a prominent French physician, Claude Sureau, argued that such research might be carefully extended to build knowledge that might address ailments beyond infertility. As Tauer put it, a case for research could be "made without sacrificing the tradition's commitments to respect human life, promote human well-being, and honor the sacred in created realities."[53]

These vocal Catholic proponents of an ethic of healing after 1998 were lay thinkers, not clerics. The 1987 instruction *Donum Vitae* had clarified the Church's absolute opposition to all destructive embryo research and reduced the room for maneuver for dissent among the clergy. In contrast to the situation from the late 1970s through the mid-1980s, when McCormick and Böckle had sat on national ethics committees that endorsed research under some circumstances, Catholics recruited to official national bodies now tended to endorse a strict antiresearch stance and equate the destruction of embryos with abortion. Prominent examples included Alfonso Gomez Lobo and Edward Pellegrino of Georgetown University, laymen who served on President Bush's Presidential Council on Bioethics, Patrick Verspieren, a French Jesuit who served on the CCNE, and Eberhard Schockenhoff, the Catholic moral theologian appointed to the German National Ethics Council. Their rejection of an "ethic of healing" echoed that of the Vatican. "Even medical findings of great value," Schockenhoff argued, "cannot invalidate ethical principles like human dignity and the related prohibition against the instrumentalization of human beings."[54]

Conservative evangelicals, too, generally did not soften their opposition to embryo-destructive research in the wake of the stem cell breakthrough. In the United States, the most powerful conservative Protestant denomination, the Southern Baptist Convention, passed a 1989 resolution reiterating the view that the "Bible teaches that human beings are made in the image

---

53. National Bioethics Advisory Commission, Ethical Issues in Human Stem Cell Research, vol. 3 (Rockville, MD: National Bioethics Advisory Commission, 1999), F-4. Tauer's observation is drawn from a background paper, ibid., D-4.

54. Eberhard Schockenhoff, "Die Ethik des Heilens und die Menschenwürde," in *Gattungsethik— Schutz für das Menschengeschlecht?* ed. Matthias Kaufmann and Lukas Sosoe (Frankfurt am Main: Lang, 2005), 343–73.

and likeness of God (Gen. 1:27; 9:6) and protectable human life begins at fertilization." The resolution asserted that "efforts to rescind the ban on public funding of human embryo research rely on a crass utilitarian ethic which would sacrifice the lives of the few for the benefits of the many." Like the Catholic Church, the Southern Baptist leaders continued to draw a tight parallel with the abortion question. They reiterated their "decades-long opposition to abortion except to save the physical life of the mother and their opposition to destructive human embryo research."[55] Conservatives and evangelicals in the United Kingdom, France, and Germany, while much fewer in number and negligible in their political influence, tended to adhere to the same line. They acknowledged the importance of healing in the Christian tradition but insisted that other research programs, in particular with adult stem cells, provided the ethically preferable way forward.

Not all Christian opposition to an ethic of healing was cast as an absolute defense of the embryo. For example, Gilbert Meilaender, a Lutheran moral theologian and member of Bush's Presidential Council, developed an ethical and theological argument against an overriding emphasis on reducing suffering. The ubiquity of arguments from compassion, he suggested, should lead one to "ponder the degree to which relief of suffering has acquired the status of trump in our moral reasoning." He posited a future conversation in which sufferers from degenerative disease would criticize those who did not do enough to save them in the present. His hypothetical response: "Perhaps we could have helped you, but only by pretending that our responsibility to do good is godlike, that it knows no limit." A more modest approach to medical ambition, he suggested, might maintain a better awareness of the redemptive dimension of suffering by rejecting what "modernity has taught us, that suffering has no point other than to be overcome by human will and technical mastery" and that "compassion means not a readiness to suffer with others but a determination always to oppose suffering as an affront to our humanity."[56] The idea that suffering was not itself an absolute evil, however deeply anchored in the Christian moral tradition, did not play a prominent role in the debate— within churches and the broader society. The leading antiresearch argument remained the parallel with abortion, even if its wider appeal diminished given the hopes placed in regenerative medicine and the fate of stockpiled surplus IVF embryos without any prospect of becoming children.

---

55. Southern Baptist Convention, "Resolution on Human Embryonic and Stem Cell Research," June 1999, http://www.sbc.net/resolutions/amResolution.asp?ID=620.

56. Gilbert Meilaender, "The Point of a Ban: Or, How to Think about Stem Cell Research," *Hastings Center Report* 31, no. 1 (2001): 9–16.

For those mainline Protestant denominations on both sides of the Atlantic open to embryo research in the 1980s and early 1990s, an embrace of embryonic stem cell research was not problematic. Given the decentralized character of Protestantism and the lack of a central teaching authority, multiple church positions coexisted, even as an emphasis on an ethic of healing became more prominent. The U.S.-based United Church of Christ provides an example. One of its leading theologians, Ronald Cole-Turner, noted in 1999 that the Church had never taken a definitive position on embryo research, although he suggested that most members did not consider embryos as persons, "believing instead that embryos have an important but lesser status." Two years later, in July 2001, an official UCC resolution explicitly embraced an ethic of healing with the biblical assertion that "Jesus set an example" by his ministry of healing and caring for the sick and disabled.[57] The healing potential of research meant that embryos utilized in experiments were perishing in a noble cause. As Karen Lebacqz, a UCC-associated thinker put it, "the fact that an embryo will be used in research does not mean that it is automatically being devalued and disrespected."[58]

Ted Peters, a leading moral theologian in the Lutheran tradition, elaborated the scriptural rationale for an ethic of healing, invoking the parable of the Good Samaritan, in which a Jew beaten by robbers and left for dead is passed by a priest and a Levite before a non-Jew, a Samaritan, comes to his aid. To oppose embryonic stem cell research, Peters argued, "risks 'passing by on the other side.' It risks failure to love one's neighbors." From his perspective, it was wrong to focus on the early embryo as a gift of God with full human dignity, the official Catholic and predominant evangelical view. "Rather than something imparted with our genetic code," he concluded, "dignity is the future end product of God's saving activity that we anticipate socially when we confer dignity on those who do not yet claim it."[59] This forward-looking perspective identified medical progress with God's will and the advancement of human dignity. It did not deny the moral status of the embryo altogether, but placed it in the broader context of God's healing plan for humanity.

---

57. "Synod OKs Federally-Funded Embryonic Stem Cell Research," *United Church News,* July 11–17, 2001, http://www.ucc.org/ucnews/julaug01/synod-oks-federally-funded.html.

58. Karen Lebacqz, "On the Elusive Nature of Respect," in *The Human Embryonic Stem Cell Debate: Science, Ethics, and Public Policy,* ed. Suzanne Holland, Karen Lebacqz, and Laurie Zoloth (Cambridge: MIT Press, 2001), 160.

59. Ted Peters, "Embryonic Stem Cells and the Theology of Dignity," in *The Human Embryonic Stem Cell Debate: Science, Ethics, and Public Policy,* ed. Suzanne Holland, Karen Lebacqz, and Laurie Zoloth (Cambridge: MIT Press, 2001), 135.

The majority of the Church of England leadership, which had set out a theological rationale for an ethic of healing in the 1980s, continued to back work with embryos in the wake of the stem cell breakthrough. Leaders including Archbishop of York John Habgood and moral theologian Gordon Dunstan had highlighted the Christian imperative of healing with reference to infertility medicine and congenital diseases, well before the horizon of regenerative medicine appeared. Their views, most fully articulated within the Church's Board for Social Responsibility, continued to predominate within the hierarchy and the rank and file. In the late 1990s, the Bishop of Oxford, Richard Harries, chair of the board at the time, expanded and adapted the imperative of healing in light of the stem cell breakthrough. In a 1999 speech he suggested that support for research was not simply "a cowardly concession to the spirit of the age." Rather it was a positive good to "interact with nature, as God's co-workers, in bringing about the health which he wills for humanity and the healthy children that he desires." Two years later, in 2001, the board published a paper that reiterated arguments of the 1980s—that the embryo before fourteen days is not an individual human being, as it can still divide and does not yet have the first foundations of a nervous system—and made an impassioned plea for embryonic stem cell research to advance a healing agenda.[60]

This was by no means a consensus view. If anything, the evangelical current within the Church of England had grown stronger since the 1980s, and several prominent bishops espoused strong prolife views that encompassed opposition to any and all embryo research. The board's 2001 paper was hotly debated at a 2003 synod of bishops, shortly after the Bishop of Wales, Rowan Williams, a research opponent, was named Archbishop of Canterbury. The board secured majority support at the synod for its proresearch position, but not without an awkward compromise. In line with an ethic of healing, the synod's communiqué referenced "the principle of the sanctity of human life which we affirm must embrace the mutuality of all life, including the sick and the dying." At the same time, on the insistence of research opponents, the document affirmed "the sanctity of the human embryo and therefore the need to treat it with profound respect." In the proceedings Williams wondered aloud how research that destroyed the embryo was compatible with its sanctity. By contrast, a prominent research supporter, the Bishop of Norwich, argued that "sanctity is the condition of being holy and we treat

---

60. "Answers to Soul-Searching Questions," *Independent,* April 26, 1999. Church of England Mission and Public Affairs Council, *Embryo Research: Some Christian Perspectives* (London: Church House, 2003).

holy people and holy places, the Holy Land and so on, with a profound care and reverence." He added: "It does not mean they are untouchable."[61]

In the United Kingdom, opposition to embryo and stem cell research was occasion for a significant ecumenical initiative—a joint statement that brought together Anglican, Catholic, Orthodox, and evangelical theologians to insist on the Christian tradition's unwavering opposition to the willful destruction of human life. In a joint statement they acknowledged the widespread view that "for most of Christian history (until 1869) the human embryo has been considered to possess only a relative value—such as might be outweighed by considerations of the general good." But they insisted that such an interpretation relied on a misreading of the tradition and that "even in the Middle Ages, when most Western Christians held that the early embryo was not yet fully human, it was held that the human embryo should never be attacked deliberately, however extreme the circumstances." Respect for the embryo was, in this reading, respect for the weakest and most vulnerable of human creatures. "Concern over the fate of embryos destined for research is inspired, not only by the narratives of the Annunciation, the Visitation and the Nativity, but also by the parable of the good Samaritan and the parable of the sheep and the goats: 'Just as you did it to one of the least of these little ones you did it to me.'"[62]

This line of argument, a minority view within the Anglican Church, remained the official position of Germany's Lutheran Church, the Evangelical Church in Germany. During the late 1980s, the EKD Council had joined with the Catholic hierarchy to oppose embryo research under all circumstances. After the embryonic stem cell breakthrough it issued a statement in May 2001 that acknowledged the centrality of healing for Christian ethics but insisted on the continued absolute protection of the embryo, because "even the smallest movement in the direction of permitting destructive embryo research crosses an important line"—the violation of human dignity set down in the constitution.[63] There were strong currents within the EKD sympathetic to an ethic of healing; a considerable minority of the Church's own ethics committee insisted in 2002 that one should consider using surplus

---

61. Church of England, *Report of Proceedings: General Synod*, July 2003 (London: Church House, 2003), 219–20, 233.

62. David Jones, "A Theologian's Brief: On the Place of the Human Embryo within the Christian Tradition and the Theological Principles for Evaluating Its Moral Status," *Ethics and Medicine: An International Journal of Bioethics* 17, no. 3 (2001): 143–54.

63. Evangelische Kirche in Deutschland, "Der Schutz menschlicher Embryonen darf nicht eingeschränkt werden: Erklärung des Rates der EKD zur aktuellen bioethischen Debatte," press release, May 22, 2001, http://www.ekd.de/presse/5220.html.

IVF embryos in research designed to heal.[64] A leading representative of this position, the moral theologian Richard Schröder, argued that "even research on emergent human life can take place in respect or awe before life and its creator."[65]

Bishop Wolfgang Huber, who took over as head of the EKD council in 2003, continued to back the Church's antiresearch stance.[66] He noted the strength of his opponents' arguments but countered that "reference to such healing possibilities cannot serve to justify actions through which a human being is no longer respected as a person, but instead is reified." A "Christian ethic," he argued, "should support alternatives to any lines of research that entailed danger of treating human beings as things."[67] In a major address before a Catholic audience in June 2004, Huber cast his strong emphasis on the protection of human dignity in all phases of life as a response to the lessons of history and the experience of Nazism and the Holocaust.[68] Support for Huber's views within the Church would erode over the course of the decade, and he softened his own stance to some degree as the policy debate deepened.

Within the Atlantic democracies, the greatest shift in a proresearch direction among mainline Protestant organizations was in France. While never unified in their approach, most church leaders had cautiously endorsed some embryo research in the 1980s and 1990s. With the embryonic stem cell breakthrough, however, the idea of an ethic of healing quickly gained ground. A 2003 statement of the French Protestant Federation (FPF) noted the tension between "therapeutic solidarity dictated by love of neighbor" and respect for life and the rejection of its instrumentalization.[69] Jean-Arnold de Clermont,

---

64. Evangelische Kirche in Deutschland, "Im Geist der Liebe mit dem Leben umgehen," *EKD-Texte* 71, August 2002, http://www.ekd.de/EKD-Texte/44633.html.

65. Richard Schröder, "Die Forschung an embryonalen Stammzellen. Argumentationstypen und ihre Voraussetzungen: Erweiterte Fassung eines Vortrags im Tübinger Stift am 20.2.2002," February 20, 2002, http://www2.hu-berlin.de/theologie/schroeder/bioethiktueb.pdf.

66. In January 2002 other Protestant theologians articulated similar views in the influential *Frankfurter Allgemeine Zeitung*. They took issue with the human-dignity argument deployed by research opponents, insisting, like Ted Peters, the idea of man in the image of God points forward toward his salvation and should not be applied as an analytical category to biological phases of life. "Pluralismus als Markenzeichen: Eine Stellungnahme evangelischer Ethiker zur Debatte um die Embryonenforschung," *Frankfurter Allgemeine Zeitung,* January 23, 2002. A similar dissenting view from the EKD position was Martin Honecker, "Embryonenschutz aus Ethischer Sicht," *Reproduktionsmedizin* 18, no. 2 (2002): 58–60.

67. Wolfgang Huber, "Wissenschaft Verantworten—Überlegungen Zur Ethik der Forschung," July 14, 2006, http://www.ekd.de/vortraege/2006/060714_rv_heidelberg.html.

68. Wolfgang Huber, "Ethik und Demokratie," June 19, 2004, http://www.kinderkrankenhausseelsorge.de/vortraege/huber/04_06_19_huber_katholikentag.html.

69. Fédération protestante de France, "Le temps est venu de réviser les lois de bioéthique," January 12, 2003, http://www.protestants.org/docpro/doc/1146.htm.

president of the FPF and a member of the CCNE, continued to acknowledge the "human character of the embryo," even as he drew a sharp line between his position and what he called the Catholic Church's "trap of the sacralization of the embryo." Research for worthy causes should be allowed for spare embryos outside of a "parental project" as long as women were not exploited for their eggs and couples gave their consent.[70]

The Ethics of Therapeutic Cloning

If the isolation of human embryonic stem cells in 1998 engaged the debate about the proper ends of research, shifting the focus from the moral status of the embryo to the struggle against degenerative disease, advances in cloning technology dramatized by Dolly's birth a year earlier posed anew the old issue of the appropriate origins of embryos for research. Those opposed to all embryonic stem cell research, even with spare embryos destined to perish in any case, naturally opposed efforts to clone embryos as a source of genetically matched stem cells. On the opposite side of the issue, those who had favored the creation of embryos for research tended to have no objection to therapeutic cloning. The main challenge was posed of those who had advocated work with spare IVF embryos but opposed the creation of embryos for research. Did the prospect of a new era of regenerative medicine justify the cloning of embryos for stem cells? For some in this group, the logic of an ethic of healing reached its limits with cloning technology, given its potential for eugenic abuses and the possibility of a slippery slope to reproductive cloning. For others, however, the combined healing potential of embryonic stem cell and cloning technologies called for new thinking.

One way out of this ethical dilemma was to recast the dominant terminology in the debate. The battle was waged on two fronts. First, many supporters of cloning embryos to derive stem cells argued that it should not be called "cloning" at all, given the term's negative association with reproductive cloning. Popular alternatives better established in the scientific literature included "nuclear substitution" and "somatic cell nuclear transfer." George Annas, for example, argued in late 1998 for a clear distinction between "the cloning of cells and tissues" and "the cloning of human beings by somatic nuclear transplantation" and for permitting the former while prohibiting the latter.[71]

---

70. Fédération protestante de France, "Révision des lois bioéthiques en 2001," November 2000, http://www.protestants.org/index.php?id=1961.

71. George Annas, "Why We Should Ban Human Cloning," *New England Journal of Medicine* 339, no. 2 (1998): 122–25.

Because the purpose was so different—future therapies, in one case, and a child, in the other—different terms should be used. The effort to avoid the term "cloning" met with only limited success. One reason was the fact that both reproductive cloning and SCNT began with the same operation: the insertion of the donor's genetic material into an enucleated egg. Another was the apparent political impetus behind the terminological debate—the effort to avoid the word "cloning" with its negative science fiction connotations.[72]

A second terminological battle went somewhat better for research supporters. It concerned whether the product of cloning was, in fact, an embryo. If it was not an embryo one could skirt the ethical quandaries associated with deliberate embryo creation. Here there were two main approaches. One was to argue that an embryo was, by definition, a product of the fertilization of an egg by a sperm; because cloning did not involve fertilization, in this reading, it did not involve the creation of an embryo. A second, more persuasive line of argument centered on a genetic difference between embryos and the products of nuclear transfer: the absence of an egg's mitochondrial DNA. Pointing to this difference, a leading stem cell researcher Rudolph Jaenisch borrowed from Paul McHugh of Johns Hopkins University, who suggested the term "clonote" for the product of SCNT.[73] "Such a distinction makes biologic sense," Jaenisch argued, "is consistent with the available evidence, and may contribute to a more rational discussion of nuclear-transfer technology."[74] Other candidates put forward were "activated egg" and "ovasome."[75]

None of the neologisms stuck. The leading scientific journals in the United States and the United Kingdom, *Science* and *Nature,* rejected terminological innovation; ultimately, the fact that the product of cloning, if implanted in a womb, might develop into a child, made it difficult to shake the embryo label.[76] Searching for alternatives to "embryo" also seemed—like the term "pre-embryo"—to be designed to duck the issue of the moral status of the embryo altogether. In France the idea that cloning did not entail embryo

---

72. Some cloning opponents also resisted the term "therapeutic cloning" partly because of the positive connotations of the term "therapeutic." Leon Kass, for example, considered the term "cloning for biomedical research" more accurate.

73. Paul R. McHugh, "Zygote and 'Clonote': The Ethical Use of Embryonic Stem Cells," *New England Journal of Medicine* 351, no. 3 (2004): 209–11.

74. See Rudolph Jaenisch, "Human Cloning: The Science and Ethics of Nuclear Transplantation," *New England Journal of Medicine* 351, no. 27 (2004): 2787–91.

75. On "ovasome," see Anne A. Kiessling, "In the Stem-Cell Debate, New Concepts Need New Words," *Nature* 412, no. 6844 (2001): 255. Kiessling coined the term while on the ethics advisory board of Advanced Cell Technology.

76. As *Nature*'s editors put it, "to suggest that [therapeutic cloning] does not involve the creation of embryos is misleading." See "The Meaning of Life," *Nature* 412, no. 6844 (2001): 255.

creation gained the most traction. Sureau, the head of the French Academy of Medicine, asserted matter-of-factly that "the result of nuclear transfer is not really an embryo," and Henri Atlan, a leading member of the national ethics committee, called it merely "an artifact of the laboratory."[77] Didier Sicard rejected Atlan's equation of the product of therapeutic cloning with "an artifact." But as the policy debate heated up, many CCNE members would come back to the idea of a distinction between therapeutic cloning and embryo creation.[78]

On balance, most participants in Atlantic debates appear to have acknowledged therapeutic cloning to be the equivalent of the creation of embryos for research purposes. This placed supporters of embryo research who had previously drawn a line at embryo creation in a difficult position. George Annas provides an example. In 1996 he, Arthur Caplan, and Sherman Elias had espoused the view that "it is the intention to create a child that makes the creation of an embryo a moral act."[79] In 1999 they saw "a considerable moral difference between creating and destroying embryos solely to obtain stem cells and destroying unwanted human embryos that will never be used for reproductive purposes to achieve benefit for those with serious diseases and disorders."[80] Several years later in the midst of the therapeutic cloning debate, however, Annas and Elias appeared to weaken their opposition to the creation of embryos for research, suggesting "the moral status of a human embryo no more depends on how or why it was created than does the moral status of a child."[81]

A clearer example of shift in perspective occasioned by the stem cell and cloning breakthroughs was Axel Kahn in France. As head of the CCNE from 1992 to 2004, Kahn had not opposed stem cell research with surplus

---

77. Claude Sureau in Senate hearings, "Auditions du 10 Novembre 1999," November 10, 1999, http://www.senat.fr/rap/r99-238-2/r99-238-24.html. He continued: "Yes it can certainly develop to become an individual, but if one follows this line of thought, every somatic cell is a potential embryo." Atlan at National Assembly hearings in November 2001, *Rapport fait au nom de la commission special,* 390. Atlan later suggested the label "pseudo-embryo" for the product of nuclear transfer and acknowledged that it could become an embryo through subsequent "uterine transfer." See his National Assembly testimony of November 25, 2008, in Alain Claeys and Jean Leonetti, *Rapport d'information fait au nom de la mission d'information sur la révision des lois de bioéthique. Auditions* (Paris: Assemblée nationale, 2010), 57–71.

78. Sicard at National Assembly hearings in November 2001, *Rapport fait au nom de la commission speciale,* 417.

79. George J. Annas, Arthur Caplan, and Sherman Elias, "The Politics of Human-Embryo Research: Avoiding Ethical Gridlock," *New England Journal of Medicine* 334, no. 20 (1996): 1331.

80. George J. Annas, Arthur Caplan, and Sherman Elias, "Stem Cell Politics, Ethics and Medical Progress," *Nature Medicine* 5, no. 12 (1999): 1340.

81. George J. Annas and Sherman Elias, "Politics, Morals and Embryos," *Nature* 431, no. 7004 (2004): 20.

IVF embryos but had drawn a line at cloning. The cloned embryo, he argued, "would in fact be a product, a thing, no matter how potentially useful." He posed the question: "What would remain of the sentiment that the human embryo deserves special consideration if it can be produced like a thing, and not in the hope of a person?"[82] At 2006 parliamentary hearings where he announced his change of mind, Kahn noted that he had not been "initially in favour of legislation authorising this experiment involving the production of cloned embryos."[83] His opposition, he insisted, had been grounded in skepticism of cloning's biomedical promise and anxiety about a slippery slope to reproductive cloning. Now that medical promise was clear and the specter of cloned babies had faded, he was in favor of pressing ahead cautiously. Kahn's interpretation of the evolution in his own thinking downplayed its most striking characteristic: the promise of healing therapies had eclipsed his earlier concerns about the instrumentalization of human life in its earliest stages.

Not everyone made the transition. Sicard, when he replaced Kahn atop the CCNE in 2004, remained opposed to cloning while open to research with stem cells derived from surplus IVF embryos. He rearticulated the argument from human dignity that had framed the French debate through the mid-1990s and called cloning in all its forms "an existential problem for humanity," condemning those for whom it is not a fundamental ethical question.[84] In Germany, too, public figures open to embryonic stem cell research, under some circumstances, continued to draw a line at cloning, less out of concern with the moral status of embryos than out of fear of a slippery slope from therapeutic cloning to reproductive cloning and eugenics. The most influential American exponent of this view was Leon Kass, the first chair of Bush's Presidential Council on Bioethics. Kass did not oppose all stem cell research with surplus IVF embryos, but he condemned research cloning as dehumanizing; there was "something deeply repugnant and fundamentally transgressive about such a utilitarian treatment of prospective human life." For him cloning represented a "total, shameless exploitation" worse than the "mere destruction of nascent life."[85]

---

82. Axel Kahn, "Le clonage humain: Engendrer un autre," *La Croix,* February 5, 1999.

83. Kahn at National Assembly hearing in Alain Claeys, *Rapport sur les recherches sur le fonctionnement des cellules humaines* (Paris: Office parlementaire d'évaluation des choix scientifiques et technologiques, 2006), 292–93.

84. Sicard at National Assembly hearings in Claeys, *Rapport sur les recherches,* 299.

85. Leon R. Kass, "The Wisdom of Repugnance," in *The Ethics of Human Cloning,* ed. Leon Kass and James Q. Wilson (Washington, DC: AEI Press, 1998), 51–52. Kass developed these arguments further in *Life, Liberty, and the Defense of Dignity: The Challenge for Bioethics* (San Francisco: Encounter Books, 2002).

The debate over therapeutic cloning in the churches paralleled controversy over embryonic stem cell research. Not surprisingly, the Vatican and leading evangelicals were strictly opposed. In June 1997, the Vatican made clear its opposition to cloning for research purposes, calling it "immoral because even in the case of a clone, we are in the presence of a 'man,' although in the embryonic stage." Some of the Catholic Church's internal critics, such as Farley, who made a case for research with stem cells derived from surplus IVF embryos, also opposed cloning for research. Others, such as Tauer and Sureau, extended their support for an ethic of healing to encompass support for therapeutic cloning. Evangelical leaders tended to side with the Vatican. In June 1997, for example, the Southern Baptist Convention passed a resolution opposing cloning that would result in "in the wanton destruction of human embryos developed for research purposes."[86] Spokesman Richard Land echoed the Vatican's argument against an ethic of healing: "We should not be the kind of society that kills our tiniest human beings in order to seek a treatment for older and bigger human beings."[87]

Not all conservative Christians opposed therapeutic cloning. An important exception was the Church of Jesus Christ of Latter-day Saints (the Mormons). Drawing on beliefs about the preexistence of souls, some Mormon thinkers argued that they entered humans not at fertilization but in the womb, once their bodies were more fully formed. It followed that experiments with embryos, including therapeutic cloning, could be justified as a means of saving lives. This dominant Mormon position, which would influence political and policy controversy in the United States, combined opposition to abortion with support for stem cell and cloning research.[88]

Mainline Protestant churches in the United States generally supportive of stem cell research were hesitant to extend an ethic of healing to cover cloning research. For example, an August 2003 general convention of the Episcopal Church reiterated its support for stem cell research, but only with embryos that would "otherwise be discarded" and "were not created

---

86. Pontifical Academy for Life, "Reflections on Cloning," June 25, 1997, http://www.vatican.va/roman_curia/pontifical_academies/acdlife/documents/rc_pa_acdlife_doc_30091997_clon_en.html; Southern Baptist Convention, "Resolution on Human Cloning," June 21, 2001, http://www.sbc.net/resolutions/amResolution.asp?ID=572.

87. Quoted in "Koreans Report Ease in Cloning for Stem Cells," *New York Times*, May 20, 2005.

88. An official statement of the Church leadership from 1970 posed the central issue: "That there is life in the child before birth is an undoubted fact, but whether that life is the result of the affinity of the child in embryo with the life of its mother, or because the spirit has entered it remains an unsolved mystery." Quoted in Rick Jepson, "Ensoulment: Stem Cells, Human Cloning, and the Beginning of Life," *Sunstone* 147 (October 2007): 71.

for research purposes."[89] A year later, an assembly of the United Methodist Church reached a similar conclusion, reiterating their 2000 stance against all cloning and warning against hubris. "We are created by God and have been redeemed by Jesus Christ," the 2004 resolution read. "It is important that the limits of human knowledge be considered as policy is made."[90] Among the liberal denominations, the United Church of Christ was most open to therapeutic cloning research, although its leadership did not set down a definitive position on the issue.

The most consequential shift in favor of therapeutic cloning was among parts of the Church of England hierarchy. During the debates of the 1980s, a majority of the Board for Social Responsibility had opposed the creation of embryos for research. In January 2001 a board majority endorsed a briefing paper supportive of therapeutic cloning under some circumstances. Its author, a leading moral theologian and board member, John Polkinghorne, asserted that "theologically one may see the human and intellectual abilities that permit us to understand and manipulate the world of which we are inhabitants as being God-given powers and a part of the imago Dei."[91] Not all of the Church leadership went along. In addition to principled opponents of embryo research, including Archbishop of Canterbury Rowan Williams, some erstwhile research backers drew a line at cloning. The most influential was the former Archbishop of York John Habgood, a prominent supporter of embryo research during the 1980s controversies. In the House of Lords in 2001, wearing what he called his "moral and theological hat," he contrasted his earlier support for embryo research with his anxiety about newer developments. Since embryos did not have "full moral status as persons," he had supported their creation, under exceptional circumstances, for infertility-related research. But cloning to support an uncertain regenerative medicine agenda made him nervous. He called it an "unending research programme, further and further removed from its original moral justification."[92]

In Germany the front against all cloning among Protestants was much stronger. The 2002 EKD ethics committee that had been split on stem cell

89. "Deputies Endorse Research on Human Stem Cells, Set Budget Priorities," *Episcopal Press and News,* August 2, 2003, http://www.episcopalarchives.org/cgi-bin/ENS/ENSpress_release.pl?pr_number=2003–188-ADeputies.

90. The UMC position on cloning was again adapted in 2008. See "Human Cloning," http://www.umc.org/site/apps/nlnet/content2.aspx?c=lwL4KnN1LtH&b=4951419&content_id={5C125586–247C-45DE-8063-EEC128BC5F89}&notoc=1.

91. John Polkinghorne, "Therapeutic Uses of Cell Nuclear Replacement," 2000. http://www.cofe.anglican.org/info/socialpublic/science/hfea/cnr.pdf.

92. United Kingdom (UK), *Parliamentary Debates.* Lords, 6th ser., vol. 621 (January 22, 2001), col. 91.

research with surplus embryos drew a line at their creation or cloning for research. (Richard Schröder was an important exception; he was among a small group open to cloning in order to build biomedical knowledge and alleviate suffering.) In February 2004, Bishop Huber greeted the announcement of the first cloning of a human embryo in South Korea—later revealed as a fraud—by noting the coincidence with the two-hundredth anniversary of the death of Immanuel Kant, "a philosopher who, like no other before him had warned against turning man into goods and thus robbing him of his dignity."[93] Later that year Huber joined the head of the German Catholic Bishops' Conference in opposing cloning for research, no matter what its healing potential.[94] Hermann Barth, an EKD vice president and a member of the National Ethics Council, rejected "ethic-of-healing arguments" surrounding therapeutic cloning, insisting that "the cloned embryo has human dignity like any other human embryo."[95]

Protestants in France, a much less influential group, were closer to the British than to the German pattern. In November 2001, the French Protestant Federation published a reflection paper that set out the different arguments on both sides of the issue. The paper sparked a debate that culminated in a January 2003 statement under the heading "The Time Has Come to Revise the Bioethics Laws." In it the FPF noted that support for cloning might "cede somewhat too quickly to the most immediate utilitarianism," but also that to reject it would be to "renounce too quickly the efforts to understand the most intimate mechanisms of life that could permit us to exercise our therapeutic solidarity in the best way possible." Jean-François Collange, then the Protestant representative on the CCNE, favored the legalization of therapeutic cloning, but the federation, in keeping with its decentralized structure, did not take a position.[96] Interestingly, a major evangelical association was openly *supportive* of therapeutic cloning, because it considered the product of cloning "cells and not an embryo, which lifts the ethical obstacle."[97]

---

93. Evangelische Kirche in Deutschland, "Klonen ist nicht zu verantworten," press release, February 13, 2004, http://www.ekd.de/presse/pm21_2004_klonen.html.

94. Evangelische Kirche in Deutschland, "Klonen ist ein Irrweg," press release, September 13, 2004, http://www.ekd.de/bioethik/presse/pm167_2004_klonen_ekd_dbk.html.

95. Hermann Barth, "Rechtfertigung durch Heilungshoffnungen?: Einige gute Gründe gegen das sogenannte therapeutische Klonen," February 2, 2005, http://www.ekd.de/vortraege/barth/050202_barth_klonen.html.

96. Fédération protestante de France, "Le temps est venu de réviser les lois de bioéthique," January 12, 2003; "Les autorités religieuses divisées sur l'exploitation thérapeutique," *Le Monde,* December 31, 2002.

97. Fédération des Eglises Evangéliques Baptistes et Union des Eglises Evangéliques Libres, "Faut-il permettre la recherche sur l'embryon humain?," press release, January 7, 2004, http://www.ueel.org/ethique/faut-il-permettre-la-recherche-sur-l-embryon-humain.html.

The extension of an ethic of healing to cloning research was most force-fully articulated by Jewish and Muslim leaders, who were more vocal in debates on both sides of the Atlantic than during the 1980s and early 1990s. For Jews, the concept of *tikkun olam* (heal the world) provided a power-ful grounding for research designed to alleviate human suffering. The chief rabbi of the United Kingdom, Immanuel Jakobovits, had drawn a line at the creation of embryos for research in 1990; a decade later, however, his suc-cessor, Jonathan Sacks, backed therapeutic cloning. In a letter to President George Bush in April 2001, Orthodox Jewish leaders emphasized that "our Torah tradition places great value upon human life" and that "the potential to save and heal human lives is an integral part of valuing human life from the traditional Jewish perspective."[98] Muslim leaders such as Dalil Boubakeur, imam of the Paris mosque and a CCNE member, expressed general con-cern that cloning technology might disrupt kinship relations, but they were generally supportive of cloning research aimed to reduce suffering.[99] In both traditions, a religiously grounded ethic of healing could be applied to stem cell and cloning research, because neither considered the early embryo a per-son; for Judaism, the threshold for full humanity was generally considered to be 40 days, and for Islam, 120 days. As with Protestantism, there was no official Jewish or Muslim position on research. But an ethic of healing was the decisive frame of reference.

As this survey of the most influential secular and religious arguments demonstrates, the cloning and stem cell breakthroughs of 1997–98 trans-formed the contours of embryo controversy. The overall frame established in the 1980s—the moral status of the embryo, on the one hand, and the potential of biomedical research, on the other—remained. But the prospect of a future era of regenerative medicine shifted the terms of debate against principled opponents of all embryo research. Catholic and evangelical lead-ers remained opposed to any destruction of embryos, and some prominent secular commentators continued to cast research with surplus embryos more as a necessary evil than as a positive good. However, more and more partici-pants in the debate, including erstwhile opponents of research, now came to see embryo, stem cell, and cloning research as a moral imperative, given its potential to alleviate human suffering. An ethic of healing, articulated in

---

98. Union of Orthodox Jewish Congregations of America and the Rabbinical Council of America, "Cloning Research, Jewish Tradition and Public Policy," press release, March 13, 2001, http://www.ou.org/public/Publib/cloninglet.htm.

99. "Recherche génétique: La science fait un nouveau pas vers le clonage thérapeutique," *La Croix*, May 23, 2005.

both a secular and a religious vein, gave embryo controversy a new cast and would shape the deliberations of national ethics committees convened to assess the issues and make recommendations for policy.

U.S. Bioethics Committees

Through the mid-1990s the U.S. experience with national ethics committees tackling embryo ethics had not been a productive one. The Ethics Advisory Board of 1978–79 had its recommendations ignored and its funding cut; Jimmy Carter's Presidential Commission skirted the embryo research issue during its 1980–83 tenure; efforts to set up a Biomedical Ethics Advisory Committee collapsed over the abortion issue in the late 1980s; and the Human Embryo Research Panel saw President Clinton criticize and Congress reject its recommendations in 1994–95. In October 1995, the Clinton administration created a new body, the National Bioethics Advisory Commission, under the chairmanship of Harold Shapiro, president of Princeton University. The eighteen-member body was weighted toward ethics professionals and included several scientists and representatives of patient-advocacy groups and the biotechnology industry—but no moral theologians. Among its prominent members were Alexander Capron, erstwhile chair of Jimmy Carter's Presidential Commission, and two former HERP members, Alta Charo and Bernard Lo.[100] The group had no plans to revisit embryo-related issues; its initial agenda was centered on genetic privacy and human-subject protections. But then cloning and stem cell breakthroughs intervened.

In late February 1997, just days after the announcement of Dolly's birth, Clinton charged the NBAC with drafting a report with cloning policy recommendations—in only ninety days. The main focus of media attention and the committee's work was to be reproductive cloning, a prospect that Clinton publicly condemned as an abomination. But his charge also alluded to cloning experiments with human embryos. "While this technological advance could offer potential benefits in such areas as medical research and agriculture," Clinton noted, "it also raises serious ethical questions, particularly with respect to the possible use of this technology to clone human embryos." The NBAC report was to include "a thorough review of the legal and ethical issues associated with the use of this technology" and "recommendations

---

100. The committee was to include at least one person in each of five categories: philosophy/theology, social/behavioral science, law, medicine/allied health professions, and biological research. See Alexander M. Capron, "An Egg Takes Flight: The Once and Future Life of the National Bioethics Advisory Commission," *Kennedy Institute of Ethics Journal* 7, no. 1 (1997): 63–80.

on possible federal actions to prevent its abuse."[101] The commission set to work immediately, held a series of public and private meetings, and heard from experts in science and bioethics, as well as Catholic, Protestant, Jewish, and Muslim representatives. The transcripts of the meetings, part of the public record, depict a lively collegial search for consensus.

A consensus did prove possible, largely because the NBAC report ended up focused almost exclusively on reproductive cloning. In the deliberations, Shapiro and his colleagues recognized cloning as a potential way to create embryos for research but opted not to address the issue. For Shapiro it was "not the time to revisit that" because he saw "no pressing reason to do so," and because the president and Congress had already decided the issue "after a very careful and thoughtful report"—a reference to the work of the HERP and the ban on public funding of embryo research with the Dickey Amendment. According to a *Washington Post* report, "at least one dissenter on the commission said they were troubled by the panel's decision not to address private sector embryo cloning." But the majority did not want to block potentially valuable research—or to complicate the task at hand and risk missing the ninety-day deadline. As one member of the commission put it, "the group could have haggled forever with scientists who would like the ban on federally funded embryo research lifted, and with activists who want the ban expanded to include private sector."[102]

The NBAC's June 1997 report, *Cloning Human Beings,* denounced reproductive cloning, joining a swelling international chorus. While it did not feature a sustained discussion of therapeutic cloning—the isolation of stem cells had not yet taken place—it included a passage that referred to the possibility: "One could imagine the prospect of nuclear transfer from a somatic cell to generate an early embryo and from it an embryonic stem cell line for each individual human, which would be ideally tissue-matched for later transplant purposes." This was, the report noted, a "a rather expensive and far-fetched scenario." Still, any effort to outlaw reproductive cloning "should be carefully written so as not to interfere with other important areas of scientific research."[103] In keeping with the terminology of many research supporters,

---

101. "President Asks for Advice on New Reality of Cloning," *New York Times,* February 25, 1997.

102. "Meeting of the National Bioethics Advisory Commission," May 2, 1997, http://govinfo. Library.unt.edu/nbac/transcripts/1997/5-2-97.pdf, 53. The NBAC's cloning report would note that "ethical concerns surrounding issues of embryo research have recently received extensive analysis and deliberation in the United States." See *Cloning Human Beings,* i. "Panel Backs Some Human Clone Work; Board Would Ban Implanting Embryos," *Washington Post,* June 4, 1997.

103. *Cloning Human Beings,* 30–31.

the text referred not to cloning embryos but to cloning "cell lines." This part of the report went unnoticed in the media; it gained new salience with the Wisconsin stem cell breakthrough just over a year later.

Immediately after that breakthrough Clinton again turned to the NBAC for recommendations on how the federal government should approach embryonic stem cell research. There followed nine months of deliberations punctuated by several hearings featuring leading scientists, bioethicists, and religious leaders. This time there was no way to finesse the question of the moral status of the embryo over and against the potentials of research. The NBAC report, published in June 1999, noted deep divisions in U.S. society. "Although we believe most would agree that human embryos deserve respect as a form of human life," there were disagreements "regarding both what form such respect should take and what level of protection is required at different stages of embryonic development." The key issue was "how to resolve the tensions between two important ethical commitments: to cure disease and to protect human life." While noting the existence of those "who believe that from the moment of conception the embryo has the moral status of a person," the commission agreed, unanimously, that research "that involves the destruction of embryos remaining after infertility treatments is permissible when there is good reason to believe that this destruction is necessary to develop cures for life-threatening or severely debilitating diseases and when appropriate protections and oversight are in place in order to prevent abuse." Such oversight would embody "the kind of respect for the embryos that most Americans would expect."[104]

A *New York Times* report highlighted some of the differences on the way to these conclusions. Given ethical concerns about embryo research in the wider society, the commission had discussed the possibility of assigning priority to stem cell tissue derived from aborted fetuses. The idea did not gain traction. A scientist on the committee, David Cox of Stanford, spoke for most of his colleagues in insisting that federal funds flow to embryonic stem cell research, which was too promising to be left unregulated in the private sector. A more contested issue was whether to recommend federal funds to derive stem cells or only approve research with cells derived in the private sector. In April 1999 the NIH had signaled its preference for the latter position—funds for research with cell lines derived elsewhere. The bioethicist Thomas Murray is reported to have recommended the NIH position to his colleagues on the NBAC: "I think we speak to a great number of Americans

---

104. NBAC, *Ethical Issues in Human Stem Cell Research,* ii, 2, 59, 67.

who have complex views and who are undecided, and many of these will find a distinction between use and derivation useful with respect to public funding." But in a straw poll, Murray received no support from his colleagues. The final report criticized the NIH position, effectively calling for a repeal of the 1995 Dickey Amendment that had banned all federal funding for research destructive of embryos. The ban, the report argued, conflicted "with several of the ethical goals of medicine, especially healing, prevention, and research."[105]

The NBAC also took up the possibility of therapeutic cloning in its 1999 report, without using the term. It noted that the "recent demonstration of cloning techniques (somatic cell nuclear transfer) in nonhuman animals suggests that transfer of a human somatic cell nucleus into an oocyte might create an embryo that could be used as a source of ES [embryonic stem] cells." For many citizens, the report acknowledged, "using embryos merely as a means to some other goal does not treat them with appropriate respect or concern as a form of human life." Less with an eye to these sensitivities than due to the early state of the science, the commission argued that the NIH itself should not yet fund such research: "Embryos created specifically for research purposes are not needed at the current time in order to conduct important research in this area."[106] On both stem cell and cloning research, then, the NBAC opposed national restrictions on work in the private sector and favored federal funding in principle, even if the time for cloning research had not come. Given that the NBAC included no principled opponents of research with embryos, its support for both research programs was not a surprise.

The next national body to take up these issues, the President's Council on Bioethics (PCB) announced by President Bush in August 2001, had a more diverse membership. While it addressed the issue of embryonic stem cell research, its most far-reaching recommendations concerned cloning. Bush was on record in favor of a total cloning ban that would encompass the public and private sectors; not surprisingly, his committee featured many of like mind. Council chairman Leon Kass was on record against all forms of cloning as an illicit exploitation of human life that harbored eugenic dangers. The council also included three prominent Catholic thinkers, all principled

---

105. "Advisory Panel Votes for Use of Embryonic Cells in Research," *New York Times,* June 29, 1999; NBAC, "Ethical Issues in Human Stem Cell Research," 69.

106. Ibid., ii, v, 71. In this, the NBAC followed the HERP September 1994 report, which supported "research involving the development of embryonic stem cells, but only with embryos resulting from IVF for infertility treatment or clinical research that have been donated with the consent of the progenitors." National Institutes of Health, *Report of the Human Embryo Research Panel*, xi–xii.

opponents of all embryo and cloning research: Robert George (Princeton), Alfonso Gomez-Lobo (Georgetown), and Mary Ann Glendon (Harvard). The PCB also included a range of proresearch voices, however, including three prominent scientists, Elizabeth Blackburn (University of California, San Diego), Michael Gazzaniga (Dartmouth), and Janet Rowley (University of Chicago). During the first half of 2002 Kass shepherded his colleagues through meetings and hearings that aired the therapeutic cloning issue from all points of view.[107]

Not unexpectedly, the committee ended up sharply divided on the cloning issue, with the scientists and Catholic members coming down on different sides. According to an account of the internal deliberations in *Science,* two neoconservatives widely believed to sympathize with the president's position, Francis Fukuyama and James Q. Wilson, proved reluctant to endorse a total public and private ban on cloning for research, given its biomedical potential. When it became clear that an up or down vote on a cloning research ban might go either way, Kass opted to organize the committee's recommendations around two alternatives: a four-year moratorium on public and private cloning research as an interval for systematic reflection on next steps; or allowance for private sector cloning research under strict safeguards. The PCB report, "Human Cloning and Human Dignity," completed in July 2002, indicated a ten to seven majority in favor of the four-year ban, including Fukuyama (but not Wilson). For the minority in dissent, an ethic of healing was the overriding concern. As they put it: "We believe that the nation should affirm and support the responsible effort to find treatments and cures that might help ameliorate or thwart diseases and disabilities that shorten life, limit activity (often severely), and cause great suffering for the afflicted and their families."[108]

The ethical debate about stem cells and cloning at the dawn of the new century continued the polarization evident during the early 1990s. The deliberations of the Human Embryo Research Panel in 1994 had seen a sharp opposition between research supporters and opponents aligned with Catholic and evangelical opposition to destructive embryo research. Its recommendations for federal funding for the creation of embryos for research had

---

107. The charter of the NBAC expired in October 2001 and was not renewed under the George W. Bush administration. Over its life span it had met some forty-eight times and generated six reports.

108. President's Council on Bioethics, "Human Cloning and Human Dignity: An Ethical Inquiry," (Washington, DC: President's Council on Bioethics, 2002). For background on the council deliberations, see Stephen S. Hall, "President's Bioethics Council Delivers," *Science* 297, no. 5613 (2002): 322–24.

generated a political backlash that culminated in a total funding ban in 1995. During the second half of the decade, the solidly proresearch NBAC sought to steer clear of the problem of the moral status of the embryo and endorsed cautious recommendations in favor of embryo research and against a total ban on research cloning. As the next chapter relates, only under the Bush administration would ethical controversy about embryo, stem cell, and cloning research fully burst onto the national political agenda.

Diverse U.K. Ethics Bodies

The United Kingdom did not have a national bioethics commission along the lines of the NBAC or the official bodies set up in France and later in Germany. Unlike other leading Atlantic democracies, however, it did have highly structured government oversight over embryo research through the Human Fertilisation and Embryology Authority that had been set up in 1991. The existence of an institutionalized policy regime, and the proresearch principles on which it rested, provided the context for ethical contestation of embryonic stem cell and cloning research into the new century.

After the announcement of Dolly's birth in February 1997, the HFEA and the Human Genetics Advisory Commission (HGAC), another government body, formed a joint working group to study the cloning issue and help formulate policy responses. The group, which included prominent research supporters such as John Polkinghorne and Anne McLaren, took up its work in June 1997. Its initial January 1998 report, which made the influential distinction between "reproductive" and "therapeutic" cloning, did not make hard-and-fast recommendations. But its proresearch bent was no secret.[109] HGAC chairman Colin Campbell stressed the group's desire to reduce "fantasies and fears" around reproductive cloning while not foreclosing "procedures that might in five years' time lead to curing of diseases."[110] Its final report, in December 1998, praised the recent Wisconsin breakthrough as heralding a new era of regenerative medicine, and called for the adaptation of the 1990 HFE Act to allow for both embryonic stem cell research and therapeutic cloning, two procedures not envisioned by the legislators at the time. "When the 1990 HFE Act was passed, the beneficial therapeutic consequences that could potentially result from human embryo research were not envisaged,"

---

109. Human Genetics Advisory Commission, *"Cloning Issues in Reproduction, Science and Medicine,"* January 1998.

110. "Laboratories Are Told They May Produce Embryo Human Clones," *Times* (London), January 30, 1998.

it pointed out. (In its final report, the working group tried, unsuccessfully, to replace their own neologism, "therapeutic cloning," with a new phrase, "therapeutic use of cell nucleus replacement." It did not stick.)[111]

The Labour government under Tony Blair sympathized with these recommendations but opted not to introduce legislation without further high-level deliberation. In June 1999 the government announced the formation of an expert group to be headed by Liam Donaldson, the United Kingdom's chief medical officer, to focus on the particularly controversial issue of therapeutic cloning. The group was dominated by scientists and physicians, most of whom were positively disposed toward research, and included Polkinghorne and the ethicist Alastair Campbell, who had both served on the HGAC/HFEA working group. The committee solicited the views of a wide range of groups and interests during late 1999 and early 2000. In May 2000 its basic proresearch recommendations were shared with government ministers and leaked to the press.[112] As widely anticipated, the Donaldson committee report supported the extension of the 1990 HFE Act to cover both embryonic stem cell research and therapeutic cloning—"for the purposes of greater knowledge about human disease and disorders and their treatment." Embryonic stem cells should, wherever possible, be derived from surplus IVF embryos. At the same time, their creation through cloning should also be legalized where "alternatives to cell nuclear replacement have been adequately considered."[113]

This ethical reasoning echoed that of the Warnock committee report a decade and a half earlier. It referred to the "special status of an embryo as a potential human being" but insisted that the "respect due to the embryo increases as it develops and that this respect, in the early stages in particular, may properly be weighed against the potential benefits arising from the proposed research." The report did acknowledge some of the particular ethical issues raised by cloning, noting that "even those who accept the current research uses of embryos might express concern about the research use of embryos created in this way." But it noted that "while research on embryos created by cell nuclear replacement does indeed involve using them as a means to an end, this

111. Human Genetics Advisory Commission and Human Fertilisation and Embryology Authority, "*Cloning Issues in Reproduction, Science and Medicine,*" Human Genetics Advisory Commission (December 1998). http://www.dh.gov.uk/prod_consum_dh/groups/dh_digitalassets/@dh/@ab/documents/digitalasset/dh_104395.pdf.

112. "Human Embryo Clones to Be Used for Research," *Times* (London), March 12, 2000.

113. UK, Department of Health, *Stem Cell Research: Medical Progress with Responsibility,* August 16, 2000, http://www.dh.gov.uk/en/Publicationsandstatistics/Publications/Publications PolicyAndGuidance/DH_4065084, 46.

can be said to apply to some degree to all research using embryos." In keeping with a utilitarian logic, the focus was squarely on the biomedical payoffs. "These benefits, if realised, would be substantial and may represent the best prospect of developing treatments for a number of degenerative disorders."[114]

One can draw a straight line from the deliberations of the Warnock committee through those of the Nuffield Council on Bioethics and the Donaldson committee. While the Warnock committee's debates were heated, and its proresearch conclusions far from unanimous, the bioethics bodies created after the passage of the 1990 HFE Act took the country's liberal research regime as their point of departure. No principled opponents of embryo research sat on either the Nuffield Council or the Donaldson committee. While they both—like the Warnock committee in an earlier era—acknowledged some moral status for the embryo and the concerns of those opposed to all research on principle, they also insisted that the prospect of a new era of regenerative medicine made it imperative to extend the existing liberal regime in new directions. The policy and politics of efforts to adapt that regime would prove contentious in the years that followed.

A Clash of German Ethics Committees

The primacy of an ethic of healing did not have the same impact on the deliberations of national ethics committees set up in Germany to address embryo and stem cell research. Like Clinton and Blair, Chancellor Helmut Kohl responded to Dolly's birth by convening a group of experts to prepare a report on cloning and its implications. The Council for Research, Technology, and Innovation, housed within the science ministry, included four religious and secular bioethicists and three scientists, among them the head of the German Science Foundation, Ernst-Ludwig Winnacker. It had a much lower profile than either the U.S. National Bioethics Advisory Commission or the U.K. joint HGAC/HFEA working group. The German council report, entitled *Human Cloning: Biological Foundations and Ethical-Legal Evaluation,* was issued in April 1997.[115] The report invoked the precedent of the Embryo Protection Law, which had explicitly prohibited cloning, and endorsed a conservative interpretation of the Constitutional Court's position, according to which

---

114. Ibid., 8. The report acknowledged the result of cell nuclear replacement as being a cloned embryo.

115. Albin Eser et al., *Klonierung beim Menschen: Biologische Grundlagen und ethisch-rechtliche Bewertung,* June 1997, http://www.freidok.uni-freiburg.de/volltexte/3691/pdf/Eser_Klonierung_beim_Menschen.pdf. Kohl had set up the Council for Research, Technology, and Innovation in 1995.

"human beings from their beginnings at fertilization fall under the protection on human dignity." The authors alluded to therapeutic cloning, which they termed cloning "to produce human embryos for purposes of diagnosis or research." Their conclusion: all cloning ran counter to "the principles of human dignity and of embryo protection" and should be banned.[116]

After the stem cell breakthrough of November 1998, two larger and more influential bodies came into being. The first was the Bundestag's Investigative Commission on Law and Ethics in Modern Medicine, created by a multi-party initiative in March 2001. It brought legislators and experts together across parties to debate the issues and make policy recommendations, and it was closely aligned with the restrictive approach embodied in the Embryo Protection Law. The second body, the National Ethics Council, was a creation of Chancellor Gerhard Schröder, who succeeded Kohl as chancellor in October 1998. Like Clinton and Blair a strong supporter of science and technology, Schröder instituted the National Ethics Council in May 2001, partly as a counterweight to the Investigative Commission, and charged it with formulating ethical analysis and policy recommendations. Both bodies reported in fall 2001 in advance of key Bundestag debates on stem cell policy—and reached strikingly different conclusions.

In its November 2001 recommendations, the Bundestag committee, under the chairmanship of the Social Democrat Margot von Renese, reaffirmed the principles set down in the Embryo Protection Law—no research destructive of embryos. All thirty-eight of the committee's members agreed that any destruction of embryos in Germany—whether linked to stem cell research or not—"remained inadmissible" (*nicht verantwortbar*) because "human life is destroyed." It noted that embryonic stem cell research was not forbidden by the Embryo Protection Law, as stem cells were not embryos in their own right. But a clear majority of twenty-six to twelve also opposed the import of stem cells as a violation of the spirit of the EPL. If it was unethical to destroy embryos to derive stem cells, so the argument went, it was wrong to import cells derived through that procedure. The minority of twelve dissented and was willing to countenance research with stem cells imported from abroad, given their healing potential.[117]

The argument of research opponents was based on a particular interpretation of constitutional norms—a central foundation of the German ethical

---

116. Ibid. On the political context for the report, see "Bonn und Vatikan gegen das Klonen von Menschen," *Die Welt*, March 9, 1997.

117. *Zweiter Zwischenbericht der Enquête-Kommission Recht und Ethik der modernen Medizin: Teilbericht Stammzellforschung*, Drucksache 14/7546 (Berlin: Deutscher Bundestag, 2001).

debate. In a swipe at the tenor of the British controversy, the committee report maintained that a utilitarian approach that did not consider the early embryo deserving of protection because it could not feel pain contradicted "constitutionally-legal anchored principles of human dignity." The majority's claim that the "teaching of constitutional law almost universally assumes" that legal protection of life begins "with the fusion of sperm and egg" was highly contentious.[118] (The Constitutional Court had always been careful to remain ambiguous on the question of whether embryonic life, like fetal life, was protected under the Basic Law.) But its inclusion in the report, based on the reading of an influential conservative scholar, reflected the strongly held ethical conviction shared by most of the Bundestag deputies, lawyers, and bioethicists on the committee—a passionate belief that the restrictive EPL embodied a deeper national moral and legal consensus.

The very different report issued by Schröder's National Ethics Council in November 2001 demonstrated the emergence of an increasingly varied ethical discourse in the country. "Although our society takes the unanimous view that the protection of human life is a primordial moral and constitutional precept," it noted, "there is disagreement on the extent of the protection to which human life is entitled during its early embryonic development." While it underscored the strength of religious opposition to the destruction of embryos, as "a likeness of God," the report insisted that faith doctrines "while deserving of respect, cannot form the basis of a universally binding secular morality and of corresponding laws."[119] By a fifteen to ten majority the council backed importing stem cells derived abroad. Just as significant was the fact that nine out of the fifteen who supported imports also thought it "ethically permissible" to derive those stem cells in Germany. In effect, this sizeable minority, which included the philosopher Volker Gerhardt and the theologian Richard Schröder, favored a revision of the EPL—a position none of the thirty-eight members of the Bundestag's Investigative Commission had endorsed.[120]

The National Ethics Committee's subsequent treatment of the cloning issue in a September 2004 report went even further. It recommended unanimously that therapeutic cloning should not be allowed in Germany *for the time being*—which was hardly surprising, given the fact that any and all embryo research remained illegal. Strikingly, however, a plurality of twelve out

---

118. Ibid., 55.

119. Nationaler Ethikrat, *Opinion on the Import of Human Embryonic Stem Cells* (Berlin: German National Ethics Council, 2001), 5, 9.

120. Ibid., 36.

of twenty-five members did not want to rule it out for good. "Given that the blastocyst, four or five days after cell nuclear transfer, is not entitled to protection of human dignity as a born human being would be," the group reasoned, "the prohibition of instrumentalization repeatedly adduced against research cloning is also untenable." Here was a break with the eugenic concerns expressed so strongly in the Benda report, the EPL legislation, and within the Bundestag Investigative Commission. While this more diverse ethical debate was to have a very limited impact on the evolution of policy, it demonstrated the waning impact of historical memory and more diverse views of constitutional constraints in German ethical discourse.[121]

The Evolution of France's CCNE

Under the impact of stem cell breakthroughs, the French debate would grow even more open and diverse than that in Germany. The evolution is easier to trace, given the existence of a single national ethics committee with a public profile. After the announcement of Dolly's birth, French president Jacques Chirac demanded an ethical review and policy recommendations on a tight timeline. The CCNE reported back to Chirac in April 1997, condemning reproductive cloning in the harshest terms and affirming that its prohibition was implicit in the 1994 Bioethics Laws, which had outlawed all embryo research. The committee noted that "an embryo might be created" through cloning to derive stem cells, but added that such experiments had not been proven beyond mice and would be illegal in France in any case. It made no further mention of the possibility of therapeutic cloning. A final section of the report referred to "nonreproductive cloning" but defined the term broadly to encompass the "nonreproductive cloning of human cells, a common and ancient practice in biomedical research and analysis." The link between cloning, stem cells, and embryo experimentation had not yet fully surfaced in the French debate.

If the CCNE was slow to pick up on the therapeutic cloning issue, it was the first national bioethics committee to tackle embryonic stem cell research. A June 1997 report laid out "recommendations regarding the possible use of techniques and therapeutic instruments which have not yet been fully developed but which it is logical to believe might well be available very soon."[122] A strong majority agreed that the healing potential of stem cells

---

121. Nationaler Ethikrat, *Cloning for Reproductive Purposes and Cloning for the Purposes of Biomedical Research* (Berlin: German National Ethics Council, 2004), 69–70.

122. CCNE, "Opinion on the Establishment of Collections of Human Embryo Cells," 3.

would legitimate lifting the prohibition on embryo research, as long as the embryos were no longer part of a "parental project," that is, were left over from IVF treatments. A plea by Olivier de Dinechin, the Catholic representative on the committee, to oppose "the reduction of the embryo to an object, to research material," went unheeded.[123] The tone of the report marked a new departure. CCNE support for embryo research had always been cast as possible in exceptional circumstances given the tragic existence of a "potential person" or the "potentiality of a person" without the prospect of becoming a child. Now the majority cast experiments with embryos without a "parental project" as a positive good, given new therapeutic horizons, while insisting that their explicit creation for research "remain prohibited."[124]

In June 1998 the minister of health, Socialist Bernard Kouchner, known to sympathize with a loosening of strictures, called on the CCNE to formulate legislative recommendations that addressed this new therapeutic horizon. The committee report, published in October 1998, covered the main provisions of the 1994 laws, touching on topics ranging from surrogacy and genetic information to organ transplantation. On the politically salient issue of embryo research, the majority recommended that "parents should be allowed to decide on the destruction of their embryos or to allow their use for research purposes after a two-year period for reflection." In view of "important prospects in the field of therapeutic research," the report suggested that new legislation should "make it possible to modify the ban" on research involving human embryos. Such research would be limited to "only frozen embryos donated by couples who have given written consent, forsaken their parental project, and have decided to put an end to conservation." The deliberate creation of embryos for research would remain banned: "Any creation de novo of human embryos for any purpose other than a parental project is still not permitted." The CCNE recommendations, which Kouchner welcomed publicly, made no reference to cloning embryos or stem cell research beyond a general invocation of the value and importance of therapeutic research.[125]

In the wake of the November 1998 stem cell breakthrough and the more real prospect of therapeutic cloning, the government again turned to the

---

123. Dinechin argued that it was more humane to let the embryos die then to use them for stem cell experiments, anticipating a key element of the debate to come. See "Une décision pragmatique du Comité d'éthique," *Le Figaro*, May 6, 1997.

124. Declan Butler, "France Is Urged to Loosen Ban on Embryo Research," *Nature* 387, no. 6630 (1997): 218.

125. CCNE, "Re-examination of the Law on Bioethics," June 25, 1998, 7–8, www.ccne-ethique. fr/docs/en/avis060.pdf. See also "Avant la révision de la loi bioéthique," *Le Figaro*, October 1, 1998.

CCNE for advice. Its January 2001 report marked a further turn in the direction of an ethic of healing. The proresearch majority reiterated the committee's earlier characterization of the embryo as "a potential human person deserving of respect by all" but insisted that, once abandoned by its parents, it had no more potential and it was wrong to "sacralize" it as a "fully human person." Here was both a not so subtle critique of the Catholic Church's position and a reassertion of the idea, developed in earlier decades, that the moral status of the embryo depended on its relationship with others. In an unusual phrase, the January 2001 opinion extended those relations beyond the parents to the society as a whole: the sacrifice of the embryo "may be viewed as an expression of virtual solidarity between parents, a life which is not to be, and those who could benefit from the research." This awkward application of the revolutionary value of solidarity to an embryo was somewhat akin to the argument, common in the United States and the United Kingdom, that one could show the embryo respect by using it up in worthy research.[126]

On the issue of therapeutic cloning, the committee posed the central question: "Do therapeutic benefits expected from the use of stem cells derived from CNR [cell nuclear replacement] embryos justify transgression of the principle on which our legislation has been based so far, according to which the creation of human embryos for any other purpose than their own development, including research, is prohibited?" After a sharp internal debate, a slight majority of fourteen out of twenty-six CCNE members affirmed the proposition. The current and future chairmen of the committee, Kahn and Sicard, were among the dissenters.[127]

The growing divisions within the CCNE about how to combine respect for the embryo with opening to new life-saving research both reflected and reinforced a sharper ethical debate in the media and among the parties. As the legislative struggle over the revision of the Bioethics Laws got underway in late 2001 and 2002, historically grounded anxiety about eugenics faded amid growing excitement about a new era of regenerative medicine. The ethical and policy struggle remained bounded by the constitutional principle of human dignity but was increasingly shaped by electoral competition and the mobilization of scientists and patient-advocacy organizations eager to liberalize the existing regime. The terms of debate established within the CCNE during the mid-1980s—how best to combine respect for the embryo

---

126. CCNE, "Opinion on the Preliminary Draft Revision of the Laws on Bioethics," January 18, 2001, 2, http://ccne-ethique.fr/docs/en/avis067.pdf.

127. "Le comite national d'éthique et le clonage," *La Croix,* February 7, 2001.

with support for biomedical research—came under continual strain. That political story is explored in the next chapter.

Conclusion

The ethical landscape that emerged in the decade after 1998 both resembled and differed from that of the previous decades. Embryonic stem cell and cloning research remained controversial mainly because it involved the destruction (and in the case of cloning, the creation and destruction) of early embryonic life. But the balance of arguments shifted. Excitement about a possible new era of regenerative medicine threw research opponents on the defensive. It became more difficult to argue that surplus IVF embryos, destined to perish in any case, should not be used in research that might save lives. And the case against the deliberate creation of embryos, which had figured prominently in debates in all four countries, now had to take into account the potential promise of therapeutic cloning. Public arguments against embryo research did not disappear. For many Catholics and evangelicals in particular, the embryo represented a human individual to be protected from destruction, no matter what the potential payoffs of research. However, the rise of an ethic of healing undermined the appeal of this argument. The discovery of IPS cells in the period from 2006 to 2008 and the prospect of an era of regenerative medicine without the destruction of embryos may eventually shift the terms of debate again. Through the end of the first decade of the new century, however, most embryonic stem cell research supporters insisted that given the uncertainty of the scientific enterprise, all promising research agendas should be pursued.

The rise of an ethic of healing did not represent a triumph of secular over religious thinking. It affected both. In the United States and the United Kingdom, where utilitarian approaches dominated among leading bioethicists, the prospect of extending embryo research beyond infertility to problems of regenerative medicine fit a concern with reducing human suffering. In France and Germany, the traditional focus on the moral status of the embryo, traditionally articulated in a philosophical and deontological vein, lost ground to a humanitarian concern with the suffering of the sick. Within faith communities, an ethic of healing came to be articulated through religious resources including Jesus' mission to heal the sick, the Jewish idea of *tikkun olam,* and the call to humanity within Islam to eradicate unnecessary suffering. The moral status of the human embryo remained a key concern, particularly for Catholics and evangelicals. But the question of what to do with growing stockpiles of frozen IVF embryos—to let them perish or use them in new, more promising lines of research—posed an additional moral conundrum.

More often than not, the rise of an ethic of healing led, not to a new debate between research supporters and opponents, but to a hardening of fronts. The terms of controversy that had developed by the mid-1980s—how to combine the moral status of the embryo with the promise of biomedical research—began to fray. More and more research supporters began to downplay or dismiss the moral status of the embryo, preferring to speak of "cells" and "tissues" for therapies, without mentioning their origins. And research opponents, rather than acknowledge the promise of embryonic stem cell research and the moral quandaries it raised, often simply asserted the scientific superiority of research with adult stem cells or IPS cells. Not many participants in the controversy took the advice of the sociologist Hans Joas to heart—that all "should admit that the new possibilities of genetic technology and the life sciences undermine their ethical certainties and that it is not easy for them to draw on their ethical and religious (or antireligious) traditions in determining out the practical approaches to the new situation."[128] Such self-critical reflection, increasingly rare in bioethical debates, would prove even rarer in the policy struggle, where the growing mobilization of parties and interest groups contributed to a polarization of embryo politics.

---

128. "Grenzen der Verfügbarkeit," *Die Zeit,* February 15, 2001.

❧ CHAPTER 4

Stem Cell and Cloning Politics

By the mid-1990s a first wave of national policy struggles over embryo research had ended. After years of controversy, first the United Kingdom and Germany and then France and the United States had instituted legal regimes between 1990 and 1995 to govern the funding and regulation of research with embryos. The policy struggles had been fierce, but the outcomes—ranging from the most restrictive regime in Germany to the most liberal in the United Kingdom—seemed relatively stable. As it turned out, these political settlements would not last long. The twin cloning and embryonic stem cell breakthroughs of 1997–98 transformed the scientific, biomedical, and ethical stakes for research and inaugurated a new phase in embryo politics. The promise of a new era of regenerative medicine reframed old debates about the moral status of the embryo and the importance of biomedical advances. It also captured the public imagination and with it the attention of their elected political leaders. On both sides of the Atlantic political battles erupted around how to remake, or at least adapt, the policy regimes forged in an earlier era. The rise of an ethic of healing recounted in chapter 3 intersected with electoral politics, interest group mobilization, and existing institutions to drive divergent policy outcomes.

In the United States, President Bill Clinton was cautious but supportive of cloning and stem cell research, while his successor, George W. Bush (2001–8), supported a total cloning ban and strictly limited federal funding for research with embryonic stem cells. In 2009 President Barack Obama liberalized U.S. policy, but only on the margins. In the United Kingdom, Tony Blair's Labour-led government extended the existing 1990 Human Fertilisation and Embryology Act to allow for both embryonic stem cell and therapeutic cloning research in 2001–2, and under his successor, Gordon Brown the cloning of animal-human hybrid embryos as a source of stem cells was legalized in 2008. The German regime changed the least. The 1990 Embryo Protection Law remained in place, and the Bundestag passed cautious measures in 2001 under Chancellor Gerhard Schröder and again in 2008 under Angela Merkel to allow for the import of some embryonic stem cells derived abroad. In France the shift was clearest. The 2004 revision of the 1994 Bioethics Laws under President Jacques Chirac reversed the total ban on destructive embryo research, allowing for the derivation of stem cells from surplus IVF embryos for a period of five years. But efforts to liberalize the French policy regime further to allow therapeutic cloning failed.

These different outcomes were, in part, a result of politics as usual—the ebb and flow of electoral fortunes and shifting government coalitions. A close examination of each case reveals different forces at work as well. Ethical contestation grew more polarized, as the terms of debate shifted away from the moral status of the embryo toward a focus on the promise of regenerative medicine. Interest group mobilization increased, as existing churches, pro-life groups, and scientific and medical associations—important players in the 1980s and early 1990s—were joined by biotechnology companies and patient-advocacy organizations with an important stake in stem cell and cloning research. Embryo politics was still mediated by the historical legacies of eugenics and abortion controversies, although these had less of an impact than in the 1980s and early 1990s. More significant was the legacy of the research regimes instituted between 1990 and 1995, which provided a common point of reference in the political struggle over new scientific and technological developments.

The United States: Polarized Stem Cell Politics

First rumblings of stem cell politics in the United States can be traced back to news of the birth of Dolly the sheep in February 1997. The day that the cloning story broke, President Clinton asked the National Bioethics Advisory Commission to come up with policy recommendations within ninety days. Two weeks later he extended the ban on federal funding for embryo research to encompass "any cloning of human beings." "Any discovery that touches upon human creation is not simply a matter of scientific inquiry," he emphasized. "It is a matter of morality and spirituality as well."[1] Like the head of the National Institutes of Health, Harold Varmus, Clinton was generally careful to distinguish between two understandings of cloning. The "cloning of human beings" stood for reproductive cloning. It differed from cloning for research, what later became known as "therapeutic cloning." Varmus's concern, shared by scientists and the biotechnology sector, was that over-hasty and general anticloning legislation would hinder stem cell research that aimed to create genetically matched cells for future patients. "I am worried about legislation that occurs in a preemptive fashion," he told a congressional committee, "before the scientific community has had a chance to respond itself."[2]

While elected leaders, interest groups, and public opinion almost uniformly denounced the prospect of reproductive cloning as an abomination, political conflict over therapeutic cloning slowly took shape. In its June 1997 report *Cloning Human Beings* the NBAC warned against a cloning ban that would restrict valuable research. In welcoming the recommendations, Clinton proposed legislation to Congress that would outlaw reproductive cloning but left open the possibility of cloning research. Without mentioning the destruction of embryos, he argued that cloning technology held "promise for producing replacement skin, cartilage, or bone tissue for burn or accident victims, and nerve tissue to treat spinal cord injury." Therefore, nothing in his proposed Cloning Prohibition Act of 1997 would prohibit "use of somatic cell nuclear transfer or other cloning technologies to clone molecules, DNA, cells, and tissues." This careful reference to "cells" and "tissues" without mention of the embryos from which they would be derived paralleled the language of the Biotechnology Industry Organization (BIO), which lobbied hard to forestall a complete cloning ban.[3]

Catholics, evangelicals, and pro-life groups and their allies in Congress began to mobilize after the *Washington Post* ran a story in early June on the NBAC's upcoming recommendations with the headline, "Panel Backs Some

1. Quoted in "Clinton Forbids Funding of Human Clone Studies," *Washington Post,* March 5, 1997; White House Press Office, "Remarks by the President on Cloning," press release, March 4, 1997.

2. U.S. Congress. U.S. House of Representatives. Committee on Science, Subcommittee on Technology, "Biotechnology and the Ethics of Cloning: How Far Should We Go?" March 5, 1997, http://commdocs.house.gov/committees/science/hsy064170.000/hsy064170_0.HTM. See also Varmus, *Art and Politics of Science.*

3. White House Press Office, "To the Congress of the United States," press release, June 9, 1997, http://clinton3.nara.gov/New/Remarks/Mon/19970609–15987.html; Biotechnology Industry Organization, "BIO Supports Bans on Cloning Humans, Seeks Medical Research Protection," press release, June 7, 1997, http://www.bio.org/news/pressreleases/newsitem.asp?id=1997_0607_01.

Human Clone Work."[4] Republican Senator Christopher Bond of Missouri introduced legislation for a total ban on cloning research in both the public and private sectors. In a February 1998 debate on the legislation, Bond noted that he had "heard from patient groups, people who are very much concerned, as we all are, about cancer, about juvenile diabetes, cystic fibrosis, Alzheimer's–the whole range of diseases." He acknowledged their concerns but insisted that "we can deal with the research without cloning a human embryo." The bill's cosponsor, Republican Senator Bill Frist of Tennessee, underscored that he did not "want to slow down science and the progress of science." At the same time, he noted that "science has been abused in the past," invoking the legacy of Nazi eugenics.[5]

In the same February 1998 debate, Democratic senators Edward Kennedy of Massachusetts and Diane Feinstein of California backed legislation that would have only banned the reproductive cloning of human beings. Kennedy cast the Bond bill as an attack on science, lamenting a "blunderbuss ban on cloning research." And in one of the first extended political appeals to an ethic of healing, he provided a preview of work with stem cells, referring to "vital medical research related to cloning—research which has the potential to find new cures for cancer, diabetes, birth defects and genetic diseases of all kinds, blindness, Parkinson's disease, Alzheimer's disease, paralysis due to spinal cord injury, arthritis, liver disease, life-threatening burns, and many other illnesses and injuries."[6] Aided by a furious lobbying effort by BIO and scientific associations, including a petition signed by twenty-seven Nobel laureates, Kennedy and Feinstein gathered the forty-plus votes they needed to prevent a floor vote on the Bond bill. Clinton praised the outcome and encouraged the Senate to take more time "to carefully craft a bill that will ban the cloning of human beings while preserving our ability to use cloning technology for morally acceptable and medically important purposes."[7]

The February 1998 Senate clash, little publicized at the time, was an early indicator of the political force of ethic-of-healing arguments. In shifting the focus away from the moral status of the embryo to the promise of "cells" and "tissues," Kennedy and Feinstein were able to broaden the proresearch

---

4. "Panel Backs Some Human Clone Work," *Washington Post,* June 4, 1997.

5. U.S. Congress, "Human Cloning Prohibition Act—Motion to Proceed," 105th Cong., 2nd sess., *Congressional Record* 144 (February 11, 1998), S600, S602.

6. Ibid., February 5, 1998, S434. The Democrats tried and failed to move their reproductive cloning ban out of committee and onto the Senate floor for a debate and vote.

7. White House Press Office, "Remarks by the President to the American Association for the Advancement of Science," press release, February 13, 1998, http://clinton6.nara.gov/1998/02/1998-02-13-remarks-by-the-president-to-aaas.html.

coalition. One pro-life Catholic senator pointed to letters from seventy-one patient groups and scientific organizations in warning against any law that might impede "valuable biomedical research." A prominent conservative from North Carolina with a daughter with diabetes insisted on a need "to investigate this issue more thoroughly so that we do not deny our citizens and our loved ones of any possible lifesaving research." And Utah's Orrin Hatch, one of the most vocal pro-life senators and a Mormon, indicated that the prospect of regenerative medicine gave him pause when considering a cloning ban. He had "profound questions about the scientific implications" of the Bond bill and its potential to block research.[8]

The question of therapeutic cloning would gain more political salience after the successful isolation of human embryonic stem cells in 1998. But that breakthrough initially raised a more basic issue—whether and how the government should support stem cell research. While the 1995 Dickey Amendment clearly prohibited the use of federal funds to derive stem cells from embryos, it said nothing about research with the cells themselves. In January 1999 lawyers from the Department of Health and Human Services (DHSS), parent to the NIH, concluded that yes, in fact, "current law permits federal funds to be used for research utilizing human pluripotent stem cells." As NIH officials began to formulate guidelines for vetting research-funding proposals, pro-life groups challenged this interpretation. In February 1999 some seventy legislators petitioned DHSS Secretary Donna Shalala to overrule the recommendation because it violated "both the letter and spirit" of federal law.[9] In March, *Science* published a letter signed by sixty-seven Nobel laureates that backed the NIH approach as a way of "protecting the sanctity of human life without impeding biomedical research that could be profoundly important to the understanding and treatment of human disease."[10]

In its July 1999 report, *Ethical Issues in Human Stem Cell Research,* the NBAC criticized the NIH approach—federal support for stem cell research but not for the derivation of those cells from embryos—as inconsistent.[11] The commission urged a repeal of the Dickey Amendment to allow the use of federal funds to create stem cell lines. In his response, Clinton aligned himself

8. Senators Connie Mack, Strom Thurmond, and Orrin Hatch in *Congressional Record,* vol. 144 (February 11, 1998), S600, S604.

9. "Government Says Ban on Human Embryo Research Does Not Apply to Cells," *New York Times,* January 20, 1999; "Ruling in Favor of Stem Cell Research Draws Fire of 70 Lawmakers," *New York Times,* February 17, 1999.

10. Robert P. Lanza et al., "Science over Politics," *Science* 483, no. 5409 (1999): 1849.

11. The NBAC criticized the "mistaken notion that the two areas of research are so distinct that participating in one need not mean participating in the other." National Bioethics Advisory Commission, *Ethical Issues in Human Stem Cell Research,* vol. 1, 71.

with Varmus and the NIH—a pragmatic recognition of continued congressional opposition to destructive embryo research. As a White House press release put it, "human stem cell technology's potential medical benefits are compelling and worthy of pursuit, so long as the research is conducted according to the highest ethical standards." It considered that "no other legal actions are necessary at this time," because it appeared that human embryonic stem cells will be available from the private sector. It concluded that "publicly funded research using these cells is permissible under the current Congressional ban on human embryo research."[12] When the NIH at last published its proposed guidelines in December 1999, scientific groups and patient advocates expressed satisfaction that the policy process was at last moving forward.[13]

There was some support for the NBAC's more comprehensive approach. In early 2000 Senators Tom Harkin, Democrat of Iowa, and Arlen Specter, Republican of Pennsylvania, proposed legislation that would have provided federal funds for the derivation of stem cells. Congressional hearings that April featuring actor Christopher Reeve (*Superman*), who had been paralyzed in a riding accident, received favorable media attention. But although the legislation was backed by a coalition of more than one hundred organizations, including the American Medical Association and the Juvenile Diabetes Foundation, it never made it beyond the committee stage.[14] Pro-life forces and their allies in Congress prevented any reconsideration of the Dickey Amendment. In the meantime, the NIH finalized its own approach. After receiving some fifty thousand public comments, it published research guidelines and a call for proposals in August 2000.

By that time, however, the presidential election campaign was in full swing, and the fate of the guidelines hung in the political balance. The stem cell issue was not prominent in the campaign; economic and social issues held center stage. But the two candidates, Democrat Al Gore and Republican George W. Bush, outlined contrasting positions on cloning and stem cells. Gore aligned himself with the NIH regulations and the Democratic platform's support for "stem cell research to make important new discoveries." The Republican platform held up the Dickey Amendment as a model and

12. White House Press Office, "Statement by Press Secretary on Human Stem Cell Research," press release, July 14, 1999, http://archives.clintonpresidentialcenter.org/?u=071499-statement-by-press-secretary-on-human-stem-cell-research.htm.

13. National Institutes of Health, "NIH Publishes Draft Guidelines for Stem Cell Research," press release, December 1, 1999, http://www.nih.gov/news/pr/dec99/od-01.htm.

14. On the mobilization of patient-advocacy organizations in the U.S. debate, see Daniel Perry, "Patients' Voices: The Powerful Sound in the Stem Cell Debate," *Science* 287, no. 5457 (2000): 1423.

praised "congressional Republicans for the steps they have taken for protection of human embryos and against human cloning."[15] While Bush supported a total ban on cloning research, his position on stem cells was less clear. An evangelical with the support of pro-life forces, Bush was sharply opposed to the use of federal funds to derive stem cells from embryos. While he did not openly promise to reverse NIH openness to research with stem cells derived without government support, scientists and their supporters had reason to be anxious. The head of a prominent coalition of patient advocacy groups noted that "a lot of my colleagues think we'll have our backs to the wall if Bush is elected."[16]

The Politics of Stem Cells under George W. Bush

On taking office in January 2001, President Bush could have immediately implemented the NIH policy developed by Clinton or refused federal funding for all embryonic stem cell research. Instead, he opted for several months of reflection, setting conservative and pro-life groups on edge. Proresearch groups sensed an opening. In January, Bush received a letter from 123 organizations, and in February, another from 80 Nobel laureates, advocating federal support for stem cell research to tackle degenerative diseases. The letters sought to strike a conciliatory tone and to isolate the question of stem cell research from that of therapeutic cloning. "While we recognize the legitimate ethical issues raised by this research," the February letter stated, "it is important to understand that the cells being used in this research were destined to be discarded in any case"—a reference to the use of surplus IVF embryos.[17] Celebrity advocates, including Christopher Reeve and fellow actor and Parkinson's victim Michael J. Fox (*Back to the Future*), drew media attention to the issue, as did Nancy Reagan, whose husband, the former president, was suffering from Alzheimer's. While in fall 2000 only about 20 percent of Americans had been following the stem cell issue, that number had grown to approximately 60 percent by the following summer, with clear majorities favoring research. Within Congress the most important proresearch shift was that of pro-life Mormon senator Orrin Hatch. After "countless hours of

---

15. Democratic Party, "The Democratic Party Platform of 2000," August 14, 2000, http://www.presidency.ucsb.edu/ws/index.php?pid=29612; Republican Party, "Republican Platform 2000," July 31, 2000, http://www.pbs.org/newshour/bb/election/july-dec00/platform4.html.

16. Daniel Perry quoted in "Biomedical Research Goes Where Candidates Dare Not," *Washington Post,* October 29, 2004.

17. "Nobel Laureates Back Stem Cell Research," *Washington Post,* February 22, 2001.

study, reflection, and prayer," Hatch recalled, "eventually I determined that being pro-life means helping the living."[18]

Research opponents, alarmed about the erosion of support in public opinion and among lawmakers, stepped up their lobbying efforts with Congress and the White House. The U.S. Conference of Catholic Bishops delivered a letter to members of the House and Senate in July 2001 that acknowledged proresearch shifts in public and elite opinion. It noted that "speculations about the possible benefits of such research, and mistaken views about the status of the human embryo, have led many to urge you to abandon your convictions."[19] None other than Pope John Paul II lobbied Bush on the issue during his first European trip in July, which included a papal audience. "A free and virtuous society, which America aspires to be," the pontiff insisted, must "reject practices that devalue and violate human life at any stage from conception until natural death."[20] The antiresearch cause got a further boost just as Bush was finalizing his position. In July 2001, U.S. IVF pioneers Howard and Georgeanna Jones, based in Norfolk, Virginia, reported that they had created embryos expressly for the derivation of stem cells. Research opponents seized on this otherwise unremarkable story—the creation of embryos for private-sector research was not new—to shift some attention away from the promise of regenerative medicine to the fate of embryos created and destroyed in labs.[21]

In his August 2001 television address to the nation, watched by about one in three Americans, Bush sought to strike a policy compromise. He first set out the opposing views on the issue, underscoring diverse religious and philosophical perspectives "within the church with people of different faiths, even many of the same faith coming to different conclusions." On the one hand, he noted that scientists believed that stem cell research offered "great promise that could help improve the lives of those who suffer from many terrible diseases—from juvenile diabetes to Alzheimer's, from Parkinson's to spinal cord injuries." On the other hand, "research on embryonic stem cells raises profound ethical questions, because extracting the stem cell destroys the embryo, and thus destroys its potential for life." The ethical stakes were

---

18. Quoted in James Randerson, "The Battle over Stem Cells," *New Scientist* 184, no. 2468 (2004): 23.

19. Quoted in "Conservatives Pressure Bush in Cell Debate," *New York Times,* July 12, 2001.

20. John Paul II, "Address of Pope John Paul II to the President of the United States of America, H. E. George Walker Bush," July 23, 2001, http://www.vatican.va/holy_father/john_paul_ii/speeches/2001/documents/hf_jp-ii_spe_20010723_president-bush_en.html.

21. Emma Young, "Human Embryos Created for Cell Harvest," *New Scientist.com,* July 11, 2001, http://www.newscientist.com/article/dn997.

high, Bush argued, for "we have arrived at that brave new world that seemed so distant in 1932, when Aldous Huxley wrote about human beings created in test tubes in what he called a 'hatchery.'" His compromise solution was to limit research funding to sixty stem cell lines *already* derived from surplus IVF embryos at the time of his speech: "This allows us to explore the promise and potential of stem cell research without crossing a fundamental moral line, by providing taxpayer funding that would sanction or encourage further destruction of human embryos that have at least the potential for life." Bush concluded his address: "I have made this decision with great care and I pray it is the right one."[22]

The initial media echo was very positive. Bush was widely praised for his compromise decision and Solomonic judgment, and snap public opinion polls registered high levels of support for his stance. The forces that had been battling on both sides of the issue were less enthusiastic. Research opponents who had favored a total ban were disappointed. The U.S. Conference of Catholic Bishops, for example, wrote: "We hope and pray that President Bush will return to a principled stand against treating some human lives as nothing more than objects to be manipulated and destroyed for research purposes."[23] On the other side of the issue, scientific organizations warned that the quality and quantity of stem cells derived before August 2001 was not sufficient to sustain viable research programs.[24] As a political matter, however, the speech settled the issue for the time being. Conservative Republicans in Congress were unwilling to take on their own president. And Democrats could still not muster enough votes to overthrow the Dickey Amendment or pass veto-proof legislation that would have allowed research with cells derived after August 2001.

As it happened, the attacks on the World Trade Center and the Pentagon on September 11, 2001, quickly relegated bioethical questions to the political margins. When embryo politics did reemerge in 2002–3, the focus returned to the cloning issue—whether to ban all cloning or only reproductive cloning, keeping its therapeutic variant legal. In April 2001, when the public controversy had swirled around stem cells, a bill to ban all cloning had passed the

22. White House Press Office, "Remarks by the President on Stem Cell Research," press release, August 9, 2001, http://bioethics.georgetown.edu/pcbe/reports/stemcell/appendix_b.html.

23. United States Conference of Catholic Bishops, "Catholic Bishops Criticize Bush Policy on Embryo Research," press release, August 9, 2001, http://www.usccb.org/comm/archives/2001/01–142.shtml.

24. American Association for the Advancement of Science, "President Bush's Stem Cell Policy: A Statement of the American Association for the Advancement of Science," August 17, 2001, http://www.aaas.org/spp/cstc/docs/01–08-17_stemstmt.htm.

House of Representatives by a vote of 265 to 175. The parallel legislation in the Senate, sponsored by Republican Sam Brownback of Kansas and Democrat Mary Landrieu of Louisiana, came up for debate in early 2002. Bush threw his weight behind a total ban in an emotional April 2002 White House meeting with cloning opponents. Invoking religious imagery, he asserted that "life is a creation, not a commodity" and that "our children are gifts to be loved and protected, not products to be designed and manufactured." Adding eugenic concerns to this pro-life stance, Bush conjured images of "embryo farms" and construed research cloning as "a significant step toward a society in which human beings are grown for spare body parts, and children are engineered to custom specifications." And he accused cloning supporters of putting science ahead of ethics. "We can pursue medical research with a clear sense of moral purpose," he warned, "or we can travel without an ethical compass into a world we could live to regret."[25]

The 2002 Senate cloning struggle was a virtual re-run of the February 1998 clash. A group of Democratic senators, including Kennedy and Feinstein, opposed the Brownback-Landrieu bill with one of their own, which would prohibit reproductive human cloning "while preserving important areas of medical research." The legislation made no mention of therapeutic cloning or of creating embryos for research, but referred instead to "nuclear transplantation" as the source of genetically matched stem cells. In the key debates, Kennedy was, as he had been in 1998, the most outspoken advocate of an ethic of healing, suggesting at one point that his legislation might eventually "empty three-fourths of the nursing home beds in Massachusetts."[26] As in 1998, opponents of a total cloning ban fell short of the sixty votes they needed to close debate and move to a floor vote in the Senate—a constellation that would recur in 2003 and again in 2004.

At least part of the success of therapeutic cloning advocates was attributable to their use of language. By referring not to cloning but to nuclear transfer transplantation and not to cloned embryos but to tissues and cells, they shifted the debate away from the moral status of embryos to the promise of research. An evolution in the editorial position of the *Washington Post* provides evidence of the success of the strategy. Responding to the 1994 recommendations of the Human Embryo Research Panel, the newspaper had argued that "the creation of human embryos specifically for research that will

25. White House Press Office, "Bush Calls on Senate to Back Human Cloning Ban," press release, April 10, 2002, http://georgewbush-whitehouse.archives.gov/news/releases/2002/04/20020410–4. html.

26. Constance Holden, "Random Samples," *Science* 295, no. 5562 (2002): 2009.

destroy them is unconscionable." Seven years later, the editors opposed efforts to outlaw therapeutic cloning because "a complete cloning ban could block many possible clinical applications of stem cell research."[27]

Research opponents, too, tended to obscure the complexity of the ethical decisions at hand. If research supporters were guilty of exaggerating the promise of embryonic stem cell research and ducking the problem of the moral status of the embryo, opponents often simply asserted that adult stem cell research was a superior scientific alternative. Brownback asserted matter-of-factly that "adult stem cell research has demonstrated a vastly greater potential to generate real treatments for real people"—a true statement in the context of already existing treatments, but questionable with respect to potential future ones. All scientists had learned in decades of work, he scoffed, was that embryonic stem cells "are very good at forming tumors."[28] As stem cells and cloning were drawn into partisan confrontation, the quality of the public policy debate declined on both sides.

The 2004 presidential campaign was one indication of this polarization. Bush's Democratic challenger John Kerry—a prochoice Catholic and supporter of both embryonic stem cell research and therapeutic cloning—pitched himself as a pragmatist and Bush an extremist. In August 2004, on the third anniversary of Bush's stem cell decision, he insisted that "here in America, we don't sacrifice science for ideology"—obscuring the fact that research supporters, too, brought their own values to bear on the policy debate. With polls showing support for embryonic stem cell research, Bush countered in one of the presidential debates that he was "the first President ever to allow funding, federal funding, for embryonic stem cell research"—even as he continued to place far-reaching constraints on it.[29]

While Bush prevailed in the election, he continued to lose support on stem cell issues in Congress. In May 2005 fifty House Republicans crossed the aisle to support lifting the August 2001 cutoff date for the derivation of stem cells to be used in federally funded research. Senate Majority Leader Frist broke ranks with Bush and supported the legislation, which passed both Houses in

27. "Embryos: Drawing the Line," *Washington Post,* October 2, 1994; "Overkill," *Washington Post,* July 31, 2001.

28. Press Office of Senator Sam Brownback, "Brownback Applauds New Stem Cell Advances," press release, November 20, 2007, http://brownback.senate.gov/pressapp/record.cfm?id=287831.

29. John Kerry, radio address August 7, 2004, quoted in "Kerry Takes on Issue of Embryo Research," *Washington Post,* August 8, 2004; White House Press Office, "Remarks by President Bush and Senator Kerry in Second 2004 Presidential Debate," press release, October 9, 2004, http://georgewbush-whitehouse.archives.gov/news/releases/2004/10/20041009-2.html.

July 2006.[30] Bush used his veto—the first of his presidency—and did so a second time when Congress passed a similar measure again in 2007.

In the meantime, increasingly frustrated research advocates had turned from the federal to the state level in search of funding and a friendlier regulatory atmosphere. The trend had begun in New Jersey and Massachusetts in 2002–3 and spread to other states. Its high point was a November 2004 ballot initiative in California to create an Institute for Regenerative Medicine. Endorsed by Governor Arnold Schwarzenegger, a Republican, and supported by a coalition of businesspeople and entertainment industry stars, the initiative passed by a large margin. It called for $3 billion in research support over ten years, including work on therapeutic cloning, as part of an effort to substitute for missing federal government funds. By the end of Bush's presidency fifteen state-run programs had combined embryonic stem cell research expenditures greater than the federal government's.

Nothing illustrated the political rise of an ethic of healing more than the 2008 election campaign in which both of the major party candidates, Democrat Barack Obama and Republican John McCain, backed an expansion of federally funded embryonic stem cell research. While their policy prescriptions were similar, they approached the issue very differently. Their most pointed exchange was at a highly publicized forum hosted by Rick Warren, a leading evangelical. Obama reiterated his support for overturning Bush's policy in order to advance "scientific research that could lead to cures," but when asked by Warren when human life deserves protection, he responded flippantly that the question was "above my pay grade." McCain, by contrast, explained his own transition from opposition to support for limited embryo research as a gradual rethinking of difficult issues. "For those of us in the prolife community," he told Warren, "this has been a great struggle and a terrible dilemma because we're also taught other obligations that we have as well"—a rare admission by a politician of the moral conundrum posed by stem cell research.[31]

On assuming office, Obama rescinded most of Bush's embryonic stem cell policy. A March 2009 executive order legalized federally funded research with cells derived after the August 2001 cutoff date. "Our government has forced what I believe is a false choice between sound science and moral values," Obama told reporters. He grounded his ethic of healing on a religious foundation. "As a person of faith, I believe we are called to care for each

---

30. "Senator Bill Frist on Embryonic Stem Cell Research," *New York Times,* July 29, 2005.

31. "Saddleback Presidential Candidates Forum," August 16, 2008, http://transcripts.cnn.com/TRANSCRIPTS/0808/16/se.02.html.

other and work to ease human suffering," he underlined. "I believe we have been given the capacity and will to pursue this research—and the humanity and conscience to do so responsibly."[32]

To the dismay of scientists, the administration subsequently clarified that only stem cells derived from surplus IVF embryos could be studied with federal funds, not those created for research purposes or through cloning technology. A further setback was a federal judge's ruling, in August 2010, that even research with embryonic stem cells already in existence violated the Dickey Amendment's ban on federal funding for experiments involving the destruction of embryos—an interpretation the administration vowed to fight in the courts. In this political and legal atmosphere, Obama did not press for federally funded research directly involving the destruction of embryos. He did not even take a position on the issue and, according to his chief domestic policy adviser, did not intend to. With the Republican takeover of Congress in the November 2010 elections, the prospects for further liberalization of U.S. policy dimmed. In the fifteen years since its first passage, the Dickey Amendment had become part of the institutional status quo. To the chagrin of research supporters in the scientific, medical, and patient-advocacy communities, only incremental changes to the existing policy regime took place.[33]

The United Kingdom: Political Opening to Stem Cell and Cloning Research

The British political struggle over cloning and stem cell research differed from the American in three major respects. First, there was a clear institutional and policy framework in place encompassing both the public and the private sectors. The Human Fertilisation and Embryology Act of 1990 had legalized embryo research—including the creation of embryos expressly for experiments—and set up a bureaucracy to regulate it. Second, and related, the more unified U.K. state made for a more structured political struggle. A Labour majority controlled both Parliament and the government during the decade following the stem cell and cloning breakthroughs, in contrast to the

---

32. White House Press Office, "Signing of Stem Cell Executive Order and Scientific Integrity Presidential Memorandum," press release, March 9, 2009, http://www.whitehouse.gov/the_press_office/Remarks-of-the-President-As-Prepared-for-Delivery-Signing-of-Stem-Cell-Executive-Order-and-Scientific-Integrity-Presidential-Memorandum/.

33. "Obama Is Leaving Some Stem Cell Issues to Congress," *New York Times,* March 8, 2009. "The Stem Cell Debate: A Federal Appeals Court Weighs in on the Ban on Embryonic Research," *Washington Post,* September 10, 2010.

U.S. pattern of divided government. While party discipline was suspended on matters of conscience like embryo research, Prime Minister Tony Blair and his successor Gordon Brown used their institutional position to frame the legislative agenda. Finally, principled opposition to all embryo research among Catholics, evangelicals, and pro-life forces, already less of a factor in the United Kingdom in the 1980s than in the United States, further receded in importance. Once Blair secured approval for the incorporation of stem cell and cloning research into the existing policy framework, political opposition to the country's liberal research regime was sustained less by moral concern with the embryo than by perceived dangers of eugenic abuses. Here a critical juncture was the government's drive in 2007–8, against considerable opposition, to allow the creation of animal-human hybrid embryos as a source of stem cells for research.

The scientific breakthroughs of 1997–98 posed a stark challenge to the HFEA framework. The 1990 law had legalized embryo research to combat infertility and congenital and chromosomal disorders, but it made no allowance for work with stem cells or cloning to address a wider range of degenerative diseases. In the wake of the Dolly announcement, the scientific establishment in the United Kingdom was initially less concerned than in the United States about a comprehensive cloning ban that would stifle future research. In March 1997, the flagship journal *Nature* raised the possibility of a moratorium on all cloning research, whether for reproductive or research purposes. Its editors did not mention stem cells explicitly but recognized that cloning might one day "generate skin grafts for burn victims, or other 'spare-part' provision." Nevertheless, they called for a moratorium, "even if it carries with it a possibility that will worry those who wish to pursue such research."[34] In contrast, Ruth Deech of the HFEA echoed the position taken by Varmus in the U.S. debate, warning against a comprehensive cloning ban that could foreclose promising avenues of research.[35] None of these issues gained much public notice, as the country was in the midst of an election campaign that centered on economic issues in which Labour under Tony Blair unseated Margaret Thatcher's successor as prime minister, John Major, in May 1997.

Blair came into office as a self-styled modernizer and named Lord Sainsbury, a close supporter with strong ties to the biotechnology industry, as science minister. On the cloning issue, the new government created a joint working group with the HFEA and the Human Genetics Advisory Committee

---

34. "Human Cloning Requires a Moratorium, Not a Ban," *Nature* 386, no. 6620 (1997): 1.

35. "MPs Warned over Panic Reaction," *Financial Times,* March 6, 1997.

to formulate recommendations. Its draft report, published in January 1998 with little public notice, inaugurated a comment period during which an initial political mobilization for and against stem cell and cloning research took place. The responses to the HFEA consultation were varied—about two hundred in all. Among scientific groups, the Royal Society referred to cloning as "embryo reconstruction" and asked that "any modification to existing legislation, or any new legislation, should be carefully drafted so as not to outlaw the potential future benefits that could be derived from research on cloned embryos."[36] On the other side of the issue, the All-Party Parliamentary Pro-Life Group focused its critique on the deliberate creation of embryos for research and on the danger of a slippery slope from therapeutic to reproductive cloning. They prefaced their statement with the phrase "I'm glad I'm not a gamma," an allusion to the human classification scheme in Huxley's *Brave New World*.[37]

The final joint HGAC/HFEA report, published in December 1998, supported the government's view that reproductive cloning was already illegal under the terms of the 1990 HFE Act, even as it advised an explicit legislative ban to remove any ambiguity. On embryonic stem cell research, it further recommended that the legitimate purposes of embryo research could be broadened to encompass the struggle against degenerative diseases. In a June 1999 response to the report, the government agreed that legislation should be considered. Rather than introduce legislation immediately, however, Blair asked Chief Medical Officer Liam Donaldson to convene an expert advisory group to "establish more clearly the evidence of potential benefits for human health of such research." Once the expert group's recommendations were published, Parliament would have an "opportunity to debate fully the issues raised, and to decide whether the proposals were acceptable." In the meantime, the government imposed a moratorium on therapeutic cloning, angering some scientists.[38]

Given the proresearch makeup of the Donaldson committee, the thrust of its recommendations was never in doubt. Sainsbury himself suggested in an interview in July 2000—before the committee report went public—that the government's position was a foregone conclusion, as "the potential medical benefits outweigh any other considerations one might have." Sainsbury

36. Royal Society, "Whither Cloning?" press release, January 1, 1998, http://royalsociety.org/Whither-Cloning.

37. All-Party Parliamentary Pro-Life Group, "Response of the All-Party Parliamentary Pro-Life Group to the HGAC/HFEA Consultation Paper 'Cloning Issues in Reproduction, Science and Medicine,'" April 1998.

38. "Human Cloning Banned in Research," *Independent,* June 25, 1999.

distanced himself from his comment after a Tory health expert accused him of "sweeping away all the complex ethical issues with complete contempt."[39] But the result of the committee's deliberations, recounted in chapter 3, was never really in doubt. The August 2000 Donaldson report recommended an extension of the 1990 HFE Act to cover both embryonic stem cell research and therapeutic cloning.

In its official response, the government welcomed the recommendations and called for the rapid introduction of new legislation to amend the 1990 HFE Act. While "the Government recognises that research involving embryos is a sensitive subject on which there are divergent views," it aligned itself with those for whom "the potential benefits of the research may be weighed against the respect due to an embryo at the very earliest stages of its development." The government response referred to therapeutic cloning as "cell nuclear replacement" but acknowledged it as a form of "research using human embryos"—in this case embryos created explicitly for research, something allowed in the 1990 legislation. To allay fears about a slippery slope between therapeutic and reproductive cloning, the proposed legislation was to include an explicit ban on the latter practice.[40]

Though the summer of 2000, the centralized structure of the British state allowed Blair, in contrast to Clinton, to channel the debate and prevent any legislative drive for a comprehensive cloning ban. With the publication of the Donaldson report and the government's introduction of legislation mirroring its recommendations, political mobilization around cloning and stem cell research began in earnest. Pro-life groups active during the 1980s controversies, including the Society for the Protection of Unborn Children (SPUC) and LIFE, another antiabortion group, sought to flood Parliament with mail and petitions criticizing any extension of HFEA regulation to cover stem cell and cloning research. Peter Garrett of LIFE objected to efforts "to create and then deliberately destroy tiny human lives."[41] The Catholic leadership also weighed in. The influential cardinal Thomas Winning of Scotland sharply criticized the Donaldson report, reiterating the official Church position that "obtaining stem cells from a human embryo is morally wrong, because it involves the destruction of a human life." He also targeted cloning: "'Therapeutic cloning' is the ultimate misnomer, for it actually means killing."[42]

---

39. Quoted in "Whitehall Split on Cloning Decision," *Guardian,* July 31, 2000.

40. UK, Department of Health, *Government Response to the Recommendations Made in the Chief Medical Officer's Expert Group Report* (London: Her Majesty's Stationery Office, 2000), 3, 5.

41. Quoted in "Experts Support Human Cloning," *BBC News,* August 16, 2000.

42. "Cardinal Condemns British Plan for Cloning," *Catholic World News,* August 16, 2000; "Cloning: A Question of Life or Death," *Glasgow Herald,* December 4, 2000.

In the media and in public opinion, these pro-life groups had less standing than in the United States. They also faced a well-organized coalition of patient-advocacy groups first forged during the successful legislative drive for the HFE Act in 1989–90. Two of the most important groups, the Association of Medical Research Charities and the Genetic Interest Group, backed the government legislation, as did other influential associations, such as the Parkinson's Disease Society.[43] As it had during the previous decade, the Church of England's Board for Social Responsibility provided additional support for proresearch forces, articulating an ethic of healing in a religious idiom. One of its leading theologians, John Polkinghorne, was a member of the Donaldson committee. And the board's chairman, the Bishop of Oxford, Richard Harries, championed the legislation.[44]

Not surprisingly, leading scientific and medical associations, including the Royal Society and the Academy of Medical Sciences, also came out in favor of adapting the HFEA framework, as did the BioIndustry Association and the Wellcome Trust, the leading private funder of research. "Broadening the scope of the research that is permitted under the law," the Trust argued, was "ethically justifiable, in view of the new understanding and treatments it could offer for conditions that affect so many people."[45] In contrast to the United States, France, and Germany, scientists could also count on the political support of a state institution—the HFEA itself. While nominally an administrative body, the authority joined in the political fray, combining appeals to an ethic of healing with the historical argument that the policy battle over the ethics of embryo research had already been fought and decided a decade earlier. In July 2000, for example, HFEA chair Ruth Deech discerned a growing consensus in favor of therapeutic cloning research "to grow new cells and tissues to help people with Parkinson's, with Huntington's, with Alzheimer's, with cancer and with burns."[46]

While Blair could rely on strategically placed allies on the government benches, the vote was not a foregone conclusion. Parliamentarians were freed from party discipline, given the moral sensitivities of the issues, and while support for embryonic stem cell research was strong, public opinion

43. Association of Medical Research Charities, "Stem Cell Research: AMRC Responds to Donaldson Report and Government Response," press release, August 16, 2000; "Experts Back Use of Therapeutic Cloning," *Times* (London), August 17, 2000.

44. "C of E says Cloning Is 'Morally Acceptable,'" *Telegraph,* December 3, 2000.

45. Wellcome Trust, "Wellcome Trust Interim Position Statement on Stem Cell Research," press release, October 2000; Biotechnology Industry Organization, "BIA Welcomes Donaldson Recommendations on Cell Nuclear Replacement," press release, August 30, 2000.

46. Quoted in "Call for a Decision on Human Cloning," *BBC News,* July 31, 2000.

remained skeptical of any form of cloning. In a November 2000 speech on the eve of a first Commons debate on his proposed legislation, Blair acknowledged strong views on all sides, praising the fact that "advances in science are debated in a moral context." While noting that "some people are opposed in principle to all forms of embryo research on ethical grounds," he pointed to "strong ethical arguments in favour so long as clear and effective regulation remains in place." Blair identified with the latter position, underscoring the potential of research to advance biomedicine. He showed little patience for opponents, even suggesting that critics of the government's approach were arrayed against science itself. "My reason for addressing you today," he declared, "is to place firmly on record my support for science and my determination not to let us slip into any form of anti-science."[47]

In introducing the legislation in the Commons debate, Undersecretary of Health Yvette Cooper placed the ethic of healing front and center. Citing numbers of those affected by degenerative disease, she wondered aloud "how many people's lives could be transformed" by embryonic stem cell research.[48] All the government was asking, she insisted, was an adjustment to the current regime to allow for such research. Other ethical questions, such as the moral status of the embryo, had been "fully aired in the House during the passage of the Human Fertilisation and Embryology Act." In the same vein, Labour spokesman Gareth Thomas posed the question: "Why should we not widen the rules" beyond IVF related research "to include promotion of advances in the understanding of other human diseases?"[49]

On the other side of the issue, members of Parliament aligned with the pro-life movement reiterated established arguments about the moral status of the embryo. Edward Leigh, for example, countered the government case, insisting that embryos, "those tiny creatures," have "rights that we must respect."[50] Just as common were two other arguments—that therapeutic cloning might lead to reproductive cloning, and that adult stem cell research provided an ethical alternative to work involving embryos. The chairman of the All-Party Parliamentary Pro-Life Group, Mary Winterton, maintained that cloning violated the "special status of the embryo" that even the 1984 Warnock committee had recognized.[51] Opposition to embryonic stem cell research was

47. Prime Minister's Office, "Speech by the UK Prime Minister, Mr. Tony Blair, at the European Bioscience Conference," January 17, 2000, http://www.monsanto.co.uk/news/ukshowlib.phtml?uid=4104.

48. UK, *Parliamentary Debates,* Commons, 6th ser., vol. 356 (November 17, 2000), col. 1179.

49. Ibid., col. 1198.

50. UK, *Parliamentary Debates,* Commons, 6th ser., vol. 357 (December 15, 2000), col. 886.

51. UK, *Parliamentary Debates,* Commons, 6th ser., vol. 356 (November 17, 2000), col. 1203.

a harder sell, given that embryo research directed toward infertility was already allowed. Member of Parliament Paul Hammond, for example, an opponent of the new legislation, nevertheless acknowledged that "it might strike some people as odd that under the terms of the current legislation it is possible to use human embryos to conduct research into contraception, but it is not possible to use them for research into degenerative diseases."[52]

Support for an extension of the purposes of the HFE Act to allow for stem cell research generated a large majority in the Commons, 366 to 174, in early December 2000. As the debate moved to the House of Lords, however, skepticism persisted, particularly with respect to therapeutic cloning. In January 2001, a group of eleven influential religious leaders, including the Archbishop of Canterbury, the two most senior Roman Catholic archbishops, an Orthodox archbishop, Protestant officials, and leaders of the Muslim, Sikh, and Jewish communities, wrote Blair a public letter of protest, warning of the possible negative consequences of the legislation for future generations. While the different signatories had diverse views on the moral status of the embryo and when it might be destroyed in research, they agreed that "these complex questions deserve to be examined in far greater detail than a brief parliamentary debate on an unamendable order would permit."[53] Blair declined to meet with the group, citing "existing diary commitments." He underscored that his government had "listened very carefully to representations made on the recommendations of the Donaldson Report and the regulations."[54]

The House of Lords took up and passed the legislation that same month, by a strong vote of 212 to 92. However, its members expressed concern with the pace of the government's approach and made final approval of the legislation conditional on a report by a Lords Select Committee on Stem Cell Research, set up in March 2001. The choice of the bishop of Oxford, Richard Harries, as chairman left little doubt as to the outcome; he was the most vocal supporter of the legislation in the Church of England. But the new body, which included distinguished scientists, ethicists, and political and cultural leaders, gave the ethical issues more serious treatment than had the Donaldson report, and effectively extended the policy debate for a full year.[55]

---

52. Ibid., col. 1184.

53. Quoted in "Ministers in Move to Avoid Defeat on Embryo Research," *Financial Times,* January 22, 2001.

54. UK, *Parliamentary Debates. Written Answers,* 6th ser., vol. 621 (February 1, 2001), col. 281W.

55. Harries was also chair of the HFEA Ethics and Law Advisory Group at the time.

The Select Committee's February 2002 report did not oppose the government's legislation, but it did address the complexity and difficulty of weighing the moral status of the embryo against the promise of biomedical research. "Even if it has not been demonstrated that the early embryo is a person," it noted, "equally it has not been demonstrated that it is *not* a person." It followed that "if there were no morally serious reasons for undertaking research on human embryos, then the mere possibility that the early embryo is a person would be sufficient reason not to do such research." At the same time, however, "if there are morally weighty reasons for doing such research a decision must be reached on the basis of arguments that fall short of proof." Noting the existence of such reasons—the suffering of people with degenerative diseases—the committee backed not just stem cell research but therapeutic cloning and the creation of embryos for research, where there is "a demonstrable and exceptional need which cannot be met by the use of surplus embryos."[56]

On the publication of the report in February 2002 and approval by the Lords, the 2001 legislation finally passed into law. Over the next several years, Blair touted the adaptation of the policy regime as an exemplary step that would improve the United Kingdom's international scientific and economic competitiveness. As he portrayed it in a May 2002 address, the process that began with the Donaldson report had led to a "lengthy discussion which gave time for all groups, including the medical charities, to make their views known, and this led to a very balanced debate in parliament, resulting in carefully framed legislation." The result, he insisted, was "an intelligent, stable regulatory regime for this crucial field."[57] While Blair alluded to "lengthy discussion," he showed little interest in the ethical complexities. In an address before the Department of Technology and Innovation in November 2004, he acknowledged ongoing controversy in passing but insisted bluntly: "We will not stop this research." Stem cell research was "just one example of a new area of science which has tremendous potential to improve quality of life and where the United Kingdom can lead the world."[58]

With the passage of the legislation and the green light from the Lords, the HFEA and the MRC stepped up their investments in embryonic stem cell research, most notably with the inauguration of a Stem Cell Bank in 2004.

---

56. UK, House of Lords, "Stem Cell Research," Sessional Papers, 2001–2, Stem Cell Research Committee, February 27, 2002, vol. 1, http://www.publications.parliament.uk/pa/ld/ldstem.htm.

57. "Full Text of Tony Blair's Speech on British Science," *Times* (London), May 23, 2002.

58. "UK Aims to Lead the Scientific World," *Times Higher Education Supplement*, November 18, 2004.

Embryo politics grew less salient. When the HFEA approved the first human cloning experiments in August 2004, the outcry was largely limited to the SPUC and other pro-life organizations. An indicator of the lack of contestation was far-reaching Conservative Party support for Blair's policy. At a 2004 party conference, Conservative leader Michael Howard acknowledged the concerns of those "fearful of meddling with what they see as the stuff of souls." But he also saw "a duty to offer hope to the millions of people who suffer devastating illnesses like Parkinson's, multiple sclerosis, motor neuron disease, Alzheimer's—and as we saw in the newspapers, possibly heart problems." He concluded, echoing Blair and Sainsbury, that "politicians must create the right framework so that the great potential of science can be harnessed for the benefit of mankind."[59]

Predictably, the SPUC attacked Howard, insisting that "promoting the killing of embryos won't help him win elections."[60] But the lack of any considerable political backlash illustrated the weakness of pro-life forces in the United Kingdom compared with the United States. Parliamentary undersecretary of state Lord Warner may have only been exaggerating slightly when he claimed in May 2004 that the United Kingdom had "achieved a national consensus" and had a "strong and effective regulatory regime in place."[61]

The Politics of Animal-Human Hybrid Embryos

When controversy again flared up during the second half of the decade, it centered not on the legality of stem cell and cloning research—still burning issues in the United States, Germany, and France—but on a new research frontier: animal-human hybrid embryos. Conceived as a way around the shortage of human eggs for therapeutic cloning experiments, the technology typically involved the insertion of human DNA into an enucleated cow or rabbit egg, its subsequent division and growth, and the isolation of stem cells. The August 2000 Donaldson report had explicitly opposed "the mixing of human adult (somatic) cells with the live eggs of any animal species," and the government had not backed the idea in the 2000–02 legislative battle. As the

---

59. "Launch of UK Stem Cell Bank," press release, May 19, 2004, http://collections.europ archive.org/tna/20060802142310/dh.gov.uk/en/News/Speeches/Speecheslist/DH_4084091; "Michael Howard Backs Stem Cell Research," *Times,* November 9, 2004.

60. "An Anti-Abortion Group Has Denounced Michael Howard," *Times* (London), November 13, 2004.

61. UK, Department of Health, "Speech by Lord Warner, Parliamentary Under-Secretary of State in the Lords," 19 May 2004.

egg shortage persisted, however, some researchers clamored for permission to work with hybrids.

The issue was raised during two extensive public consultations relating to the future of the HFEA and human reproduction, one led by the House of Commons Science and Technology Committee in 2003–4 and another by the Department of Health in 2005–6. The House committee gave its conditional backing to stem cell research with hybrids in 2006. But a December 2006 Department of Health white paper remained skeptical, noting "considerable public unease with the possible creation of embryos combining human and animal material, and particularly to the prospect that such entities could be brought to term." The paper proposed "that the creation of hybrid and chimera embryos in vitro, should not be allowed" but might be enabled at a future date.[62] In justifying the restrictive conclusion, Health Minister Caroline Flint reiterated her overall support for embryo research but cautioned that "we are also minded by the moral compass of how those technologies are used." She called hybrids "a good example of where developments have moved on but we are not in a place where we can say 'yes we can do this now.'"[63]

Flint's negative stance sparked an immediate uproar among researchers and their supporters. In January 2007 the London *Times* published a public letter from leading scientists, including several Nobel Prize winners, denouncing the white paper. Blair himself distanced himself from its recommendations, and from Flint. He admitted to the existence of "difficult" issues surrounding the creation of embryos that are mostly human but have a small animal component." But he added: "I'm sure that research that's really going to save lives and improve the quality of life will be able to go forward."[64] In April, leading patient-advocacy organizations, including the Association of Medical Research Charities, the Genetic Interest Group, and the Parkinson's Disease Society sent Blair an open letter urging him to support research with animal-human hybrids.[65] The House Science and Technology Committee quickly set up an additional inquiry that concluded in May that the government proposals

62. UK, Department of Health, *Review of the Human Fertilisation and Embryology Act* (London: Her Majesty's Stationery Office, 2006), 25.

63. Quoted in "Why are Ministers Opposed to Hybrids?" *BBC News,* January 5, 2007.

64. Quoted in "Blair Relents on Labour's Embryo Research Attitude," *Birmingham Post,* January 6, 2007. See also "Nobel Scientists Urge Fertility Watchdog to Back Hybrid Embryos," *Times* (London), January 10, 2007.

65. Association of Medical Research Charities and Genetic Interest Group, "Letter to the Prime Minister about the Creation of Hybrid Embryos for Research," April 5, 2007, http://www.amrc.org.uk/tabs_news-2007_letter-to-the-prime-minister-about-the-creation-of-hybrid-embryos-for-research.

were "unnecessarily prohibitive" and recommended "opening the door to research using human-animal chimera or hybrid embryos."[66]

The government's draft legislation, published in May 2007 by the Department of Health, ultimately came down in favor of the controversial research. The Human Tissue and Embryos (Draft) Bill covered a range of topics, including an expansion of preimplantation genetic diagnosis. Most significantly in political terms, it now deemed hybrid research "necessary"—in contrast to the white paper of just six months earlier. Gordon Brown, who replaced Tony Blair in June as prime minister and was also known for his proresearch views, backed the bill. In September 1997 the HFEA announced its strong support for hybrid experimentation. The queen's speech of November 2007, which is traditionally drafted by the prime minister, mentioned the rationale for the new legislation: "A Bill will be brought forward to reform the regulation of human embryology and to ensure that Britain remains at the forefront of medical research." As under Blair's leadership, the themes of technological competitiveness and an ethic of healing dominated government thinking. Brown steered clear of the question of the moral status of hybrid embryos.[67]

As they had at earlier junctures, the Catholic Church and the pro-life movement led criticism of the proposed legislation. The Vatican denounced hybrid research as a "monstrous act against human dignity."[68] While internally divided on the issue, the Anglican Church lent some official support to the legislation. A report of the Mission and Public Affairs Council, the successor to the Church's Board for Social Responsibility, reiterated the view that embryos should not be deliberately created for research but insisted that therapeutic cloning, with or without the creation of a hybrid, was something else: the creation of embryos to save lives. The derived cells "might be used therapeutically to help a sufferer from a disease like Alzheimer's or Parkinson's." While supportive of hybrid research, the Mission acknowledged sensitivities around the issue and urged caution. "The most stringent restrictions should be in force to prevent such a hybrid being brought to birth."[69]

---

66. UK, House of Commons, Science and Technology Committee, *Government Proposals for the Regulation of Hybrid and Chimera Embryos* (London: Her Majesty's Stationery Office, 2007), 48.

67. On the HFEA's position, see Andy Coghlan, "Are Human-Animal 'Cybrids' Really Possible?" *New Scientist* 195, no. 2621 (2007): 15; "Queen's Speech 2007 in Full," *BBC News,* November 6, 2007.

68. "Vatican attacks human hybrids as 'monstrous act against human dignity,'" *Daily Mail,* September 7, 2007.

69. Church of England Mission and Public Affairs Council, "Response from the Church of England Mission and Public Affairs Council to the Call for Evidence from the Joint Committee on the Draft Human Tissue and Embryos Bill," June 2007, http://www.cofe.anglican.org/info/socialpublic/science/hfea/humantissue.pdf.

Like Blair in the legislative battles of 2000–2002, Brown aligned himself closely with proresearch forces intent on broadening the range of permissible experiments under the HFE Act. In early 2008, after the legislation had passed the Lords and before it went before the House of Commons, Brown apparently considered going further than Blair had in imposing party discipline on the vote—an effort he eventually abandoned, in part so as not to alienate the Catholic ministers in his government.[70] In a newspaper article in May 2008 on the eve of the Commons debate, Brown cast the legislation as a "moral endeavour" for a worthy end. "If we want to sustain stem cell research and bring new cures and treatments to millions of people," he asserted, "I believe admixed embryos are necessary." The new Conservative leader, David Cameron, adhered to the same line. Seeking the mantle of modernizer, he too portrayed the legislation as a pragmatic adaptation of a proven institutional framework, insisting that "the law needs updating."[71] The high degree of consensus diverged sharply from the polarized embryo politics in the United States.

In the decisive Commons debate, Secretary of State for Health Alan Johnson claimed that the need for research with hybrid embryos was "recognised by scientists across the world as an essential building block for establishing cures for many life-threatening diseases, such as multiple sclerosis, Parkinson's and Alzheimer's."[72] As they had in 2000–02, research supporters invoked the institutional status quo of the HFEA. They insisted that the political battle over embryo research had been settled in 1990 and that cloning and stem cell research had been given the green light in 2002. To support hybrid research, in this view, only meant adjusting the current research regime and increasing its effectiveness. Kenneth Clarke, who had helped to shepherd the HFE Act through Parliament almost two decades earlier, lauded it as "that rather successful and groundbreaking piece of legislation." He insisted that "the judgment of 14 days or the emergence of the primitive streak has held up well for the past 18 years and we should stick to it." Clarke did address the Catholic Church's official stance on treating the embryo as a person from conception, if only to dismiss it. "I respect the Roman Catholic view," he told his colleagues, "but I do not believe that every Roman Catholic shares it. The House needs to establish a consensus."[73]

---

70. "Brown Softens Stance on Cloning to Head Off MPs' Revolt," *Independent,* March 24, 2008.

71. "Brown Urges Embryo Bill Support," *BBC News,* May 18, 2008; "MPs Vote for Human-Animal Hybrid Embryos," *Telegraph,* May 19, 2008.

72. UK, *Parliamentary Debates,* 6th ser., vol. 475 (May 12, 2008), cols. 1067–68.

73. Ibid., col. 1094.

Edward Leigh spoke for antiresearch forces, as he had in the 2000 Commons debates. At issue, he insisted, was less the moral status of the embryo than the fundamental question of human dignity. Where the legislation's supporters saw the pragmatic extension of an existing regulatory framework, he saw a sharp departure. "We do not have to be Christians to believe that we are all created in God's image," he told his colleagues. "We can surely accept that embryos contain the genetic make-up of a complete human being and that we cannot and should not be spliced together with the animal kingdom."[74] Ultimately, the effort to ground opposition to the bill in a sense of anxiety or repugnance, overlaid by religious sensitivities, failed. Brown did lose some support within his own Labour Party. For example, Transport Secretary Ruth Kelly, a Catholic, resigned in protest over the bill and was among sixteen Labour MPs who voted against it. Nonetheless, a strong majority, encompassing most Conservative members, backed the legislation, which passed by a vote of 336–176 in its final reading May 2008. Among the supporters was David Cameron, who would succeed Brown as Prime Minister in May 2010.

The outcome of the U.K. cloning and stem cell controversies points to the enduring institutional force of the 1990 policy settlement. By creating a durable framework that allowed embryo research under certain conditions, the HFE Act framed political responses to new technological developments. Extending the institutional framework aligned with the priorities of both Tony Blair and Gordon Brown, proresearch prime ministers whose Labour Party controlled the legislative agenda. Arguments about an ethic of healing, first developed in the United Kingdom in the late 1980s in support of the first push to legalize embryo research, drove further legislative innovation forward two decades later. Once the destruction of embryos in research under carefully limited circumstances became part of the institutional status quo, it was more difficult to argue against the extension of that research beyond infertility to degenerative diseases. Research supporters successfully cast work with animal-human embryos not as a risky new departure but as a practical necessity, given the lack of embryos for cloning experiments.

Germany: The Struggle over Stem Cell Imports

Embryo politics in Germany over the same period was very different. While the United Kingdom maintained and extended its liberal embryo research

---

74. UK, *Parliamentary Debates,* 6th ser., vol. 476 (May 19, 2008), col. 28.

regime, Germany adapted its much more restrictive legal framework. Just one month after reunification in December 1990, the Bundestag had passed the Embryo Protection Law, which included a comprehensive and criminal ban on the creation or destruction of embryos for research. Historical anxieties about eugenics and consensus around the principle of human dignity enshrined in the Basic Law had generated broad support for the EPL from Christian Democrats on the right to secular Social Democrats and Greens on the left. The stem cell and cloning breakthroughs at the end of the decade did not spark a political challenge to that regime. The EPL clearly ruled out the derivation of stem cells from embryos in Germany, as well as cloning experiments, which legislators had explicitly prohibited in 1990. Scientists, patient-advocacy organizations, and legislators could have called for the revision of the EPL in the decade after 1997–98, and some isolated voices did. But the political struggle ended up centered on a much narrower issue—the permissibility of importing embryonic stem cells that had been derived abroad.

Not surprisingly, the Dolly announcement of February 1997 did not spark a therapeutic cloning controversy in Germany parallel to the one in the United States and the United Kingdom. A broad revulsion against the idea of any cloning was reinforced by the Nazi legacy. The daily *Die Welt* remarked that "human cloning would fit perfectly into Adolf Hitler's world view" and thanked God the technology had not been available at the time. The respectable newsweekly *Die Zeit* asked how long it would be until "a new Einstein, Lollobrigida, or even Hitler populates the brave new world?" Among the first German politicians to pick up the issue was science minister Jürgen Rüttgers. He used the opportunity of a March 1997 audience with Pope John Paul II at the Vatican to underscore that Germany had been "the first country to put into place a legal prohibition against cloning"—a core provision of the 1990 Embryo Protection Law. He emphasized that he and the pope agreed on the importance of a worldwide prohibition based on the German model.[75]

Rüttgers sounded the same themes in a first Bundestag debate on the issue that same month, professing shock at U.S. discussions about the ethics of reproductive cloning, which reminded him of "Nazi barbarism," and amazement at the "casual tone" of the British debate.[76] The sentiment was widely shared across the parties. Herta Däubler-Gmelin, a leading Social Democrat, went so far as to suggest that a cloning ban might be incorporated

---

75. "Bonn und Vatikan Gegen das Klonen vom Menschen," *Welt am Sonntag,* March 9, 1997.

76. Bundestag, *Verhandlungen des deutschen Bundestages, Stenographischer Bericht,* ser. 13 (March 21, 1987), 15129.

into the German constitution.[77] The distinction between reproductive and therapeutic cloning that characterized the U.S. and British debates early on played almost no role in the discussion—in part because both were clearly illegal under German law. The closest mention was by Maria Steindor, an SPD deputy, who asked, "What happens when cloned embryos come into discussion as spare organ parts inventories, not in the form of living human beings but in the form of a certain kind of individually reprogrammed cell culture that can be cultivated into organs or organlike matter?" None of her colleagues took up this awkwardly phrased scenario, and Steindor herself condemned it. At the close of the debate the Bundestag unanimously passed an unambiguous and comprehensive anticloning declaration.[78]

In contrast to the United States and the United Kingdom, even the scientific leadership was part of this chorus. In a February 1997 article in the *Frankfurter Allgemeine Zeitung,* head of the German Research Foundation (DFG) Ernst-Ludwig Winnacker praised the EPL, suggesting that that "in retrospect it appears a blessing to have put in place legal foundations for the protection of embryo and egg cells long before these developments." He recalled that "research freedom is certainly one of the rights protected in the constitution," but added that "it was and is never absolute." Winnacker cited the principle pioneered by bioethicist Hans Jonas—that technological advances should be occasions to think through and prevent their potential negative future consequences. Unlike the head of the U.S. National Institutes of Health, Harold Varmus, Winnacker made no mention of a possible link between cloning and stem cell research. Neither did leading patient-advocacy organizations or the German Medical Association, which, unlike its U.S. and U.K. counterparts, labeled all cloning "incompatible with the ethical principle of human dignity and the protection of embryos that follows from it."[79]

Chancellor Helmut Kohl's first major public statement on the cloning issue came in October 1997, several months after the science ministry's Council on Research, Technology, and Innovation issued its own blanket condemnation of cloning, as recounted in chapter 3. In a speech in Strasbourg he explained why Germany could not sign on to a European Bioethics Convention that did not include prohibitions on embryo and cloning research. "Looking back to a dark page of our history where barbarity ruled during the Nazi period,

---

77. Ibid., 15124.

78. Ibid., 15126. For the declaration, see Bundestag, *Verbot des Klonens von Menschen,* Drucksache 13/7243 (Berlin: Deutscher Bundestag, 1997).

79. "Wir wollen keine Menschen klonen," *Frankfurter Allgemeine Zeitung,* February 28, 1997; "Beschlussprotokoll des 100. Deutschen Ärztetages," May 27–30, 1997, http://www.bundesaerztekammer.de/downloads/beschlussprotokoll_100_daet_eisenach_1997.pdf.

Germans take this issue very seriously," he said. "Scientific research, human rights, and basic ethical standards are inseparable." For Germans, he argued, "this is a particular responsibility against the background of the Nazi regime's barbaric deeds."[80] Kohl's suggestion that all Germans shared his historically informed anxieties was an exaggeration. His main political rival at this point, the technology-friendly governor of Lower Saxony, Gerhard Schröder (SPD), styled himself as a pragmatic innovator in the Clinton and Blair mold. Still, in the election campaign that culminated in an SPD-Green victory in October 1998, Schröder did not openly question the Embryo Protection Law or raise the possibility of revisiting it in the near future.

The coincidence of Schröder's electoral victory and the Wisconsin stem cell breakthrough in November 1998 gradually opened the German debate. The German media, like its counterparts elsewhere, waxed enthusiastic about the prospect of a new frontier of regenerative medicine. But how should Germany approach embryonic stem cells as a policy issue, given that any destruction of embryos for research was a criminal offense? The situation was somewhat analogous to the United States, with its federal ban on destructive embryo research. As in the United States, a restrictive policy regime ruled out the derivation of stem cells but not necessarily research with stem cells produced elsewhere—in the U.S. case, mainly in the private sector, and in the German case, abroad. Some German researchers began to plead openly for such a research trajectory. The head of the German Cell and Tissue Society, for example, expressed the hope in December 1998 that "scientists in Germany, too, could work with human embryonic stem cells in pursuit of the goal of tissue and organ replacement."[81]

The DFG, the publicly funded source of most of the country's basic research support for the life sciences, was initially more cautious. In August 1998 Winnacker had lamented that German discussions "in the area of so-called bioethics are often marked by anxiety and irrationality." In January 1999, he responded to consideration of therapeutic cloning in the United Kingdom by underscoring that "the DFG still stands behind the Embryo Protection Law."[82] This caution extended to the question of research with stem cells derived outside the country's borders. In March 1999 a DFG commission

---

80. Quoted in "Kohl Mahnt den Westen zur Hilfe für Osteuropa," *Süddeutsche Zeitung,* October 11, 1997.

81. Quoted in "Medizinisches Klonen bietet Chance," *Focus,* December 14, 1998.

82. "Risiken der Wissenschaft," *Die Tageszeitung,* August 22, 1998; Deutsche Forschungsgemeinschaft (DFG), "Statement des DFG-Präsidenten, Professor Ernst-Ludwig Winnacker, zum Klonen menschlicher Embryozellen," press release, January 1999, http://www.dfg.de/download/pdf/dfg_im_profil/reden_stellungnahmen/archiv_download/emb_klon_stat_99.pdf.

recommended that, given "legal and ethical concerns," there was no need to support such experiments "at this time." In part because Germany was already among the leaders in morally unproblematic adult stem cell research, the DFG adopted a wait-and-see attitude. It set up a major research program on "stem cells" in May 1999, without specifying whether embryonic stem cells might someday be part of it. With the exception of the uproar caused by the philosopher Peter Sloterdijk's July 1999 lecture, "Rules for the Human Zoo," which had sketched a future of genetic selection and enhancement, there was little public engagement with the ethics of new life science technologies.

By early 2000 the DFG had begun to reconsider its skeptical approach to embryonic stem cell research. In March 2000, two months after the NIH published its draft guidelines for stem cell research proposals in the United States, Winnacker sent up a trial balloon in an article in the country's leading daily, the *Frankfurter Allgemeine Zeitung*. After an overview of embryonic stem cell research abroad, he mentioned that "German scientists are asking themselves whether, if they cannot produce these cells, they can simply import them from abroad." He viewed the legal issue as open, "as it has not been clarified whether such a path would represent a violation of the Embryo Protection Law." In opposition to scientists who wanted an immediate green light, he argued that a Bundestag clarification of the situation was "a precondition for the use of human embryonic stem cells."[83] A further critical juncture was an August 2000 application by neuroscientist Oliver Brüstle for DFG for funds to support research with stem cells derived abroad. Noting the publication of the Donaldson report in the United Kingdom that month, Brüstle insisted publicly that such imports were critical if Germany was not to be left behind in stem cell science.[84]

These changes of attitude in the German scientific community, and the advance of research abroad, led Schröder to stake out a more public position for change. In a November 2000 Bundestag debate he noted policy changes in the United States and the United Kingdom and called for parliamentary consideration of the stem cell issue in its economic, emotional, and ethical dimensions.[85] The following month he wrote a much-quoted article suggesting that Germany should break with its reticent approach to cutting-edge

83. "Stammzellen—Verheißung für die Biomedizin: Therapeutische Visionen und ethisch-rechtliche Grenzlinien," *Frankfurter Allgemeine Zeitung*, March 29, 2000.

84. "Gute Nacht, Deutschland?" *Frankfurter Allgemeine Zeitung*, August 18, 2008; "Auf Forschungszug aufspringen," *Focus*, August 21, 2000.

85. Bundestag, *Verhandlungen des deutschen Bundestages*, ser. 14 (November 29, 2000), 13219.

science. "A policy of ideological blinders and principled bans would not only be unrealistic," he argued, "it would also be irresponsible" in light of the biomedical potential of stem cell research. While he acknowledged the EPL as a legal foundation and did not call openly for its revision, he suggested that "regulations about reproductive medicine should continually be evaluated as to their scientific and ethical suitability." In an interview with *Stern* in January 2001, when reminded that his "friend" Blair had backed therapeutic cloning, Schröder lamented the alliance in Germany between "hostility to progress" on the left and "conservative fundamentalism" on the right.[86]

An interview with the *Frankfurter Allgemeine* in early May 2001 marked Schröder's fullest exposition yet of the need for a new departure. While he argued that the EPL was a proven framework that should remain for the time being, he questioned whether the German constitution offered the embryo absolute protection. While it was a bearer of human dignity, that dignity was not absolute—or else the Constitutional Court would not have tolerated Germany's abortion regime. What Germany needed, Schröder argued, was a more wide-ranging debate, less overshadowed by the demons of the past. He disputed that "we as Germans must approach these issues much more cautiously" because of the negative legacy of Nazi scientists and doctors, an unsettling argument because it "questioned the quality of our social order" decades after Hitler. If Germans could not trust themselves not to repeat a terrible past with its eugenic abuses, he argued, German democracy was in terrible shape indeed.[87]

Schröder's effort to test the readiness for change provoked sharp criticism from within his party, the Christian Democrats, and Greens—and some support from the more research-friendly Free Democratic Party. The issue might have died had the DFG leadership not completed the turn in its thinking. In a major May 2001 policy statement precipitated in part by Brüstle's application for funding, the DFG acknowledged that "work with human embryonic stem cells is becoming more interesting." It laid out several possible steps, beginning with the import of stem cells derived abroad. Should the eventual supply from abroad prove insufficient, the statement continued, Germany should adapt the EPL to allow the derivation of stem cells from surplus embryos within the country, numbered at "about a hundred." The creation of embryos for research should remain forbidden, the DFG insisted, and therapeutic cloning was rejected "for various scientific and ethical reasons." The

---

86. "Was Tun—Herr Schröder?" *Stern,* January 11, 2001.
87. "Die Notwendigkeit der Abwägung stellt sich immer wieder neu," *Frankfurter Allgemeine Zeitung,* May 3, 2001.

German regulatory regime should remain strong so that the "door to embryo research opened up by the introduction of artificial reproduction not
become a slippery slope." While the DFG continued to insist that adult stem
cells "be given preference" over embryonic stem cells, this was a major new
departure.[88]

The DFG statement sparked a year-long political struggle over stem cell
imports. Research minister Edelgard Bulmahn, a close ally of Schröder's, suggested that the proposed "far-reaching changes" be discussed widely, and
requested that the DFG suspend its consideration of Brüstle's application
pending legislative action.[89] That wider discussion began immediately. The
Bundestag's Investigative Commission on Law and Ethics in Modern Medicine took up the issue during spring 2001, as did a new German ethics
council created by Schröder with the express goal of broadening the German
debate. The deliberations of both bodies were recounted in chapter 3.

Research opponents found a powerful ally in German president Johannes
Rau. While his office was largely ceremonial, Rau—a Social Democrat like
Schröder—could use it as a platform to weigh in on critical issues of the day.
Two weeks after Schröder's interview and the DFG statement, Rau gave a
highly publicized speech in Berlin entitled: "Will Everything Turn Out for
the Best?" In a thinly veiled attack on Schröder's pragmatic focus on innovation without "ideological blinders," Rau called for the careful ethical
interrogation of new life science discoveries and their applications. He acknowledged that "diseases that were understood to be invincible now might
be healed" but insisted that "the lofty goals of scientific research should not
determine the point at which human life should be protected." Rau praised
the German commitment to embryo protection, insisting that "taboos are
not a relic of premodern societies" and that "you do not have to be a Christian" to see a tension between scientific possibilities and the constitutional
norm of the "inviolability of human dignity." The German historic experience carried a universal message, he insisted. The Holocaust and Nazi eugenics were a living warning that "nothing should be placed above the dignity
of an individual human being."[90]

---

88. DFG, "Empfehlungen der Deutschen Forschungsgemeinschaft zur Forschung mit menschlichen Stammzellen," press release, May 3, 2001, http://www.dfg.de/aktuell/stellungnahmen/
dokumentation_1.html.

89. Alison Abbott, "Stem Cell Research in Doubt as Funders Clash with Government," *Nature*
411, no. 6834 (2001): 119–20.

90. Bundespräsidialamt, "Wird Alles Gut?—Für Einen Fortschritt Nach Menschlichem Maß," press
release, May 18, 2001, http://www.bundespraesident.de/Reden-und-Interviews/Reden-Johannes-Rau-
,11070.41073/Wird-alles-gut-Fuer-einen-Fort.htm?global.back=.

A Bundestag debate at the end of May gave Schröder a chance to respond—
and the parties an opportunity to join in the fray. "I think the ethic of healing
and helping deserves as much respect as respect for creation," Schröder told
his colleagues. He also defended himself against Rau's charge of an exces-
sive emphasis on innovation and competitiveness—what Rau had termed
"pure economism"—and insisted leaders should acknowledge the economic
consequences of policy choices, even in ethically sensitive areas. Perhaps sens-
ing his position was in the minority, Schröder did not propose anything
more sweeping than stem cell imports; the EPL should not be changed "too
quickly."[91] Angela Merkel, who had emerged as Kohl's successor atop the
Christian Democratic Union (CDU), took an antiresearch line. She began
her address: "Human life begins with the mixing of egg and sperm," a statement she "grounded in Christian responsibility before God." Like most of
the speakers—CDU as well as SPD and Green—she opposed stem cell imports as "incompatible with the spirit of the EPL."[92] Representatives of the
Free Democrats, who had officially backed legal changes to "allow for stem
cell research" early in the month, were among the small minority backing
not only imports but a loosening of the strictures of the Embryo Protection
Law itself.[93]

By summer the debate had narrowed to the question of whether Germany
should pass a stem cell law, alongside the EPL, to either permit or prohibit the
import of stem cells derived abroad. There was nothing like the proresearch
mobilization that took place in the United States and the United Kingdom.
Having staked out a position, the DFG opted to leave matters to elected
leaders and was cautious and diplomatic in its statements. (Hubert Markl of
the Max Planck Society was the country's only prominent scientific leader
openly to advocate not only stem cell imports but a revision of the EPL
and a regime along British lines.)[94] Medical and patient-advocacy groups,
too, generally adopted cautious stances. The German Medical Association
made adult stem cell research its top priority.[95] The Multiple Sclerosis Society, among the most influential patient-advocacy groups, did cautiously call

91. Bundestag, *Verhandlungen des deutschen Bundestags,* ser. 14 (May 31, 2001), 16893.

92. Ibid., 16901–2.

93. This was also the context of Nida-Rümelin's intervention. "Dr. Julian Nida-Rümelin zur
Bio-Ethik:'Wo die Menschenwürde beginnt,'" *Tagesspiegel,* January 3, 2001.

94. Hubert Markl, "Freiheit, Verantwortung, Menschenwürde: Warum Lebenswissenschaften
mehr sind as Biologie," June 22, 2001, http://www.mpg.de/pdf/jahrbuch_2001/jahrbuch2001_
009_024.pdf.

95. Bundesärztekammer, "Beschlussprotokoll des 104. Deutschen Ärztetages vom 22–25. Mai
2001 in Ludwigshafen: Forschung mit humanen embryonalen Stammzellen," May 2001, http://
www.bundesaerztekammer.de/page.asp?his=0.2.23.2618.2619.2626

for "as much freedom of research as necessary." But it, too, stopped short of pushing for any revision of the EPL, not to mention any advocacy of therapeutic cloning.[96] Perhaps the sharpest contrast with the United Kingdom and the United States was the biotechnology industry, whose peak association in Germany did not even stake out a public position. The fact that these groups had no close ties to embryonic stem cell researchers—a nonexistent group in Germany—contributed to their caution, as did public opinion polls that still showed widespread opposition to destructive embryo research.[97]

A further, basic difference with policy struggles in other countries was the prominence of constitutional constraints. The German Supreme Court had agreed, in its abortion rulings of 1975 and 1993, that unborn human life fell under the constitutional protection of human dignity. However, it had not been specific about whether that protection began with fertilization or later, with implantation. Legal experts aligned with research opponents claimed that dignity extended back to fertilization and that any relaxation of the EPL would therefore be unconstitutional. They pointed in particular to part of the 1993 ruling that stated that "irrespective of how the different phases of prenatal development can be assessed from the biological, philosophical, even theological standpoint and irrespective of how they have been judged historically, in any case what is involved are the indispensable stages of development of individual human life." The court's conclusion: "Wherever human life exists, it should be accorded human dignity."[98] Research supporters countered that the court's language did not rule out the possibility that an individual human life actually begins with implantation. In their perspective, research with early embryos under carefully controlled conditions was constitutional. These legal debates spilled over into the political fray in 2001, when two prominent figures, a member of the Constitutional Court, Jutta Limbach, and a former federal president and jurist, Roman Herzog, publicly opposed the view that any destructive embryo research would necessarily be deemed unconstitutional.[99]

---

96. Deutscher Multiple Sklerose Gesellschaft, "Zur Bedeutung der Stammzellen: Forschung für die Therapie der Multiplen Sklerose," press release, July 2001.

97. Interview with Gerhard Schröder, "Die Notwendigkeit der Abwägung stellt sich immer wieder neu," *Frankfurter Allgemeine Zeitung,* May 3, 2001; Verband Forschender Arzneimittelhersteller, "Forschung mit humanen Stammzellen," press release, April 30, 2001; Bundesverband der Pharmazeutischen Industrie, "Embryonenforschung erst nach Experimenten an Säugetieren und adulten Stammzellen," press release, January 24, 2002.

98. *Bundesverfassungsgericht,* 2 BvF 2/90, May 28, 1993, http://www.bverfg.de/entscheidungen/fs19930528_2bvf000290en.html

99. Jutta Limbach, "Medizin und Gewissen," *Die Zeit,* May 24, 2001. Former Supreme Court justice and former federal president Roman Herzog argued that "the right of those with heritable

To some extent the legal debate was academic; a liberalization of the EPL itself was not on the table. But the more limited issue of stem cell imports also roused emotions on both sides. As in the United States, where a simultaneous debate was raging, the issue was whether the use of stem cells derived from embryos involved moral complicity in their destruction. In his August 2001 decision, George W. Bush approved federal funding for research with stem cells derived before that cutoff date in order to reduce the incentives for any future embryo destruction. Around the same time, as the Bundestag debates approached, the idea of allowing the import of cells derived before a certain cutoff emerged as a possibility. In its November 2001 report, the Bundestag's Investigative Commission set out the alternatives: an import ban in keeping with "the spirit" of the EPL, and an import allowance that would specify the date by which the stem cells had to be derived—referred to as "the Bush model." In the imports scenario, cells would have to be derived from surplus IVF embryos and could only be used in research for "medical findings of great value"—a phrase traceable to the 1985 Benda Commission report.[100]

The growing ranks of those opposed to research in principle but open to the possibility of imports alarmed Protestant and Catholic leaders. During the first part of the year, the Christian Democrats, at least, had seemed to be strongly anti-import. At a June 2001 meeting, for example, Evangelical Church in Germany and CDU leaders had reiterated that position.[101] In December the EKD leadership applauded the Investigative Commission's strong opposition to "destructive embryo research" and called it a "self-contradiction" to allow imports under those circumstances.[102] The German Catholic Bishops' Conference was even more outspoken. Days before the major Bundestag debate in late January 2002, it released a statement that expressed "concern" about the growth of support for imports of embryonic stem cells from abroad. Imports "involved the killing of embryonic humans, which fundamentally contradicts the Christian ethos" as well as the "spirit

diseases to be saved by further research also has the value of human life on its side." Roman Herzog, "Ich warne vor absoluten Verboten," *Die Welt,* May 28, 2001. For an overview of legal opinion prepared for the Bundestag Investigative Committee, see Wolfram Höfling, "Verfassungsrechtliche Aspekte der Verfügung über menschliche Embryonen und 'humanbiologisches Material,'" May 2001, http://www.bundestag.de/gremien/medi/medi_gut_hoe.pdf.

100. Benda Commission, *Working Group on In Vitro Fertilisation, Genom Analysis, and Gene Therapy Report* (Bonn: Federal Ministry for Research and Technology, 1985).

101. Evangelische Kirche in Deutschland, "CDU und EKD Sprachen über Bioethik und Zu-wanderungspolitik," press release, June 1, 2001, http://www.ekd.de/bioethik/5228.html.

102. Evangelische Kirche in Deutschland, "Der menschliche Embryo ist keine bloße Biomasse," press release, December 7, 2001, http://ekd.de/presse/pm124_2001_stammzellen.html.

of the Embryo Protection Law."[103] In a joint statement on the eve of the vote, Cardinal Karl Lehmann and EKD Council chair Manfred Kock, the leaders of both Churches, insisted that the EPL and the Basic Law guaranteed "unlimited protection for life from the moment of conception" and flatly rejected any embryonic stem cell imports.[104]

As the decisive January 2002 Bundestag debate approached, three main legislative proposals emerged. The largest single group of legislators, drawn from the Social Democrats, the Christian Democrats, and the Greens, rallied behind the restrictive proposals endorsed by the Investigative Commission— a ban on the import of embryonic stem cells into the Federal Republic. A much smaller group, centered on the Free Democrats, supported a revision of the EPL to allow the derivation of stem cells, and was even willing to countenance therapeutic cloning in Germany. A third compromise proposal upheld the principle of no destructive embryo research in Germany and outlawed the import of embryonic stem cells in principle, but allowed for exceptions if the cells were derived before a January 1, 2002, "cutoff date" and the research served "medical findings of great value" or progress against degenerative diseases. In contrast to the United States, the proposed cutoff-date model would bind both the public and the private sectors.[105]

Across the parties, opponents of all embryonic stem cell research drew on a combination of religious and secular arguments, with the emphasis on the latter. One Christian Democrat grounded his defense of the embryo not just in the "Christian image of the human being" but also in the "great traditions of the Enlightenment." Along the same lines, an SPD spokesman equated the derivation of stem cells with the "killing of a human being," reasoning that "we were all once an embryo." Germany, he insisted, should remain a model of principled opposition to unethical practices in science and bioethics—a role many had come to respect and admire. A Green spokesperson, in keeping

---

103. Deutsche Bischofskonferenz, "Erklärung des Vorsitzenden der Unterkommission Bioethik der Deutschen Bischofskonferenz, Bischof Dr. Gebhard Fürst, zum Votum des Nationalen Ethikrates vom 29 November 2001," press release, November 30, 2001, http://www.alt.dbk.de/aktuell/meldungen/2903/index.html.

104. Evangelische Kirche in Deutschland, "Kirchen Schreiben an Bundestagsabgeordnete," press release, January 17, 2002, http://www.ekd.de/print.php?file=/presse/pm6_2002_kirchenbrief_mdbs_menschenschutz.html. See also the Protestant Church's negative response to the DFG recommendations in May 2001, http://www.ekd.de/EKD-Texte/2086_5220.html.

105. "Schutz der Menschenwürde angesichts der biomedizinischen Möglichkeiten–Kein Import embryonaler Stammzellen," *Drucksache 14/8101* (Berlin: Deutscher Bundestag, 2002); "Keine verbrauchende Embryonenforschung: Import humaner embryonaler Stammzellen grundsätzlich verbieten und nur unter engen Voraussetzungen Zulassen," *Drucksache 14/8102* (Berlin: Deutscher Bundestag, 2002); "Verantwortungsbewusste Forschung an embryonalen Stammzellen für eine ethisch hochwertige Medizin," *Drucksache 14/8103* (Berlin: Deutscher Bundestag, 2002).

with the party's general skepticism of technology, warned of a slippery slope. If imports were allowed, a change in the EPL would naturally follow, and Germany ultimately would move into the field of "embryo production."[106]

The linchpin of the debate was whether support for imports could be squared with high levels of embryo protection. Merkel was now among the emergent Bundestag majority for whom it could be. She continued to reject all "destructive embryo research" and to insist on the "absolute priority" of work with adult stem cells. But she was now willing to support the import of already existing embryonic cells under "strict conditions." Such a compromise, she suggested, would uphold the letter of the German law while opening Germany to policy discussions and scientific projects unfolding abroad. "Because we in Germany want to be able to use these therapies," she argued, the country should not oppose the imports of cells altogether.[107] Andrea Fischer of the Greens, Schröder's health minister from 1998 to 2000, also backed stem cell imports while reiterating her absolute opposition to the deliberate destruction of embryos. "From the mixing of sperm and an egg the embryo develops as a human being," she argued. But the use of cells from embryos that had already been destroyed did not involve complicity in their destruction. Fischer also emphasized eugenic concerns. "If we begin to use human beings as means to an end, no matter how noble the end," she argued, the result might be "what Habermas calls a self-instrumentalization of the species."[108]

The third main proposal, in favor not just of imports but of revising the EPL to allow for the derivation of stem cells in Germany itself, was spearheaded by the Free Democrats. FDP leader Wolfgang Gerhardt articulated a secular perspective centered on the compatibility of research in Germany with human dignity and with the principle of freedom of research. He argued against a position "connected with religious convictions" and in favor of trust in the German scientific leadership and the DFG. In an interesting twist on the negative legacy of Nazism, he argued that without the high professional and ethical standards of the German scientific community, "the country and its research capacity would not have come back from the catastrophe of its history." Frozen embryos in Germany—what he referred to simply as "collections of cells"—should be made available for research "in order to gain

---

106. Bundestag, *Verhandlungen des deutschen Bundestags,* ser. 14 (January 30, 2002), 21193–21235.

107. Bundestag, *Verhandlungen des deutschen Bundestages,* ser. 14 (January 31, 2002), 21217, 21207. Merkel did not refer, as she had in the May 2001 debate, to "Christian responsibility" or a "Christian image of humanity" in making her case.

108. Ibid., 21203, 21204.

some knowledge and therefore help people." Schröder seems to have personally sympathized with this position but aligned himself with the limited import position, apparently for political reasons. In his own contribution to the Bundestag debate he remarked on the complexity of the emerging controversy in which "supporters and opponents of stem cell research" do not fall into the "usual categories of Right and Left" or religious affiliation.[109]

The most striking and unexpected element of this complexity was a group of prominent Protestant Christian Democrats who came out in favor of both importing cells and deriving them in Germany. Peter Hintze, a Lutheran pastor and former CDU general secretary, insisted that "as Christians we should save people, not principles." And former CDU chairman Wolfgang Schäuble, confined to a wheelchair by a would-be assassin's bullet, emphasized that the constitutional principle of the "inviolability of human dignity" also applied to the promise of research. He advocated a space of "diverse ethical and religious convictions" in which scientists should be able to conduct their research responsibly. He also warned against German dismissals of the more open debates and liberal policies in other Atlantic democracies. If other states "come to different conclusions with respect to stem cell research," he pointed out, "we should be cautious about evaluating these as violations of the inviolability of human dignity."[110]

After proponents of a complete research ban failed to amass a majority, the import compromise prevailed in a contested vote of 340 to 265. Research with imported stem cells derived from surplus IVF embryos abroad before a January 1, 2002, cutoff date was to be permitted, after careful scientific and ethical review. With final parliamentary approval in April 2002, the Central Ethics Commission for Stem Cell Research was created within the Ministry of Health to evaluate research proposals.[111] A year's worth of controversy had seen considerable movement in the political landscape; some openness to embryonic stem cell research had emerged, as had a first, cautious debate about perhaps revising the EPL in the future. Compared with the United Kingdom and the United States, however, the overall approach to embryo research remained restrictive. Religious and secular arguments for embryo protection, reinforced both by the negative legacy of Nazi eugenics and the "human dignity" norm of the Basic Law, continued to frame the debate.

---

109. Ibid., 21196.
110. Ibid., 21197.
111. Bundesministerium der Justiz, "Gesetz zur Sicherstellung des Embryonenschutzes im Zusammenhang mit Einfuhr und Verwendung menschlicher embryonaler Stammzellen," *Bundesgesetzblatt Jahrgang 2002,* no. 42, June 29, 2002, http://www.bmbf.de/pub/stammzellgesetz.pdf.

Therapeutic cloning, hotly debated elsewhere, did not make it onto the national political agenda.

Efforts to Broaden the German Debate

After the narrow reelection of his Social Democrat–Green coalition in September 2002, Schröder did encourage several efforts to further widen the debate to encompass the Embryo Protection Law itself—with no success. In September 2003 he gave a major address lamenting "limits" on biotechnology in light of international competitive pressures. A month later his SPD minster of justice, Brigitte Zypries, publicly revived the idea that the embryo might not be protected under the human dignity provisions of the Basic Law. She insisted that as long as it was in the petri dish, the embryo had only the "abstract possibility" of developing into a person and that this "was not enough for the imputation of human dignity" at a constitutional level. Zypries emphasized that she did not consider the embryo "simply a lump of cells" that scientists could manipulate at will. She drew a line at therapeutic cloning and was careful not to call openly for a repeal of the EPL. But her intervention as justice minister on a key issue broadened the German policy debate.[112]

The reaction was strongly negative. A CDU press release charged Zypries with making "*Menschen zu Material*"—human beings into things. In her own SPD, her predecessor as justice minister accused Zypries of an irresponsible new departure, and a Green parliamentary leader criticized her "nonchalant approach to the constitution." Not surprisingly, the established churches were up in arms. Bishop Gebhard Fürth, the Catholic representative on the National Ethics Council, suspected a deliberate campaign to undermine the EPL, or at least get the question of its revision onto the political agenda. "This is an alarm signal," he said of the speech by Zypries, "with the goal of undermining protection for the embryo."[113] Zypries did have her supporters in the Schröder administration. And she could invoke many jurists who backed her

---

112. Bundesministerium der Justiz, "Bundesjustizministerin Zypries beim Humboldt-Forum 'Vom Zeugen zum Erzeugen? Verfassungsrechtliche und rechtspolitische Fragen der Bioethik': Wir brauchen eine Spezifikation der Werte," press release, October 29, 2003.

113. "Neuer Streit zum Embryo-Schutz," *Frankfurter Rundschau*, October 30, 2003; "Grüne über Zypries erbost," *Frankfurther Rundschau*, October 31, 2003; "Bischof warnt vor neuer Biopolitik," Associated Press, November 3, 2003. On the controversy, see also "Leben gegen Leben," *Die Zeit*, November 6, 2003.

view that constitutional law did not rule out destructive embryo research. In political terms, however, her trial balloon proved a nonstarter.[114]

During the last two years of his chancellorship, Schröder continued his efforts to broaden the German debate, with limited success. In September 2004 the National Ethics Council released a report with majority recommendations for changing the EPL to allow stem cell derivation and cloning research in Germany. While not openly backing the recommendation, Schröder praised the fact that the council's work continued to provide "important impulses for the societal debate in Germany that certainly can be carried out more broadly than it has been to up to this point." For other party leaders, the council's recommendations went much too far; the Bundestag refused to consider any changes in the Embryo Protection Law.[115] Schröder's last major intervention as chancellor was a June 2005 speech on innovation. In the past, he noted, "researchers who had supported research with embryonic stem cells were defamed as without conscience and self-important." Such criticism was now unacceptable, as those researchers are working to "help others and heal illnesses." Schröder asked, "Can there be any more wonderful task?" Germany, he insisted, should develop a new research culture "without chains, but not without boundaries." Like his earlier efforts to broaden the debate, this one drew a chorus of criticism. The head of the Green parliamentary group referred to any destructive embryo research, colorfully, as "cannibalism dressed up as science policy."[116]

When Schröder lost the September 2005 elections, the CDU-SPD government under Chancellor Merkel soon confronted a new issue—whether to update the cutoff date in the 2002 Stem Cell Law. German scientists, like their counterparts in the United States, were anxious to gain access to newer, better cell lines for their experiments. The new research minister, Annette Schavan of the CDU, initially ruled out any such revision, as did the SPD's chief science spokesperson.[117] The scientific community's frustration with

---

114. Matthias Herdegen's influential commentary on the Basic Law warning against the "inflationary" usage of the human dignity provisions, in line with Zypries's argument, sparked a drawn-out debate. See, for example, "Menschenwürde nicht diskutabel," *Frankfurter Allgemeine Zeitung,* September 27, 2007.

115. Nationaler Ethikrat, *Wortprotokoll: Niederschrift über den öffentlichen Teil der Sitzung, 23. September 2004* (Berlin: Nationaler Ethikrat, 2004).

116. Bundesregierung, "Rede von Bundeskanzler Gerhard Schröder anlässlich der Verleihung der Ehrendoktorwürde der Universität Göttingen," press release, June 14, 2005, http://www.bundesregierung.de/Content/DE/Bulletin/2001__2005/2005/06/__Anlagen/nr-58-1858077,property=publicationFile.pdf.<; Volker Beck quoted in "Schröders Stammzellen-Vorstoß löst Empörung aus," *Der Spiegel,* June 14, 2005.

117. "Schavan bremst Stammzellenforscher," *Die Welt,* July 25, 2006.

the status quo culminated in a major DFG statement in November 2006 officially petitioning the government to change the Stem Cell Law. "As a result of the legal framework conditions," the DFG leadership argued, "science in Germany can only make a limited contribution to this field."[118] Lifting the cutoff date for imports was imperative. Significantly, the statement did not call openly for a revision of the EPL and the derivation of embryonic stem cells within Germany. In contrast to leading scientific officials in the United States and the United Kingdom, German researchers also did not press for therapeutic cloning—less out of principle, perhaps, than out of awareness of political constraints.[119]

At first it looked as if the DFG initiative would go nowhere. Within two hours of its publication Schavan rejected the idea of revising the import cutoff date, insisting it was critical not to provide any incentive for the destruction of embryos.[120] But the reception among other leading Christian and Social Democrats was more positive. In May 2007 the Bundestag's multiparty Committee for Education, Research, and Technology invited research supporters to make their case. One witness after another condemned the 2002 Stem Cell Law for putting German scientists working with international research teams in potential legal jeopardy.[121] Legal experts Matthias Herdegen and Reinhard Merkel argued that given the state's obligation under the Basic Law to protect both the life and the health of its citizens, stem cell research was imperative. Herdegen acknowledged that the human embryo had some dignity under the constitution. Nonetheless, it was a dignity not absolutized but instead weighed against both potential benefits of research and the constitutional value of scientific freedom.[122]

In the face of scientific pressure and some mobilization by patient advocates and their allies in Germany, Schavan softened her position. In May 2007 she wondered aloud whether there were alternative ways to "link up the protection of life and the expectations of researchers."[123] With Merkel's support she settled on the idea of moving the cutoff day forward as a means of increasing

118. DFG, "DFG Puts Forward New Recommendations for Stem Cell Research," press release, November 10, 2006.

119. One important exception was Hubert Markl, head of the Max Planck Society. See *Markl,* "Freiheit, Verantwortung, Menschenwürde."

120. "Wissenschaftler beklagen Kriminalisierung der Embryonen-Forschung," *Die Welt,* November 11, 2006.

121. Bundestag, *Ausschuss für Bildung, Forschung und Technikfolgenabschätzung, 34. Sitzung, 09. Mai 2007, Protokoll 16/34* (Berlin: Deutscher Bundestag, 2007).

122. Ibid., 56–57.

123. Quoted in "Wissenschaftler fordern tief greifende Änderungen am Stammzellengesetz," *Die Welt,* May 10, 2007.

the supply of cell lines from abroad available to German researchers—a move that appalled party conservatives. During fall 2007, in the run-up to the first parliamentary debates on the issue, divisions among Christian Democrats broke out into the open.[124] At a December 2007 party conference, a motion to rule out any liberalization of the Stem Cell Law was narrowly defeated; Merkel, Schavan, and other supporters of moving the cutoff date forward five years prevailed.[125] Catholic leaders decried the retreat from the CDU's traditional focus on embryo protection. Robert Zollitsch, head of the German Bishops' Conference, insisted that "no one has the right to healing that depends on the complete reification of a third party."[126]

The Catholic hierarchy was also alarmed by the Protestant leadership's evolution in a more liberal direction. The head of the EKD, Bishop Wolfgang Huber, had signaled his position in a 2006 speech suggesting that a "glance at German history" showed the dangers of "trampling on human dignity." In the same speech, however, he had insisted that a one-time shift in the cutoff date was desirable, given the healing potential of stem cell research.[127] A November 2007 synod ratified the idea, placing the EKD in the remarkable position of supporting the extension and liberalization of a law it had originally opposed. The strong Catholic-Protestant alliance of the previous two decades dissolved. There had been joint Catholic-Lutheran statements in favor of the EPL in 1990 and against the Stem Cell Law in 2002. There would be no joint statement in the run-up to the climactic Bundestag debate this time around.[128]

As the final April 2008 Bundestag debate neared, controversy centered on three opposing proposals, each with some cross-party support. One group of deputies sought to prevent any liberalization of stem cell imports, while another group sought to eliminate the idea of a cutoff date altogether. A third proposal, backed by Merkel and Schavan—to adapt the 2002 Stem Cell Law

---

124. Evangelische Kirche in Deutschland, "Lockerung der Stammzellforschung von Bischof Huber befürwortet," press release, February 11, 2008, http://www.ekd.de/aktuell_presse/news_2008_02_11_1_rv_sz_interview_stammzellen.html.

125. "Zwischen Stammzellen und Stammwählern; Die CDU hat sich für eine Liberalisierung der Embryonenforschung ausgesprochen—und gefährdet ihre Identität," *Frankfurter Allgemeine Zeitung,* January 20, 2008.

126. Deutsche Bischofskonferenz, "Erklärung des Vorsitzenden der Deutschen Bischofskonferenz, Erzbischof Dr. Robert Zollitsch, zur Debatte über das Stammzellgesetz am 11.04.2008," press release, April 10, 2008, http://www.dbk.de/nc/funktionen/suche/?tx_solr[q]=zollitsch+stammzell gesetz&id=69.

127. Wolfgang Huber, "Wissenschaft verantworten—Überlegungen zur Ethik der Forschung," July 14, 2006, http://www.ekd.de/vortraege/2006/060714_rv_heidelberg.html.

128. "Kulturkampf um Stammzellen," *Die Welt,* January 16, 2008.

by moving the cutoff date for embryonic stem cell imports to include those derived before May 1, 2007—garnered the most political support.[129]

In the Bundestag debate, all sides sought to position themselves as the party of continuity. Schavan insisted that changing the cutoff date for imports did not alter the foundational German approach to embryo research. "We are not discussing the Embryo Protection Law," she told her colleagues. "It is the foundation for all the reflections we are engaged in. It is not up for debate." Shifting the cutoff date represented a "further development of the law, not a liberalization." On the other side of the issue, Maria Böhmer of the CDU, a minister of state in the Chancellor's Office and research opponent, accused Schavan and her allies of an unjustified break with the 2002 Stem Cell Law, which had institutionalized a cutoff date so as not to incentivize any further destruction of embryos. Shifting the date, she argued, would constitute "an ethical change of course and a dam break in embryo protection." Along the same lines, the Green parliamentary leader charged that any relaxation of the regulations would violate the human dignity provisions of the constitution, and another opponent asserted that "there is not a single study that proves the utility of research with human embryonic stem cells." He held up adult stem cells and IPS cells as the morally unproblematic and scientifically superior alternative.[130]

The polarized debate was followed by three votes. The proposal to outlaw any further embryonic stem cell imports into Germany failed by a vote of 118 to 442, as did the proposal to eliminate a cutoff date altogether, by a vote of 126 to 443. The proposal to shift the cutoff date for imports passed with 346 votes for, 228 against.[131] Since the first debates on the Stem Cell Law in early 2002, the tide had turned against research opponents as a result of scientific advances, shifts in public opinion, and the fissure within and across the major churches. Viewed from a broader comparative context, however, it is not change but continuity that is most striking in the German case. The 1990 Embryo Protection Law remained in place, as did prohibition of stem cell imports in principle set down in the 2002 law. The allowance for imports under exceptional circumstances, extending to encompass cells derived

---

129. Bundestag, *Keine Änderung des Stichtages im Stammzellgesetz—Adulte Stammzellforschung fördern, Drucksache 16/7985* (Berlin: Deutscher Bundestag, 2008); Bundestag, *Gesetz für eine menschenfreundliche Medizin—Gesetz zur Änderung des Stammzellgesetzes, Drucksache 16/7982* (Berlin: Deutscher Bundestag, 2008); Bundestag, *Gesetz zur Änderung des Stammzellgesetzes, Drucksache 16/7981* (Berlin: Deutscher Bundestag, 2008).

130. Bundestag, *Verhandlungen des deutschen Bundestages,* ser. 16 (April 11, 2008), 16286–87, 16289–90, 16304–05.

131. Ibid., 16309–317.

before May 2007, did give German researchers access to more cells. But they could still not derive them in Germany, let alone experiment with therapeutic cloning. And because legislation covered both the public and private sectors—on the British model—German scientists did not have the option available to their American colleagues of working with biotechnology firms or state governments to conduct research in those more sensitive areas.

Patterns of German politics and the structure of the German state help to explain this outcome. As in the United Kingdom, the fusion of executive-legislative power gave the government greater leverage to shape the policy agenda. Germany's system of multiparty coalitions undercut the power of the chancellor, however, as powerful parliamentary parties with considerable autonomy shaped legislative outcomes. As a result, both Schröder and Merkel had limited impact on the policy struggle. Ultimately, however, it was the very different institutional legacy of the EPL that shaped political responses to new scientific and technological breakthroughs. The absence of embryo research in the Federal Republic meant there was no constituency of researchers eager to move into stem cell or cloning research. Most saw the EPL as a starting point for thinking about stem cell research, a consensus framework not to be tampered with. The 2002 Stem Cell Law and the start of stem cell research in Germany did mobilize researchers and the DFG around the prospect of its further extension and liberalization in 2007–8, but despite the efforts of Schröder and some of his allies, the Embryo Protection Law—and its widespread identification with the constitutional norm of human dignity—provided a durable and restrictive framework for embryo research in the country.

France: A Cautious Opening to Embryonic Stem Cell Research

The stem cell and cloning debate in France resembled the German one in certain respects. As in Germany, a restrictive regulatory regime served as a point of departure. The 1994 French Bioethics Laws had outlawed all experimentation with human embryos, except in the effectively nonexistent case of research designed to help the embryo itself. The politics of the 1994 settlement had differed from the German case in several ways. In France, supporters of embryo research in the service of biomedical progress had appeared in the ascendant in the ethical controversies and policy struggles of the early 1990s, until a 1993 electoral sweep brought conservatives to power and moved the legislation in a more restrictive direction. The political swings continued in the years after 1994, in contrast to the more incremental shifts in the German political struggle. What continued to distinguish both countries from the

United States and the United Kingdom, however, was the absence of political polarization around the abortion issue and the persistence of human dignity as a frame of reference.

In France, as elsewhere, the news of Dolly's birth in February 1997 was an occasion for media speculation about human cloning and its possible abuses. *Le Monde* led its coverage with the claim that "a considerable and disquieting line has just been crossed in the history of biology and the instrumentalization of reproduction."[132] President Jacques Chirac reacted quickly, as had Bill Clinton. He wrote a public letter to the head of the National Consultative Ethics Committee, Jean-Pierre Changeux, noting that the breakthrough raised "ethical questions of the greatest importance for mankind." Invoking the 1994 legislation, he recalled that "our country was the first to inscribe certain bioethical principles in its positive law." Chirac noted that the 1994 laws had been intended to prevent eugenic abuses and asked the CCNE to insure that cloning was covered. (It had not been mentioned explicitly in the text.) In contrast to Clinton, Chirac did not limit his call for a ban only to reproductive cloning. He was more broadly concerned to "avoid any risk of the utilization of these cloning techniques on humanity."[133]

Like their German colleagues, French scientists and ethicists did not bring up the prospect of therapeutic cloning at this early stage—in fact they may not have been fully aware of it. In a series of interviews and statements in early 1997, the physician and bioethics expert Jean-François Mattei approached cloning solely as a matter of reproduction. When asked about the possible scientific uses of cloning technology, he referred not to stem cells but to the "shocking and nonsensical" scenario of cloned "doubles who could play the role of organ reserves."[134] Axel Kahn, the prominent French biologist and a leading member of the CCNE from 1992 to 2004, was virtually alone among French scientific leaders in raising the therapeutic cloning issue early on. In an article in *Nature* in March 1997 that roundly condemned reproductive cloning, he mentioned the possibility of future "fabrication of an embryo in order to use its cells for therapeutic goals." Unlike leading American and British scientists who weighed in at this juncture, he stridently

132. "Des chercheurs sont parvenus à cloner un mammifère adulte," *Le Monde,* February 25, 1997.

133. Letter of February 28, 1997, quoted in "M. Chirac saisit le Comité d'éthique sur le problème du clonage des mammifères," *Le Monde,* March 1, 1997.

134. "'Il faut prévenir les manipulations aberrante,'" *La Croix,* March 1, 1997. Mattei also wrote an essay in *Le Monde* on cloning that did not mention any possible connection with stem cells, as did Jacques Testart. See "Mythe et réalité," *Le Monde,* March 5, 1997; "Procréer ou reproduire?" *Le Monde,* March 18, 1997.

opposed the procedure. Invoking Kant and the principle of human dignity, he argued that human life "should never be thought of only as a means, but always also as an end."[135]

Chirac met personally with a CCNE delegation in late April and publicly praised its report and its recommendations, in particular its "vehement, categorical, and definitive" criticism of human cloning, which he called a "degrading attack on human dignity."[136] He did not pick up on the report's suggestion that "an embryo might be created" through cloning to derive stem cells; the CCNE itself suggested that such a development was far off and would be illegal in France in any case. The closest thing to a therapeutic cloning controversy in France at this juncture was a June 1997 statement from the French National Academy of Sciences opposing reproductive cloning while "leaving the way open to research that might find beneficial applications." The French failure to engage the issue at an early stage was partially due to the fact that the country's scientists, like their German counterparts, did not already have embryo research programs in place.

The revision of the 1994 Bioethics Laws, called for by statute every five years, would eventually provide an opportunity for debate about both embryonic stem cell research and therapeutic cloning. Initially, however, controversy centered on the efforts of French researchers and their political allies to reform the restrictive regime that the conservative majority had instituted in 1994. The National Academy of Medicine broached the topic in 1996 and passed a formal resolution in June 1998 that referred to research on fertilization, cryopreservation, and implantation as a "medical obligation" in order to build knowledge about infertility and for broader therapeutic ends. Claude Sureau, a Catholic physician and leader of the academy, backed the resolution, even as he noted "wide divergence" among its members on the issue.[137] A leading professional association, the National Order of Physicians, published recommendations the same month along the same lines. Both organizations drew a line at the creation of embryos for research, although the physicians also suggested that nonreproductive cloning "may not be without interest."[138]

---

135. Axel Kahn, "Clone Mammals... Clone Man," *Nature* 387, no. 6635 (1997): 754. See also his interview "Ethique: 'Il faut un consensus international contre le clonage,'" *La Croix,* May 2, 1997.

136. Quoted in "Chirac en campagne contre le clonage," *Le Figaro,* April 30, 1997.

137. "Maîtriser la Santé: La loi met des verrous à la recherche sur l'embryon," *Le Monde,* October 17, 1996; "L'embryon pourrait être objet de recherche," *La Croix,* November 2, 1998.

138. Conseil National de L'Ordre des Médecins, "Révision des lois de bioéthique," Bulletin de l'Ordre National des Médecins (July 1998). See also Sureau's June 1998 testimony at National Assembly hearings, in Alain Claeys and Claude Huriet, *Rapport sur l'application de la Loi no. 94–654 du 29 juillet 1994. Audition* (Paris: Office parlementaire d'évaluation des choix scientifiques et technologiques, 1999), 5–7.

The minister of health, Bernard Kouchner, welcomed these reports, as well as the CCNE's June 1998 recommendations that, given "important prospects in the field of therapeutic research, new articles might well be drafted when the law is up for revision at the end of 1999 which should make it possible to modify the ban on embryo research."[139]

The November 1998 Wisconsin stem cell breakthrough created further momentum for a future liberalization of the French regime. The idea of "therapeutic research," already raised by the CCNE and the Science and Medicine academies earlier in the year, took on greater significance. The renowned biologist Charles Thibault lamented that, despite the promise of stem cells, "in the current legal situation it is not possible to sacrifice an embryo in the interests of society."[140] Other organizations joined the pro-research chorus. In June 1999 the National Consultative Commission on Human Rights, a prestigious government-appointed body, concluded that "studies should be carried out on surplus embryos that are no longer part of a parental project," given that the development of "embryonic therapies requires experiments."[141]

Within France's secular political culture, the Church had few resources with which to counteract the momentum for some liberalization of the 1994 laws.[142] Olivier de Dinechin and his predecessor as the Catholic representative on the CCNE, Patrick Verspieren, criticized the widening chorus of organizations open to embryonic stem cell research.[143] But their voices were muted by the absence of a pro-life movement, historical tensions with the Protestant community, and the thoroughly secular ethos of public life. In recognition of that ethos, lay Catholic leaders opposed to research tended to articulate their views without reference to the Church or its teachings. The most well-known conservative on bioethics issues, Mattei, who had championed the 1994 laws as a bioethics spokesman for the government majority, self-consciously avoided religious arguments. In a secular country, he told

---

139. Comité Consultatif National d'Ethique (CCNE), "Re-examination of the Law on Bioethics," June 25, 1998, www.ccne-ethique.fr/docs/en/avis060.pdf.

140. Quoted in "Juristes et chercheurs se penchent sur l'embryon," *La Croix,* November 16, 1998.

141. Conseil d'Etat, *Les Lois de la bioéthique: Cinq ans après* (Paris: La Documentation française 1999), 15, 9.

142. On the very secular tenor of the French debate, in contrast to the United States, see Thomas Banchoff, "Stem Cell Politics, Religious and Secular: The United States and France Compared," in *Democracy and the New Religious Pluralism,* ed. Thomas Banchoff, 301–321 (Oxford: Oxford University Press, 2007).

143. See, for example, "Pour l'Eglise, un crime contre la dignité d'êtres humains," *Le Monde,* October 1, 1998; "La science convoite les embryons," *La Croix,* January 17, 1999.

an interviewer, embryo controversy "leaves the strictly religious domain and enters that of human dignity." The French situation was sharply different from the American, where "the president swears upon a Bible."[144]

By March 1999, when the government asked the Council of State to make legislative recommendations, it was already clear that the five-year timetable for revision of the 1994 laws would not be upheld. The complexity of the issues was part of the reason; three major ministries, those of science, health, and justice, were by now engaged in drawn-out consultations concerning the legislation. The new stem cell issue added to the complexity, which was now overlaid by the political rivalry between the Conservative Chirac and his prime minister, the Socialist Lionel Jospin. Within this configuration of "cohabitation," Jospin and his health minister, Kouchner, favored a liberalization of the 1994 regime. Mattei carved out a conservative position on the issue aligned with the status quo of the 1994 Bioethics Laws. The fact that Chirac was up for reelection in 2002, and that Jospin was to be his likely opponent, further sharpened tension between both men, their parties, and their science experts. Throughout this period, controversies over embryo research, stem cells, and cloning played a very minor political role alongside economic, social, and foreign policy questions. But on scientific and bioethical questions, too, the pressures of French electoral politics sharpened the policy struggle.

Jospin had encouraged the Council of State to be bold in its recommendations, not just on stem cells, but also on cloning. Conditions under which both kinds of research might be authorized "deserved deep reflection."[145] In its November 1999 recommendations, the Council of State was generally cautious. In line with the approach of the CCNE, it drew distinctions between embryos that enjoyed full dignity as the "consecration of a parental project" and those that, once abandoned, might be used up for the worthy social goal of biomedical progress. Perhaps anticipating the criticism that the moral status of an embryo should not depend solely on the plans of its parents, the Council called for "gradual protection adapted to each moment in its development." This gradualist approach, the report argued, was not "a capitulation to utilitarianism or to economic imperatives"—a reference to

---

144. Mattei at November 1999 National Assembly hearings, in Alain Claeys and Claude Huriet, *Rapport sur le clonage, la thérapie cellulaire et l'utilisation thérapeutique des cellules embryonnaires* (Paris: Office parlementaire d'évaluation des choix scientifiques et technologiques, 2000). For his views at the time, see also Jean-François Mattei, "Vers une révision des lois 'bioéthiques'?" in *Les lois bioéthiques à l'épreuve des faits: Réalités et perspectives,* ed. Briggitte Feuillet-Le Mintier, 330–41 (Paris: Presses Universitaires de France, 1999).

145. Lionel Jospin, "Allocution en clôture du colloque Biovision sur la politique de développement des biotechnologies, à Lyon (Rhône)," March 29, 1999, http://lesdiscours.vie-publique.fr/pdf/993000885.pdf.

the U.S. and U.K. debates. The Council opposed the creation of embryos for research and therapeutic cloning, whatever their biomedical potential, as the embryo "should never be considered as a thing susceptible to instrumentalization, but as a potential human person."[146]

Within this general framework, the Council's report suggested several alternatives for legislators. One proposed revision to the Bioethics Laws might allow couples to donate their embryos for different kinds of worthy research, while another would restrict that research to work with embryonic stem cells. Other variations concerned whether to open research in general, or only for a provisional period of five years. All of the Council's proposed legislative scenarios included an absolute ban on the creation of embryos for research: "The conception of human embryos in vitro for research or experimentation purposes is prohibited."[147] The Council's cautious opening to research, its report concluded, was an effort to "find an equilibrium between advances in the life sciences" and "the principle of safeguarding the dignity of the human person," which the Constitutional Court had made a "constitutional principle" in its ruling on the 1994 Bioethics Laws.[148]

As the government ministries worked with the cabinet and leading parliamentarians to draft the legislation, research supporters tried to keep therapeutic cloning on the agenda with the argument that it did not involve the creation of embryos. In November 1999 Sureau wondered aloud whether "a cell that had undergone nuclear transfer, in other words a clone, is a human embryo or remains a human cell?" He added, "If it is a cell, nothing can oppose its being used in experiments."[149] Along similar lines the National Human Rights Commission reiterated its absolute opposition to the creation of embryos for research but considered cloning to generate stem cells another matter altogether. It suggested that lawmakers keep an open mind concerning the application of cloning technology to "elements of the human body," given its therapeutic promise.[150]

These efforts to skirt the problem of the moral status of the embryo by describing therapeutic cloning as the creation of cells and tissues, without reference to their origin, initially only drew the attention of experts. Axel Kahn was the most prominent critic. In early 1999 he had insisted that

---

146. Conseil d'Etat, *Les Lois de la bioéthique,* 9, 17.

147. Ibid., 44–45.

148. Ibid., 94.

149. Sureau quoted in "Les lois de bioéthique attendront jusqu'en 2001," *La Croix,* November 17, 1999.

150. Commission nationale consultative des droits de l'homme, *Avis portant sur la révision des lois de 1994 sur la bioéthique,* June 29, 2000, http://www.cncdh.fr/article.php3?id_article=262.

therapeutic cloning involved the production "of human embryos with the sole goal of preparing therapeutic material."[151] In August 2000 he used the occasion of the Donaldson report in the United Kingdom to reiterate the point. Kahn scorned British openness to therapeutic cloning as further evidence of a utilitarian Anglo-Saxon approach for which "everything that diminishes suffering and augments happiness is acceptable." For "continental Europeans," he countered, "the overriding principle is that of respect for human dignity."[152] *Le Monde* noted strong opposition to the British report from a Vatican spokesman and favorably quoted German minister of health, Andrea Fischer: "The argument from utility is never enough.... There is a great danger if we permit embryos to become material for scientists."[153]

The political and policy conflict over embryo, stem cell, and cloning research began in earnest in November 2000, when Jospin finally presented the outlines of his government's proposed legislation in a public address before the CCNE. He made a passionate plea for a repeal of the embryo research ban given the potential of embryonic stem cells, which he labeled "cells of hope," to revolutionize medicine. This was all in keeping with the November 1999 Council of State report and the CCNE opinions of the preceding years. But Jospin unexpectedly went further, suggesting that France be open to the creation of stem cells through "the transfer of somatic cells," an oblique reference to therapeutic cloning. Jospin refused to use the term cloning to describe such a transfer, so as to distinguish it sharply from reproductive cloning. He also refused to describe the product of nuclear transfer as an embryo, following the logic of Sureau and the Human Rights Commission. While Jospin recognized the existence of public anxieties about new technologies, he recalled that people had gotten used to the birth of Baby Amandine. By implication, they could get used to therapeutic cloning as well.[154]

Recognizing that he was breaking new ground, Jospin made a preemptive attack on his religious and philosophical critics through a passionate insistence on the independence of science from faith and a call for a rational public debate: "Should motivations deriving from philosophical, spiritual, or religious principles lead us to deprive society and the sick of the possibility of

---

151. Quoted in "Le clonage humain: Engendrer un autre," *Le Monde*, February 5, 1999.

152. Quoted in "Clonage: Jusqu'ou l'homme peut-il modifier l'homme?" *L'Humanité*, September 16, 2000.

153. "La décision de Londres sur le clonage humain condamnée par Berlin et le Vatican," *Le Monde*, August 19, 2000.

154. Lionel Jospin, "Allocution devant le Comité consultatif national d'éthique pour les sciences de la vie et de la santé," press release, November 28, 2000.

therapeutic advances?"[155] Given the role of philosophical and ethical ideals in French political discourse, Jospin could not have intended to denounce them altogether. What irked him was not principles in general but a particular understanding of human dignity, articulated in a religious idiom by the Church and in a secular idiom by the Council of State, that opposed the deliberate creation of human life for research purposes. Jospin acknowledged a role for "fundamental values," as long as they did not "render impossible" necessary advances in biomedical knowledge and practice.

Following on the speech, the government put forward a proposed legislative framework in December 2000 that included provisions for therapeutic cloning. Initially the media did not pick up on the issue, in part due to what *Le Monde* called "the surprisingly ambiguous terms" Jospin used to make his case, eschewing the words "therapeutic cloning" altogether.[156] Gradually, however, criticism mounted from religious and some secular circles. In December 2000 testimony before a parliamentary commission, Verspieren took issue with Jospin's use of terminology, in particular his willingness to "violate the fact that nuclear transfer leads to the creation of an embryo."[157] Axel Kahn remained another vocal critic. Writing in *Libération* in early December, he suggested that one should not "refuse to mention what one is talking about, that is to say the production, for research and therapeutic purposes, of human embryos obtained through the cloning method." If therapeutic cloning should prevail, it would be preferable for people to use clear terms and "conclude that the real benefits for the sick justify a certain reification of potential persons."[158]

Despite these criticisms, Jospin's legislative push for therapeutic cloning appeared to be on track as the year began. In January he received a mixed vote of confidence from the CCNE in its official response to the government's proposed legislative framework. The committee reiterated its position taken in March 1997 and again in June 1998: research with surplus IVF embryos could be justified, both for infertility and stem cell research. More significantly, a narrow majority of fourteen of its twenty-six members endorsed the principle of therapeutic cloning, apparently swayed by the argument that it did not involve the deliberate creation of embryos for

---

155. Ibid.

156. "Clonage thérapeutique, l'annonce inattendue," *Le Monde,* December 7, 2000.

157. Charles Bernard and Alain Claeys, *Rapport d'information de la mission d'information commune préparatoire au projet de loi de révision des lois "bioéthiques" de juillet 1994,* vol. 3, *Auditions* (Paris: Office parlementaire d'évaluation des choix scientifiques et technologiques, 2001), 506.

158. "Le clonage thérapeutique est-il légitime?" *Liberation,* December 5, 2000.

research and was therefore permissible.[159] That same month the Human Rights Commission reiterated the same argument, first articulated in its June 2000 report—despite the public protest of one of its members, the archbishop of Paris, Jean-Marie Lustiger. It backed therapeutic cloning in principle, but suggested its authorization might still be premature, given the promise of embryonic stem cells derived from surplus IVF embryos, as well as work with adult stem cells and cells from umbilical cord blood.[160]

In early February the therapeutic cloning issue moved onto the national political stage. Chirac, who had said little on bioethical questions since his blanket denunciation of cloning in 1997, launched a high-profile attack on Jospin's proposed legislation. Though a practicing Catholic, Chirac did not rule out embryonic stem cell research altogether, noting that "the perspectives opened by cellular therapies can justify an evolution in approach." He suggested an openness to relaxing the prohibition on embryo research in the 1994 laws, given the potential of regenerative medicine. However, he remained categorically opposed to cloning, for it was "necessary to maintain the absolute prohibition on the creation of embryos for scientific ends." France, he insisted, in a veiled critique of the British Parliament's recent approval of therapeutic cloning, "cannot let a utilitarian conception of the human being prevail that would challenge even the foundations of our civilization and threaten human dignity."[161]

With the presidential election just over a year away, the conflict put Jospin and Kouchner in a difficult position. In April 2001, as public opinion was trending against cloning, the government announced the need for more time to complete its full draft of the legislation, sparking criticism from Mattei and other parliamentarians.[162] June marked a critical turning point. The Council of State published a legal commentary on the proposed legislation critical of its cloning provisions as a violation of the constitutional principle of human dignity and insisting that therapeutic cloning did in fact entail the creation of embryos for research. Within a week Jospin finally relented. He dropped cloning from the government's legislative proposals, even as he expressed hope that lawmakers would keep an open mind in the future.[163] The draft law that went forward called for a cautious opening to embryo and stem

159. CCNE, "Opinion on the Preliminary Draft Revision of the Laws on Bioethics."

160. Commission nationale consultative des droits de l'homme, *Avis portant sur l'avant-projet de loi tendant à la révision des lois relatives à l'ethique biomédicale,* January 25, 2001, http://www.cncdh.fr/IMG/pdf/01.01.25_Avis_Ethique_biomedicale_.pdf.

161. Présidence de la République, "Allocution de M. Jacques Chirac Président de la République à l'occasion de l'ouverture du forum mondial des biotechnologies," press release, February 8, 2001.

162. "Le gouvernement ajourne la réforme des lois de bioéthique," *Le Monde,* April 19, 2001.

163. "Bioéthique: Jospin s'interdit de bouleverser le cadre légal avant la présidentielle," *Les Echos,* June 21, 2001.

cell research with surplus IVF embryos out of "solidarity that society owes to those suffering incurable diseases," and for the creation of an agency for procreation, embryology, and human genetics reminiscent of U.K.'s Human Fertilisation and Embryology Authority.[164]

The six months between the publication of the draft law and its first reading in the National Assembly, in January 2002, saw unprecedented political mobilization around bioethical questions. Religious groups gained greater visibility. The Catholic Bishops' Conference under Lustiger produced a statement in June 2001 greeting the elimination of cloning provisions but denouncing any liberalization of the 1994 laws. The bishops rejected the view that an embryo abandoned by its parents had a lesser moral status, insisting on its "unique value no matter how it is obtained." Its deliberate destruction should not be countenanced, even to produce cells that "certain people refer to as 'cells of hope'"—a pointed reference to Jospin.[165] French Protestants, Jews, and Muslims were generally more supportive of research and open to the possibility of therapeutic cloning. The French Protestant Federation published a report in November 2001 that presented contrasting positions for and against embryo research, without staking out an authoritative position. A leading French rabbi, René Sirat, noted his tradition's emphasis on an ethic of healing—and that "the position of the Catholic Church is not the position of Judaism." The Muslim representative on the CCNE, Dalil Boubakeur, supported embryonic stem cell research and was critical of therapeutic cloning, while noting a variety of views within Islam.[166]

Scientific, medical, patient-advocacy, and industry groups also mobilized around a proresearch agenda. Two publicly funded laboratory networks, the Centre National de la Recherche Scientifique (CNRS) and the Institut National de la Santé et de la Recherche Médicale (INSERM), home to ambitious adult stem cell research programs, also went on record in support of embryonic stem cell research. In January 2002 the National Academy of Medicine reiterated its early support for work with surplus IVF embryos, insisting that those without a "parental project" fell outside the medical profession's ethical obligation to be treated as patients, even if "such research implies a sacrifice

---

164. Assemblée nationale, "*Projet de loi relatif à la bioéthique,*" June 20, 2001, http://www.assem blee-nationale.fr/11/projets/pl3166.asp.

165. Conférence des évêques de France, "L'embryon humain n'est pas une chose," press release, June 25, 2001, http://www.eglise.catholique.fr/conference-des-eveques-de-france/textes-et-decla rations/lembryon-humain-nest-pas-une-chose.html.

166. Fédération protestante de France, "A propos du clonage: Eléments de débat et de réflexion," November 15, 2001, http://www.protestants.org/?id=1731. Sirat and Boubakeur testified at National Assembly hearings on the topic in November 2000. See Bernard and Claeys, *Rapport d'information,* 417–28, 471–83.

of the embryo."[167] The giant among French patient-advocacy groups, the French Muscular Dystrophy Association (AFM), began to shift its attention toward stem cells and therapeutic cloning in 2000, and sided with Jospin in his struggle with Chirac early in 2001. It continued to publicly back therapeutic cloning even after Jospin dropped it from his proposed legislation.[168] The AFM's chief scientific adviser called for consideration of therapeutic cloning out of "respect for the suffering human being and the solidarity of society toward people afflicted with major diseases," and the organization would share stories of suffering with legislators as the political conflict sharpened.[169] France Biotech, the country's leading biotechnology industry interest group, also weighed in for both stem cell and cloning research.[170]

When the National Assembly debate finally opened in January 2002, three months before the presidential election scheduled for that April, proresearch forces were ascendant. Research minister Roger-Gérard Schwartzenberg set the tone with an opening address praising the healing potential of embryonic stem cell research and attacking those for whom the embryo was sacred and therapeutic cloning objectionable. "It is impossible to use rational arguments against this objection, which depends on one's ethical, philosophical, or spiritual view of the nature of the embryo," he lamented. Following Jospin's lead, Schwartzenberg asked, "In a lay republic, can the legislator privilege one philosophical or religious conception over another?" Because the "law is the expression of the general will"—an axiom within the French political tradition—policy should follow a "universal ethics" and an "ethics of life." From Schwartzenberg's perspective, the consultations of the previous years, including those of the Science and Medicine academies and the Council of State, pointed to an emerging consensus in favor of embryo research. The restrictive research regime set up in 1994 was blocking progress.[171]

The opposition leader and shadow health minister, Mattei, did not question the premise of Schwartzenberg's argument—that legislators should abstract from particular philosophical and religious traditions and reflect and act in the public interest. But for him, reason led in a different direction. He insisted that the embryo represented not a part of the human body but

167. Academie Nationale de Médecine, "Communiqué concernant le projet de loi relatif à la bioéthique," January 8, 2002.

168. "L'AFM mise sur les cellules souches," *Les Echos,* March 13, 2001.

169. "Le clonage thérapeutique derize les sages," *Le Figaro,* February 8, 2001; Association Française contre les Myopathies, letter to National Assembly deputies (manuscript), January 24, 2003.

170. France Biotech, "France Biotech souhaite que la recherche médicale sur les cellules souches et le clonage thérapeutique puisse se développer en France avec une réglementation stricte," press release, January 10, 2002.

171. *Assemblée Nationale, Compte rendu integral* (January 15, 2002), 481–88.

a "human person in becoming." To use surplus embryos to derive stem cells for therapies, he insisted, would be to instrumentalize human life.[172] Another lay Catholic and outspoken research opponent, Philippe Villiers, accused the bill's supporters of "scientific clericalism." Like Mattei, he rejected any ethical distinction among embryos that are or are not part of a parental project: "The intention of the parents or of the researchers in no case changes the nature of the embryo." For Villiers the reification of the embryo had "something morbid about it and contrary to civil peace."[173]

While Mattei, Villiers, and other opponents of the government's legislation were careful not to invoke explicitly religious arguments, they were nevertheless accused of doing so. Among the most vocal critics was the Socialist Henri Emmanuelli, a proponent of therapeutic cloning who associated research opponents with the "Roman Catholic Apostolic religion."[174] Schwartzenberg was more circumspect. During the debate he noted that parliamentarians did not share the same "spiritual, moral, and ethical" conceptions. "We legislate in general fashion, for the whole of the nation," he insisted. "By virtue of the principle of *laïcité*," he continued, "it seems difficult to privilege one ethical, philosophical or religious conception over another." The goal was to get as close as possible to "an ethic in conformity with the values of the French Republic."[175]

The outcome of the debate and vote in January 2002 demonstrated the political strength of the proresearch position and the triumph of ethic-of-healing arguments. Socialist and Communist deputies, divided over the 1994 Bioethics Laws, now voted unanimously in favor of the new departure. So too did the Green Party, in sharp contrast to their German counterparts. In discussing the bill, a leading Green deputy skipped over embryo research questions altogether and focused on the legislation's other provisions.[176] Conservative opposition to embryo research had also eroded. A majority of Chirac's Rally for the Republic (RPR) abstained on the vote, as did the centrist French Democratic Union (UDF). Some prominent conservatives voted for the legislation, including future president Nicolas Sarkozy. The final vote was 325 to 21, with 151 abstentions. Interestingly, even Mattei's Democratic Party (DP) had abstained rather than vote against the bill. His official reason: the upcoming elections might reverse majorities and allow for the drafting of new, more restrictive legislation.[177]

---

172. Ibid., 508.
173. Assemblée Nationale, *Compte rendu intégral* (January 16, 2002), 578.
174. Assemblée Nationale, *Compte rendu intégral* (January 17, 2002), 715.
175. Assemblée Nationale, *Compte rendu intégral* (January 15, 2002), 517.
176. Chantal Robin-Rodrigo in Assemblée Nationale, *Compte rendu intégral* (January 16, 2002), 550.
177. Assemblée Nationale, *Compte rendu intégral* (January 22, 2002), 15–20.

Electoral Shifts and Policy Revisions

The April 2002 presidential elections and the June 2002 parliamentary elections that followed did in fact alter the course of the legislation. The Socialist Party, with Jospin at its head, suffered a catastrophe. In the first round of the presidential ballot Jospin was outpolled by Jean-Marie Le Pen, the Far Right candidate, who went on to lose by a large margin to Chirac in the second round. The conservative RPR-UDF-DP alliance secured a majority in parliament in the legislative elections that followed. Jean-Pierre Raffarin was elected prime minister, and Mattei was named minister of health. As he had a decade earlier, Mattei took over bioethics legislation in midstream—after its initial consideration and approval by a center-left National Assembly. In 1993–94 Mattei had successfully shifted course, replacing provisions that allowed for embryo research under restricted circumstances with the total ban that eventually became law in 1994. Over the course of a second protracted struggle, from 2002 to 2004, things worked out differently.

A less visible sideshow in France concerned the legality of embryonic stem cell imports. As in Germany, those imports had not been forbidden—or even foreseen—in the existing research regime. As the political battle over the revision of the 1994 laws dragged on from 1999 into 2001, French researchers began to press for access to imports, much like their frustrated German counterparts. When leading scientific figures, including four Nobel Prize winners, published a November 2001 petition backing the government's proposed legislation, they included a plea to allow French scientists to work with imported stem cells in the interim. After the Bundestag approved imports in 2002, the calls from the French scientific community grew louder. Schwartzenberg was initially cautious. He wanted to wait for parliamentary consideration of the Bioethics Laws as a whole, out of respect for the "the fundamental rules of democratic debate."[178]

Not willing to wait for the new law to be finalized, scientists kept up the pressure. The head of INSERM, Christian Brechot, circulated a brochure in March 2002 arguing for lifting strictures on French scientists, and the CNRS pushed for funding of a project of Jacques Hatzfeld, who, like Oliver Brüstle in Germany, wanted to extend his work with mouse stem cells to embryonic stem cells. Schwartzenberg finally announced that he was willing to move ahead through the constitution of a "committee of the wise" to examine the

---

178. "La recherche bloquée sur les cellules souches," *Figaro,* November 17, 2001; "Polémique sur l'usage des cellules souches humaines," *Le Monde,* November 16, 2001; "Paris hostile à des exportations de cellules embryonnaires," *Le Monde,* February 1, 2002.

issue, with members including Anne Fagot-Largeault, Claude Sureau, and Charles Thibault, all prominent research supporters. Not surprisingly, the committee backed imports.[179] After the elections but before leaving office, Schwartzenberg authorized imports, insisting that the January 2002 debate and vote were enough of a mandate.[180] Pro-life forces, including the Right-to-Life Alliance, petitioned the Council of State to reverse the policy. Their argument, like that of research opponents in the United States and Germany, was that the use of embryonic stem cells, whatever their origin, was ethically and legally tantamount to participating in the destruction of embryos.[181]

Ultimately, the issue was decided in parliament. Mattei decided to block any imports until the new majorities in the Assembly and the Senate had completed their revisions of the 1994 laws. The government's position on the revisions—and the legislation passed through the Assembly in January—was initially shrouded in uncertainty. Mattei indicated he would not pursue a complete overhaul. Would he try to scale back the legislation, as he had in 1992–93, to preclude research on the human embryo? If that was politically impossible, what was the alternative? Having criticized the legislation so sharply in the January 2002 debate, he had put himself in a bind. Moreover, his colleague the new research minister, Claudie Haigneré, was known to be sympathetic to embryonic stem cell research, and Chirac himself had never come out publicly against it.

Research proponents, determined to avoid a repeat of 1993–94, when an electoral shift had favored a restrictive turn in the Bioethics Laws, mobilized in favor of the legislation that had passed the Assembly. Leading scientific, medical, and patient-advocacy groups made a public case both for work with surplus IVF embryos and for therapeutic cloning. In a joint communiqué dated June 2002, the Academy of Medicine and the Academy of Sciences expressed frustration "about the blockage of research in France" and called for final passage of the bill approved by the National Assembly that January. The communiqué distinguished between stem cells of "embryonic origin" and those "obtained through nuclear transfer," and approved both as well as continued support for adult stem cell research.[182] During the spring and

179. "L'importation de cellules souches embryonnaires va être autorisée," *Le Monde,* March 28, 2002.

180. "La France autorise l'importation de cellules souches issues d'embryons humains," *Le Monde,* May 5, 2002.

181. "Cellules souches embryonnaires: Importation suspendue," *Le Figaro,* November 15, 2002.

182. Académie des sciences de l'Institut de France and Académie Nationale de Médecine, "Recommandations de l'Académie des sciences et de l'Académie Nationale de Médecine relatives à l'utilisation de cellules souches embryonnaires humaines," June 10, 2002, http://www.academie-sciences.fr/actualites/textes/cellules_souches_10_06_02.pdf.

summer of 2002, the AFM convened two highly publicized panels—one of experts, the other of families stricken by muscular dystrophy—to discuss their healing hopes for both stem cell and cloning research.[183] Mattei, who faced a hail of criticism at one of the AFM events, appeared to be rethinking his position. On a television talk show in October 2002 he mused aloud about how difficult it was to reconcile "absolute respect for life" with biomedical advances that have always involved "transgressions."[184]

In November, just two months before the Senate was to address the legislation, Mattei made further hints that his views were evolving. In an interview in *Le Monde* he noted that the January 2002 vote in the National Assembly had produced "a very large majority" in favor of some research with surplus IVF embryos. "We are going to naturally make some modifications" to the legislation, he suggested, "but they will probably not be of the kind to unravel this consensus."[185] In Senate committee testimony in December he acknowledged he was looking for ways to maintain the principle that embryo research should remain illegal while allowing carefully calibrated exceptions. Unlike the legislation passed in January 2002, the reform of the 1994 laws he advocated would maintain the existing ban in principle but allow research for five years on a "derogatory and transitory" basis. Surplus IVF embryos would be used only to derive stem cells, not for research into infertility or other areas, and embryo production for research—and therapeutic cloning—would remain illegal.[186]

With support of conservative senators, the legislation passed by the Assembly was amended along the lines Mattei suggested in January 2003. In opening the final Assembly debate on the Senate version of the legislation in December 2003, Mattei emphasized the constitutional imperative of "respect for human beings from the beginning of life" and admitted that he had "long hoped" that embryonic stem cell research could be avoided. "But the reality of the demands for the research," he had become convinced, necessitated the authorization of research "under certain conditions." Mattei acknowledged this was a change: "I do not want to hide the fact that this solution represents an ontological disruption [*bouleversement*]."[187] But he insisted that the new

---

183. "Les scientifiques français plaident en faveur des cellules souches," *Les Echos,* June 25, 2002.

184. "Jean-François Mattei gagne ses galons à la télévision," *Le Figaro,* October 24, 2002.

185. "Le Comité d'éthique joue son role," *La Croix,* November 27, 2002.

186. Sénat, "Audition de M. Jean-François Mattei, ministre de la santé, de la famille et des personnes handicapées," December 12, 2002, http://www.senat.fr/commission/soc/soc021214.html#toc9.

187. Assemblée Nationale, *Compte rendu intégral* (December 9, 2003), 11994.

direction was continuous with the approach set down in 1994: that research remain illegal in principle, with exceptions now made for surplus IVF embryos. In presenting the same legislation, Haigneré emphasized change rather than continuity. She insisted that "research utilizing embryonic stem cells of human origin is in fact unavoidable" and even held out the possibility that one day, should it become necessary scientifically, the government might take up the question of therapeutic cloning.[188]

From the point of view of the Socialist opposition and some members of the center-right parties, Mattei's evolution had not gone far enough. They viewed the principled opposition to embryo research in the new legislative draft as an unacceptable reversal of what had passed in January 2002. In December 2003, at the outset of the Assembly's debate on the Senate's proposed amendments, Schwartzenberg criticized the government for delaying the legislation and for "disfiguring" the "consensus text" passed almost two years earlier. "All of society must contribute to making suffering and death recede," he insisted. "That is an ethical imperative that the health minister seems to forget." When the Assembly finally took up the bill, Schwartzenberg pushed the argument further, emphasizing the rights to health care and to scientific freedom.[189] In the debate itself, he referred to the "pre-embryo" to describe the early embryo and insisted it was not yet a "potential human person." Here and elsewhere he took aim at the Catholic Church as the enemy, dismissing its argument about the early embryo as unacceptable dogma: "One cannot confuse an article of faith with an article of law." Another Socialist even cast the legislation as "laws of moral order"—a reference to the altar-throne alliance of an earlier era in French history.[190]

The French Catholic Church was disappointed by Mattei's willingness to countenance embryo research, if only under narrow circumstances and for a window of five years. In a statement in late January 2003, Jean-Pierre Ricard, president of the French Bishops' Conference, lamented that with the legislation embryos would be reduced to the status of objects: "For the first time a human being in gestation will be legally treated as a thing."[191] Without

---

188. As Haigneré put it in Senate hearings in early 2003, "transgression of the principle of the protection of human life from its beginnings does not appear acceptable in light of the available scientific facts" that had not yet "demonstrated the feasibility of therapeutic cloning." See Pierre-Louis Fagniez, *Rapport fait au nom de la commission des affaires culturelles, familiales et sociales sur le projet de loi, adopté par le Sénat, relatif à la bioéthique* (Paris: Assemblée nationale, 2003): 20.

189. "Pour le PS, le texte proposé à l'Assemblée constitue une 'régression,'" *Le Monde,* December 10, 2003.

190. Assemblée Nationale, *Compte rendu intégral* (December 9, 2003), 12014, 12020.

191. Conférence des évêques de France, "Pas d'exception au respect dû à l'embryon humain," January 27, 2003, http://www.eglise.catholique.fr/conference-des-eveques-de-france/textes-et-declarations/pas-dexception-au-respect-du-a-lembryon-humain-.html.

criticizing Mattei or the government by name, he warned that any embryo research would contravene the principle of human dignity. In a revealing interview in *L'Express* in December 2003, on the eve of the final debate in the Assembly on the Senate draft, Mattei addressed his Catholic critics. "In a Republic, the principle of *laïcité* must prevail," he said, adding that "as an elected official, I am not bearer of my personal convictions, I try to know and understand the evolution of our society."[192] Other lay Catholics in the Assembly, too, stuck to secular arguments. Even Christine Boutin, a member of the Pontifical Academy of Sciences, made no mention of Church teaching. Instead, she cast the issue of embryonic life as one of human rights and social solidarity. "Our social cohesion depends on the fate we reserve for the weakest," she argued.[193]

When the legislation finally passed in the Assembly with the votes of the ruling parties and was endorsed by a joint Assembly-Senate committee in July 2004, five years of extended political and policy controversy came to an end. The three Bioethics Laws of 1994 were now folded into the Bioethics Law of 2004. As it had in 1994 the Constitutional Court gave its blessings to the legislation. A national regulatory organization was set up, the French Biomedicine Agency. It authorized the first import of embryonic stem cells to France in September 2004 and solicited first proposals for research involving the derivation of stem cells from surplus IVF embryos soon after. This was a significant new departure but no clean break from the policy regime instituted in 1994. Experiments with embryos remained illegal in principle and were authorized only for five years. The creation of embryos for research, therapeutic cloning, and any destruction of embryos for purposes other than the derivation of stem cells remained forbidden.

During the years that followed, embryonic stem cell and cloning research remained an object of political contestation, not least because the Bioethics Law was slated to come up for a another planned revision at the end of the decade. Cloning proponents kept up the pressure. In May 2005, encouraged by news of the purported therapeutic cloning breakthrough in South Korea, Schwartzenberg introduced legislation from the opposition benches to permit the practice.[194] The following month ten leading scientists including Claude Sureau backed the legislative proposal.[195] As recounted in chapter 3,

---

192. "La Bioéthique selon Mattei," Mattei *L'Express,* December 4, 2003.

193. Assemblée Nationale, *Compte rendu intégral* (December 9, 2003), 12026.

194. "Clonage thérapeutique: Schwartzenberg appelle à ne 'pas désespérer' maladies," Agence France-Presse, May 25, 2005. Text of proposed legislation reprinted in Pierre-Louis Fagniez, *Cellules souches et choix éthiques* (Paris: Assemblée nationale, 2006), 235–41.

195. "Dix scientifiques appellent à autoriser le clonage thérapeutique," *Le Figaro,* May 25, 2005.

even Axel Kahn of the CCNE, long a principled opponent of cloning research, adjusted his position. In light of these shifts a December 2006 report authored by the Socialist Alain Claeys on behalf of a parliamentary commission suggested it was now "possible to reach a political agreement on the authorization of therapeutic cloning." Given the promise of regenerative medicine, Claeys dismissed the problem of the moral status of the embryo as a matter for public discussion and called it instead an issue for "the most intimate sphere of each individual."[196]

The Catholic Church and its allies sought to counter these trends, with little success. In a June 2006 address to the National Assembly, Lustiger's successor as the country's senior prelate, Archbishop André Vingt-Trois, criticized the rise of an ethic of healing, calling it "an illusory dream to imagine that human life could develop beyond any illness." Therapeutic hopes connected with embryonic stem cell research, he insisted, were still "largely hypothetical." Vingt-Trois skirted the difficult question of what to do with more than 160,000 frozen embryos in France, some of which might be made available for regenerative medicine research.[197] His most high-profile intervention was an attack on the AFM and its popular annual telethon, held each December. While he acknowledged the group's success in raising awareness and promoting research, he insisted that "just because the telethon is a generous enterprise does not mean that one should give it a blank check," given its support for human embryo research.[198]

While the attack on the telethon proved a public relations disaster, twin scientific developments—the revelation of South Korean cloning fraud and the discovery of IPS cells—undercut political momentum for a further liberalization of the French research regime. In another shift in his position, Kahn now suggested that therapeutic cloning "does not make much sense anymore," in view of the possibility of creating genetically matched cells for therapies through IPS technology.[199] The Academy of Medicine and the Academy of Sciences maintained their support for therapeutic cloning but stopped pressing the issue. In parliamentary testimony in 2008 Sureau placed more emphasis on expanding research with surplus IVF embryos.[200] The French Biomedicine

196. Alain Claeys, *Rapport sur les recherches sur le fonctionnement des cellules humaines* (Paris: Office parlementaire d'évaluation des choix scientifiques et technologiques, 2006), 92, 9.

197. Fagniez, *Cellules souches,* 210–13. On the accumulation of frozen embryos in France, see "Embryons congelés: Le choix délicat des parents," *Le Figaro,* November 5, 2009.

198. "Mgr Vingt-Trois: Pas de chèque en blanc pour le Téléthon," Agence France-Presse, November 27, 2006.

199. Alain Claeys and Jean Leonetti, *Rapport d'information fait au nom de la mission d'information sur la révision des lois de bioéthique. Auditions* (Paris: Assemblée nationale, 2010), 37–48.

200. Ibid., 253–68.

Agency, a strong advocate for scientists, acknowledged that the initial success of IPS technology undermined the case for therapeutic cloning. At the same time, it was open to a liberalization of nuclear transfer technology as well as to the creation of embryos for research on the British model.[201]

The position of conservative President Nicolas Sarkozy, who succeeded Chirac in May 2007, was uncertain. He was a Catholic who surprised French intellectuals by insisting on a public role for religion in French life. But on embryo stem cell research his views did not mirror those of the Church leadership: he had voted for the Jospin government's January 2002 legislation. As the reconsideration of the Bioethics Law planned for 2009–11 took shape, he did not stake out his own position. On the occasion of a visit by Pope Benedict XVI in September 2008, he noted that "the important and rapid progress of science in the domains of genetics and procreation poses delicate philosophical questions for our societies." It was, he suggested, "the responsibility of politics to organize a framework for reflection" on challenging issues.[202] In that spirit Sarkozy initiated an Estates-General for Bioethics, a series of public meetings across the country during the first half of 2009 designed to bring together experts and citizens to discuss key issues as a precursor to the revision of the Bioethics Law. The final report of the Estates-General, delivered to Sarkozy in July 2009, pointed both to widespread hope about regenerative medicine and to ethical concerns about the instrumentalization of early human life, but it did not make any hard-and-fast recommendations.[203]

As it had during earlier legislative cycles, the Council of State played a major role in structuring the legislative debate. Its April 2009 report and recommendations included a call to legalize embryo research on a permanent basis, ending the five-year probationary period instituted in 2004. Pointing to the fact that most proposals that passed scientific muster had been approved by the French Biomedicine Agency, the Council suggested that an endorsement of embryo research in principle under certain circumstances would provide a positive signal for scientists working on medium- and long-term projects. On the question of the origins of embryos and the purpose

201. *Bilan d'application de la loi de bioéthique du 6 août 2004* (Paris: Agence de la biomédecine, 2008), 76.

202. Présidence de la République Française, "Visite en France de Sa Sainteté le pape Benoît XVI: Allocution de M. Le Président de la République Française," September 12, 2007, http://www.elysee.fr/president/les-actualites/discours/2008/visite-en-france-de-sa-saintete-le-pape-benoit-xvi.2085.html.

203. Etats généraux de la bioéthique, "Rapport final: Etats généraux de la bioéthique," July 1, 2009, http://www.etatsgenerauxdelabioethique.fr/uploads/rapport_final.pdf.

of research, the Council pleaded for continuity on the basis of the 2004 revision of the 1994 Bioethics Laws. Research should still be directed toward a therapeutic end, and no embryos should be "conceived for research"—a formulation intended to rule out therapeutic cloning.[204]

In December 2009 parliamentary testimony, Mattei's successor as minister of health, Roselyne Bachelot, suggested that the government would not follow the Council of State's advice on the full legalization of embryo research.[205] The practice should remain illegal in principle and be approved on a case-by-case basis, without unnecessary delays. The legislation she presented in October 2010 reiterated this cautious approach, while dropping the five-year probationary period for the arrangement.[206] Broad support for at least maintaining, if not extending, the modest liberalization of the 1994 laws adopted in 2004 demonstrated a pattern of continuity and incremental change in France. As parliament geared up for revisions to the established policy regime, slated for completion in 2011, differences remained. But a cautious approach to research with surplus IVF embryos and a reluctance to endorse their creation for research represented strong elements of continuity in French embryo politics.

Conclusion

A comparison of embryo politics across leading Atlantic democracies reveals very different outcomes during the decade after 1997–98. The U.S. government continued to restrict the use of federal funds for research involving the destruction of embryos, including the derivation of stem cells and therapeutic cloning, while allowing both practices to continue in the private sector and at the level of the states. In the United Kingdom, a liberal regime of stem cell research and therapeutic cloning was instituted. On the opposite extreme, the German government continued to oppose any destruction of embryos for research purposes and only approved the import of stem cells derived abroad before a certain date. The French government went the furthest in changing its position, allowing the derivation of embryonic stem cells for therapeutic ends in 2004, for a period of five years.

---

204. Conseil d'Etat, *La révision des lois de bioéthique* (Paris: La Documentation françiase, 1999), 9.

205. Claeys and Leonetti, *Rapport d'Information,* 1159.

206. "Le projet de loi bioéthique présenté mercredi en Conseil des ministres," Agence France Presse, October 19, 2010.

Familiar political factors help to explain these outcomes—the interplay of interest group pressures and electoral fortunes. The rise and fall of elected leaders with particular ethical approaches to research shaped the evolution of government policy, as did the mobilization of key interest groups, including scientists, churches, biotechnology companies, and—increasingly—patient-advocacy groups. Party and interest group politics do not tell the whole story, however. In each of the four countries, both proponents and opponents of liberalizing existing research regimes were constrained by those very same regimes. Existing institutions embodied the outcome of the previous phase of embryo politics, from the late 1980s through the mid-1990s—clashes that most national leaders, whatever their positions, generally showed little inclination to revive. The policy status quo provided a shared frame of reference, favoring incremental over radical change.

This institutional legacy helps to explain the high degree of continuity in the decade after 1997–98. While Barack Obama abolished most of George W. Bush's restrictions on federal funding of embryonic stem cell research, he did not challenge the Dickey Amendment, which prevented federal funding of activities involving the deliberate creation and destruction of embryos. Tony Blair, Gordon Brown, and their conservative challengers lined up behind the HFEA and supported its adaptation to allow for embryonic stem cell and cloning research. Gerhard Schröder backed an overhaul of the restrictive embryo research regime but said so only obliquely, seeking instead to introduce liberalization slowly—with little success. The force of the institutional status quo proved strong in France as well. There, provisions for the regular updating of the 1994 Bioethics Laws provided opportunities for incremental change on an existing institutional foundation.

Through these developments the tenor of ethical contestation in Atlantic democracies shifted. By and large, there was consensus about what was at stake—the destruction of embryos and the hope for life-saving therapies. But the revolutionary promise of stem cell research effectively transformed the familiar terms of debate. The moral status of the embryo, the center of gravity in the debates of the 1980s and 1990s, receded in political salience, even in the United States, where Catholics and evangelicals were a powerful political force, and in Germany, where the historical legacy of Nazi eugenics still informed the policy struggle. The prospect of reducing human suffering through stem cell therapies promoted the rise of an ethic of healing that cast established questions in a new light. Might not thousands of surplus IVF embryos, destined to die in any case, be used up instead for potentially life-saving research? Did therapeutic cloning, whatever its biomedical promise, nevertheless represent the deliberate creation and destruction of embryos for research? How should democracies combine respect for the embryo with support for biomedical progress under new circumstances?

Unfortunately, participants in the policy debates proved less willing to address such difficult ethical questions than they had during the first era of embryo politics, through the mid-1990s. Rather than tackle the moral conundrums in a spirit of modesty that admitted to its complexity, politicians, churches, and interest groups tended to stake out fixed and unreflective positions. Research supporters increasingly dismissed the problem of the moral status of the embryo as irrelevant, and research opponents often refused to acknowledge the biomedical potential of embryonic stem cell research. Each side questioned the ethical seriousness of the other. The increasing politicization of ethical controversy undercut the quality of public debate. The future of embryo politics will largely depend on whether and how robust ethical contestation informs policy struggles going forward.

Conclusion

We are just over four decades into a new era. In the years after 1968, the living human embryo moved out of the darkness of the womb and into the light of the laboratory for the first time. Over the next four decades further breakthroughs included the first child born by in vitro fertilization, the cryopreservation of embryos, the derivation of embryonic stem cells, and the first cloned human embryo. The future trajectory of research with embryos is uncertain. Some researchers will continue to focus on stem cells, infertility, and early human development. Others will turn to frontier technologies such as preimplantation genetic diagnosis and, further into the future, genetic enhancement. The analysis of embryos and their selection for a growing number of genetic characteristics via PGD is already a reality. The enhancement of traits through intervention in the genome, if someday successful, could mark a turning point in human evolution.

Ethical and policy struggles, and not just science and technology, drove the direction of embryo research in the United States, the United Kingdom, Germany, and France over its first four decades. Clashes over the moral status of the embryo and the imperative of biomedical progress, embedded in national histories, institutions, and electoral and interest group competition, shaped the evolution of policy regimes ranging from the most liberal in the United Kingdom to the most restrictive in Germany.

These different components of embryo politics will likely persist into the future. Historical and institutional legacies will provide a point of departure for countries wrestling with new technological developments. Electoral competition and the mobilization of interest groups such as the biotechnology industry and patient-advocacy organizations will shape the political fate of policy alternatives. Ethical arguments about the moral status of the embryo and the promise of biomedical research will persist.

How central ethics will be to the future of embryo politics is far from clear. When life begins, deserves protection, and can be destroyed to advance biomedical knowledge emerged as a public issue by the mid-1980s and informed the policy struggles that produced first embryo research regimes from 1990 to 1995. With the cloning and stem cell breakthroughs of 1997–98, however, the quality of public ethical debate declined. Excited by a research program that could help millions, research supporters often sidestepped the problem of the moral status of the embryo. Research opponents, for their part, often refused to acknowledge the therapeutic potential of embryonic stem cell research. Mutual recriminations increasingly displaced an acknowledgment of the complexity of the ethical issues at hand.

The polarization of debate need not continue into the future. Revolutionary changes in the life sciences have been and will always be a reason to pause and reflect. Wherever we come down on the moral status of the embryo or the importance of research, citizens and leaders should ask big questions and assume responsibility for their stances. Principled adherents of opposing views should not have to temper their positions or seek compromise for its own sake. Nonetheless, all should acknowledge the complexity of the challenges posed by new developments to their established religious and philosophical traditions. They should interrogate their own views, as well those of their opponents, in constructive dialogue. French president François Mitterrand put it eloquently in December 1983. "The greater the pace of change, the greater the temptation of the unknown, and the more we should take time," he said, "time for moderation, for exchange and reflection, that is, time for moral reasoning."[1]

Four Decades of Embryo Politics

This book has argued that the governance of embryo research in four leading Atlantic democracies is best explained in terms of ethical contestation,

---

1. Présidence de la République, "Allocution de M. François Mitterrand, Président de la République, à l'occasion de la mise en place du Comité consultatif national d'éthique pour les sciences de la vie et de la santé," December 2, 1983, http://lesdiscours.vie-publique.fr/pdf/837208100.pdf.

national historical and institutional legacies, and electoral and interest group competition. A comparison of the four country cases across two key phases, 1968–96 and 1997–2008, reveals three overarching trends: the rise and decline of a structured public debate about the moral status of the embryo and the value of biomedical research; the fading of deeper historical legacies and the rise of more recent institutional constraints as frames for policy struggles; and increasing political salience of embryo, stem cell, and cloning research amid electoral and interest group mobilization. The intersection of these related trends has shaped the evolution of research regimes in all four countries and transformed the shape of embryo politics over time.

The Evolution of Ethical Contestation

After an initial post-1968 decade in which IVF controversy revolved around eugenic anxieties, safety, and human sexuality, the moral status of the embryo and limits on its scientific use emerged as a key ethical issue. Science and technology helped to drive this development. The move from the first fertilization of an egg in 1968 to the first embryo transfer efforts in the early 1970s to the birth of the first IVF child, Louise Brown, in 1978, probably saw the creation, observation, and discarding of hundreds rather than thousands of embryos. Only after IVF became routine and the freezing of embryos was introduced in the mid-1980s did the number of embryos available for research increase. As the media picked up on the issue, the emerging debate among philosophers and moral theologians in the nascent field of bioethics came to the attention of a wider public. Governments turned to ethics committees for guidance. Amid "a wide diversity in moral feelings," the U.K.'s Warnock committee argued in its 1984 report, there must be "*some* barriers that are not to be crossed, *some* limits fixed, beyond which people must not be allowed to go."[2]

After extensive deliberations, the four most important national committees framed the ethical stakes in comparable fashion and came up with strikingly similar policy recommendations. The Ethics Advisory Board in the United States (1979), the Warnock committee in the United Kingdom (1984), the Benda Commission in Germany (1985), and the National Consultative Ethics Committee (CCNE) in France (1986) all acknowledged both the moral status of the embryo as a developing form of human life and the promise of biomedical research into fertility and other areas. The EAB insisted on "profound respect" for the embryo but also that "this respect does not necessarily

---

2. United Kingdom, Department of Health and Social Security, *Report of the Committee of Inquiry into Human Fertilisation and Embryology* (London: Her Majesty's Stationery Office, 1984), 2.

encompass the full legal and moral rights attributed to persons." For the Warnock committee, embryos deserved "some added measure of respect beyond
that accorded to other animal subjects," but such respect "cannot be absolute." The Benda Commission approached the embryo as "a human subject
in its early form of development," whose status could "be carefully weighed
against the paramount importance of modern genetic research for the health
of mankind." For the French National Consultative Ethics Committee, the
embryo was a "potential human person" to be protected in principle but
sacrificed under exceptional circumstances.[3]

The deliberations within each committee demonstrated the difficulty of
arriving at consensus, given the diversity of religious and philosophical view-
points represented, including Kantian concerns about the instrumentalization
of human life and the utilitarian focus on the alleviation of suffering through
biomedical advances. Still, majorities across the committees reached remark-
ably similar conclusions: under carefully regulated conditions, embryos created for procreation and left over from IVF treatments might be utilized in
experiments to improve treatments for infertility and related ailments. The
Benda Commission went slightly further, supporting research that extended
beyond infertility to address "medical findings of great value." And the Warnock committee endorsed the creation of embryos expressly for research—by
a narrow margin. On balance, though, all four bodies approached ethical
dilemmas and formulated policy recommendations in similar ways.

Starting in the late 1980s, as embryo research became an object of political
struggle, ethical controversy—and the work of national ethics committees—
became more polarized. A debate initially dominated by scientists, philosophers, and theologians now broadened to include the Catholic hierarchy
and many evangelicals opposed to destructive embryo research under any
circumstances, as well as scientific and medical professionals concerned about
the safety and effectiveness of IVF as an infertility treatment. The confrontation was especially fierce in the United States, where the 1994 Human
Embryo Research Panel's support for the deliberate creation of embryos for
research provoked a barrage of criticism from the Catholic Church and its

---

3. Ethics Advisory Board, *Report and Conclusions: HEW Support of Research Involving Human In
Vitro Fertilization and Embryo Transfer* (Washington, DC: Department of Health, Education, and Welfare, 1979), 101; UK, Department of Health and Social Security, *Report of the Committee of Inquiry
into Human Fertilisation and Embryology*, 3, 2; Benda Commission, *Working Group on In Vitro Fertilisation, Genom Analysis and Gene Therapy Report* (Bonn: Federal Ministry for Research and Technology,
1985), 6–7, 58; Comité Consultatif National d'Ethique (CCNE), "Opinion on Research and Use of
In-Vitro Human Embryos for Scientific and Medical Purposes," December 15, 1986, http://www.
ccne-ethique.fr/docs/en/avis008.pdf.

pro-life allies. But it also was evident in the United Kingdom, where Anne McLaren, a leading scientist and member of the Warnock committee, lashed out against "fundamentalists" in 1990.[4]

Amid this polarization, the basic framework for ethical contestation that had emerged by the mid-1980s generally persisted. Voices as diverse as the utilitarian bioethicist Peter Singer and Pope John Paul II acknowledged both the moral status of the embryo and the promise of research as key issues—even while reaching very different conclusions. "The human embryo is a member of the species *Homo Sapiens,*" Singer wrote in 1990, while insisting that it could be used in research as long as it was incapable of feeling pain. For Pope John Paul II, by contrast, biomedical research was a positive good, but human life was a gift of God to be welcomed and nurtured from fertilization onward.[5] These and other research proponents and opponents reached sharply divergent conclusions but agreed broadly on the terms of debate.

This running argument began to break down with news of the embryonic stem cell and cloning breakthroughs of 1997–98. The prospect of a new era of regenerative medicine cast the fate of thousands of surplus IVF embryos in a new light, while the promise of therapeutic cloning to aid victims of Alzheimer's, Parkinson's, and other degenerative diseases made the creation and destruction of embryos in research seem less objectionable to many. Here was an occasion to reflect anew on how to combine respect for the embryo with solidarity with the sick. Instead, the debate within and across ethics committees and legislatures degenerated too often into charges and counter-charges. Research opponents typically refused to acknowledge the promise of embryonic stem cells or to reflect on what should be done with thousands of frozen embryos available for research that were destined to perish in any case. Research supporters, for their part, tended to dismiss the question of the moral status of the embryo by referring simply to "stem cells" or "cloned cells" with no mention of their origin.

The careful analysis and framing of policy alternatives typical of the national committees of the 1970s and 1980s gave way to a cacophony of different bodies, often stacked in support of one side or the other. One set of committees, dominated by scientists, doctors, and secular bioethicists,

---

4. Anne McLaren, "Research on the Human Conceptus and Its Regulation in Britain Today," *Journal of the Royal Society of Medicine* 83, no. 4 (1990): 212.

5. Singer's phrase, originally published in 1982, is in Peter Singer and Helga Kuhse, *Unsanctifying Human Life* (Oxford: Blackwell, 2002), 184. See Pope John Paul II, "Address of John Paul II to Members of the Pontifical Academy of Sciences," October 23, 1982, http://www.vatican.va/holy_father/john_paul_ii/speeches/1982/october/documents/hf_jp-ii_spe_19821023_pont-accademia-scienze_en.html.

came to overlapping conclusions. The National Bioethics Advisory Council in the United States (1999), the Donaldson committee in the United Kingdom (2000), the German National Ethics Council (2004), and the CCNE in France (2001) all supported the derivation of stem cells from surplus IVF embryos, while differing over therapeutic cloning. The President's Council on Bioethics set up by President George W. Bush in 2001 was more cautious on research, as was a select committee set up by the House of Lords that same year. In Germany, a Bundestag investigative commission in 2001 rejected even the idea of importing embryonic stem cells derived elsewhere, while in France, a 2006 parliamentary commission report was more supportive of both embryonic stem cell and therapeutic cloning than was the CCNE.

Within the committees themselves there was less genuine deliberation and questioning than in the earlier era. Public and private expert hearings typically brought together representatives of different positions, but many if not most committee members appear to have taken up their work with their minds already made up. Scientists and their allies generally showed little concern with the moral status of the embryo, while embryo research opponents downplayed the promise of embryonic stem cell research. The 2006 French parliamentary commission on stem cells, for example, insisted that the embryo's fate was not a quandary for the polity but belonged mainly "to the most intimate sphere of each individual." The contrast with the CCNE's seminal 1986 report, which reflected in detail on the broader ethical and other implications of the embryo's status as a "potential human person," was striking.[6] On the other side of the issue, Catholic members of different committees were careful not to stray from the Church's principled opposition to research under all circumstances. Almost completely absent were Catholic moral theologians of the stature of Richard McCormick (Ethics Advisory Board) and Franz Böckle (Benda Commission), who had once wrestled with how best to uphold the moral status of the embryo and support life-giving research.

Shifting Historical and Institutional Legacies

This first trend—the rise and fall of a productive ethical debate setting the moral status of the embryo against the promise of research—unfolded alongside a second: a shift in the way that historical and institutional legacies

6. Alain Claeys, *Rapport sur les recherché sur le fonctionnement des cellules humaines* (Paris: Office parlementaire d'évaluation des choix scientifiques et technologiques, 2006), 9.

shaped policy outcomes. In all four countries the rise of the embryo as a focus of ethical contestation by the mid-1980s intersected with previous political and policy legacies—the liberalization of abortion in the United States and the United Kingdom and eugenics and the legacy of Nazism in Germany and, to a lesser degree, in France. During the 1980s Catholic and evangelical leaders in the United States were able to fold embryo research into a politically potent pro-life agenda; in the United Kingdom they tried, but failed. In Germany, Nazi eugenics and the legacy of the Holocaust provided a powerful rallying point for opponents of embryo research; in France, the Nazi legacy and a constitutional commitment to human dignity initially favored a cautious approach to research as well.

In the United States, the pro-life movement gradually took up the embryo research issue in the 1980s, less than a decade after the 1973 *Roe v. Wade* Supreme Court decision that legalized abortion. Republican presidents, unwilling to offend an important part of their constituency, refused to implement the proresearch recommendations of the EAB. In the United Kingdom, where Catholics and evangelicals were less of a force, an initial surge of pro-life mobilization in the mid-1980s was overtaken by a strong proresearch coalition that included scientists, patient advocates, and most of the leadership of the Church of England. In Germany and France, the Nazi experience and the focus on human dignity embedded in postwar constitutional orders favored those suspicious of embryo research as an instrumentalization of human life and possible step down a slippery slope to a eugenic future. In all of the cases except the United Kingdom, once the embryo moved onto the political agenda the force of historical legacies pushed policy in a more restrictive direction than ethics committees had advocated.

During the second phase of embryo politics, from the late 1990s onward, these deeper historical legacies had less immediate political impact. Pro-life mobilization was not as powerful, in part because destroying embryos for the sake of regenerative medicine appeared to many to stretch the abortion parallel, especially in the case of surplus IVF embryos without any prospect of becoming children. In Germany and France, where abortion had never framed the debate, the deeper legacy of the Nazi past faded, obscured both by the passage of time and by the emergence of the new, hopeful frontier of regenerative medicine. The German ethical debate gradually broadened to include the possibility of loosening the restrictive Embryo Protection Law. In France, research supporters shifted the focus on human dignity from the embryo to the victims of degenerative disease and construed the destruction of embryos to derive stem cells as a case of what the CCNE termed "virtual

solidarity between parents, a life that is not to be, and those who might benefit from research."[7]

If national historical legacies had less of an impact during the second
phase of embryo politics, more recent institutional legacies mattered more.
The policy regimes forged from 1990 through 1995 constrained the efforts
of research supporters to open up embryonic stem cell and therapeutic research. A political logic was in play. Opponents of far-reaching liberalization
could argue that the existing policies represented the outcome of a legitimate
political process that should be respected. Moreover, national leaders tended
to see few political benefits in revisiting the divisive ethical controversies
that had culminated in the status quo. In Germany, for example, research
supporters within the major parties were reluctant openly to challenge the
1990 Embryo Protection Law. In France, the 2004 revisions of the 1994
National Bioethics Laws marked only an incremental departure: permission
to derive embryonic stem cells for an exceptional and provisional five-year
period. President Barack Obama also followed this cautious political logic.
On coming to power in 2009 he relaxed George W. Bush's stem cell policy
but did not seek to overturn the Dickey Amendment that outlawed the use
of federal funds for the derivation of embryonic stem cells—to the chagrin
of many of his supporters.

One should not overestimate the path-dependent effects of existing institutions.[8] Opposition to far-reaching change in Germany and France remained linked back to deeper historical legacies of Nazism and eugenics.
Obama's decision not to press for a repeal of the Dickey Amendment was a
function of the overall political constellation, not just the force of the institutional status quo. In order fully to grasp trends in the evolution of embryo
politics, including the push to liberalize established policy regimes and the
limits it encountered, one must also bring in electoral and interest group
competition.

Growing Political Salience

A key difference between the first and second phases of embryo politics was
the increased political salience of stem cell and cloning research. In the late
1970s and early 1980s the emergence of the moral status of the embryo as an

---

7. CCNE, "Opinion on the Preliminary Draft Revision of the Laws on Bioethics," January 18,
2001, http://ccne-ethique.fr/docs/en/avis067.pdf.

8. For a fuller discussion see Thomas Banchoff, "Path Dependence and Value-Driven Issues:
The Comparative Politics of Stem Cell Research," *World Politics* 57, no. 2 (2005): 200–30.

issue for national ethics committees took place without much public notice or political controversy. The EAB in the United States labored in relative obscurity in 1978–79; its recommendations were drawn into abortion politics only later. The birth of the first IVF children—1978 in the United Kingdom, 1981 in the United States, and 1982 in Germany and France—and the subsequent deliberations of the Warnock and other national ethics committees generated some media attention. Only with the legislative struggles that began in 1985 in the United Kingdom and later emerged in other countries did embryo research register as a political issue for parties and interest groups.

Through the mid-1990s its political salience remained sharply circumscribed. Many Catholic and evangelical leaders and allied pro-life groups were mobilized around the embryo research issue, as were some scientific and medical associations and—particularly in the United Kingdom—an emerging patient-advocacy community. For parties and elected officials more concerned with economic and social questions, however, IVF and embryo research were a sideshow. The leadership of both the Conservative and Labour parties in the United Kingdom was broadly proresearch; the issue did not serve to differentiate one from the other. The two major German parties, the Christian Democrats and the Social Democrats, were generally skeptical of embryo research, while the left wing of the SPD and the smaller Green Party were radically opposed. The German Free Democrats were proresearch in orientation but had less political influence.

The issue had greatest political salience in the United States and France, for several related reasons. It tended to map onto the left-right split in each country, which in turn was reinforced by a religious-secular divide. The election of Bill Clinton in 1992 created an opening for research supporters that closed again after the Republican takeover of Congress two years later and the passage of the restrictive Dickey Amendment in 1995. In France, laws allowing for some embryo research passed a first parliamentary hurdle in early 1992 but were derailed when the Socialist government lost power to a center-right coalition that put its stamp on the restrictive 1994 laws. In neither country did the embryo issue rival the major economic, social, and foreign policy controversies of the day. Nevertheless, in both, electoral swings between the Left and the Right shaped policy outcomes.

Salience grew in all four countries with the cloning and stem cell breakthroughs and hopes for a new era of regenerative medicine. Interest group mobilization broadened in support of research, given its potential. Scientific and medical associations were more aggressive in making their case and could now count on the support of a broad array of patient-advocacy groups hoping for cures for a wide range of degenerative diseases afflicting millions.

A new wave of biotechnology companies eager to help develop and market new stem cell therapies joined this proresearch mobilization. The media picked up on letters and statements by Nobel Prize–winning scientists in favor of stem cell and cloning research and the personal testimonials of celebrities, including Christopher Reeve (star of *Superman*) and Michael J. Fox (star of *Back to the Future*). On both sides of the Atlantic, the Catholic Church and its allies in the pro-life movement found themselves increasingly on the defensive, as more and more denominations, as well as Jewish and Muslim communities, lent their support to embryonic stem cell and therapeutic cloning research.

The groundswell of interest group mobilization in support of research, covered sympathetically in the media and mirrored in public opinion trends, had a political impact. Powerful groups, including the American Biotechnology Industry Organization, the French Muscular Dystrophy Association, and the British Parkinson's Disease Society lobbied parties and legislatures for a liberalization of existing research regimes, with some success. A broad proresearch coalition benefited John Kerry in his effort to unseat George W. Bush in the 2004 presidential election, and a concerted AFM campaign in 2002–4 helped to convince enough conservative French legislators to countenance some embryonic stem cell research in the revisions to the Bioethics Laws. In the United Kingdom, Parliament may not have endorsed the creation of human-animal hybrid embryos without pressures applied by the Parkinson's Disease Society and its allies.

The greater political mobilization around stem cell research and the polarization it generated reinforced the impoverishment of public ethical debate. Confident that political momentum was with them, scientific, medical, biotechnology, and patient-advocacy groups were loath to admit that the research they so passionately supported raised any moral dilemmas at all. One cannot blame those with a stake in research for taking a one-sided view designed to mobilize public opinion and move elected officials. But where political leaders adopted this approach, critical moral issues were obscured. As early as February 1998, for example, Senator Edward Kennedy praised cloning research with "the potential to find new cures for cancer, diabetes, birth defects and genetic diseases of all kinds." But he made no mention of the cloned embryos that would serve as a source of cells. Neither did Tony Blair in setting out his support for therapeutic cloning on the eve of a critical House of Commons debate in October 2000, nor French prime minister Lionel Jospin in a programmatic speech on the topic the following month that described the procedure simply as the "transfer of somatic cells."[9]

---

9. Prime Minister's Office, "Speech by the Prime Minister at the European Bioscience Conference," press release, November 17, 2000.

For their part, research opponents in the policy struggle often refused to acknowledge the biomedical promise of embryonic stem cells and insisted dogmatically that adult stem cells and—after 2006—IPS cells held greater scientific potential. Senator Sam Brownback, Republican of Kansas, for example, one of the fiercest opponents of embryo research in Congress, asserted matter-of-factly that "adult stem cell research has demonstrated a vastly greater potential to generate real treatments for real people"—a true statement in the context of already existing treatments, but questionable with respect to the potential future ones. After "25 years of embryonic stem cell research in animal models and a decade of work with human embryonic stem cells," he contended on the Senate floor, "what we have learned about embryonic stem cells is that they are very good at forming tumors."[10]

Like other opponents of embryo research, Brownback bypassed the question of the fate of thousands of frozen embryos left over from IVF treatments and whether they might be utilized in research directed toward regenerative medicine. One could argue that it made more sense to use those embryos in life-giving research rather than to discard them. Or one could insist that it was more humane to let them thaw and die. Instead of working through the ethical debate, research opponents tended to equate all embryonic stem cell research with abortion—whatever the sources of the embryos or the purpose of the research. In a definitive 2008 statement, the Vatican reiterated its opposition to the use of frozen embryos in research, while acknowledging the problem of what to do with them. Their fate was a "situation of injustice which in fact cannot be resolved."[11] The idea of embryo adoption as a way out of the dilemma, supported by Brownback and others, did not find much resonance on either side of the Atlantic.

The clearest evidence of how the politicization of embryo and stem cell research abetted the obfuscation of the ethical issues was a tendency on each side to refuse to engage the substantive arguments of the other. Research supporters often denounced their opponents as antiscience. "My reason for addressing you today," Blair said in his speech before the Commons vote in October 2000, "is to place firmly on record my support for science and my determination not to let us slip into any form of anti-science." In his speech the following month, Jospin questioned whether "philosophical, spiritual, or

10. Press Office of Senator Sam Brownback, "Brownback Applauds New Stem Cell Advances," press release, November 20, 2007, http://brownback.senate.gov/pressapp/record.cfm?id=287831.

11. Congregation for the Doctrine of the Faith, *Instruction Dignitatis Personae on Certain Bioethical Questions,* December 12, 2008, http://www.vatican.va/roman_curia/congregations/cfaith/documents/rc_con_cfaith_doc_20081208_dignitas-personae_en.html#_ftn36.

religious principles" should get in the way of scientific progress and the alle-viation of suffering. In March 2001, Chancellor Schröder attacked the "ide-ological blinders" blocking scientific progress in Germany, and Kerry taunted Bush in August 2004 with the implied accusation: "Here in America, we don't sacrifice science for ideology."[12] In all these cases, research supporters set up a false opposition between reason, on the one hand, and ideology on the other—not acknowledging that their stances, too, were linked back to particular philosophical and religious positions. The hopes raised by regen-erative medicine made it politically expedient to cast the issue, wrongly, as one of science against its enemies.

Research opponents, too, fell into the trap of dismissing their opponents as ideologues of a different stripe—uncritical cheerleaders for science. "Ad-vances in biomedical technology must never come at the expense of human conscience," Bush told his supporters at an anticloning forum in February 2002. "We can pursue medical research with a clear sense of moral purpose or we can travel without an ethical compass into a world we could live to regret." Rather than critique the ethical compass that many therapeutic cloning supporters did have—their unwavering enthusiasm for embryonic stem cell research out of solidarity with the victims of degenerative disease—Bush and other cloning opponents questioned their moral seriousness. Accusa-tions of bad faith on both sides negated opportunities to acknowledge and explore the ethical trade-offs and their policy implications.[13]

There were examples of thoughtful political interventions that explored the issues in more of their complexity. In a stinging rebuke to Jospin in Feb-ruary 2001, French president Chirac insisted that the perspectives opened up by embryonic stem cell research required a "profound debate." A "utili-tarian conception of the human being" should not be allowed to prevail, he declared, but neither should "humanity be deprived of the possibility of re-ducing suffering" over time. "To address these questions," he pointed out, "is the responsibility of politics." During his unsuccessful run for U.S. president in 2008 John McCain openly spoke of the difficult ethical trade-offs. "For those of us in the prolife community," he told a national audience at a public

---

12. Prime Minister's Office, "Speech by the UK Prime Minister, Mr. Tony Blair, at the Eu-ropean Bioscience Conference," January 17, 2000, http://www.monsanto.co.uk/news/ukshowlib. phtml?uid=4104;Lionel Jospin, "Allocution devant le Comité consultatif national d'éthique pour les sciences de la vie et de la santé," November 28, 2000; John Kerry, radio address August 7, 2004, quoted in "Kerry Takes on Issue of Embryo Research," *Washington Post,* August 8, 2004.

13. White House Press Office, "President Bush Calls on Senate to Back Human Cloning Ban," press release, April 10, 2002, http://georgewbush-whitehouse.archives.gov/news/releases/ 2002/04/20020410–4.html.

forum, embryonic stem cell research had been "a great struggle and a terrible dilemma because we're also taught other obligations that we have as well."[14]

Such acknowledgement of moral complexity was relatively rare in embryo politics. In the United Kingdom, where research supporters were in the ascendancy, there was little political reason to address the concerns of those often dismissed as "pro-lifers." And in Germany, where research supporters were outnumbered, there was less of an open engagement with the promise of embryonic stem cell and cloning research. In France and the United States, left-right and religious-secular tensions often militated against a constructive debate. In the American context, many embryonic stem cell and cloning-research advocates derided their opponents as fundamentalists and were accused, in turn, of relativism and secular humanism. In France it was the memory of Catholic Church power, more than its reality, that polarized the discussion. Research backers accused their opponents of pushing a religious agenda, even though the Church's impact was probably marginal and research opponents were extremely careful to couch their arguments in philosophical, not religious terms.

Transnational Linkages and the Primacy of the National

The three trends—the rise and fall of a constructive public ethical debate; the decline of deeper historical legacies and the rise of new institutions as a context for controversy; and greater political salience—all underscore the centrality of the nation-state as the context for embryo politics over its first four decades. At first glance, this might seem curious. Embryo and IVF research was an international enterprise from the outset, incorporating teams of researchers not only in the major Atlantic scientific powers, but also in Australia, Canada, Israel, elsewhere in Europe, and in the rising scientific powers of Asia. The ethical stakes also had a universal dimension, encompassing questions of life, death, and suffering that cut across countries and religious and philosophical traditions. Why, then, did the ethical and political controversies traced in this book have such a strong national character?

There were in fact a variety of transnational linkages. The pioneering work of Edwards and Steptoe, for example, received funding from the

---

14. Présidence de la République, "Allocution de M. Jacques Chirac Président de la République à l'occasion de l'ouverture du forum mondial des biotechnologies," press release, February 8, 2001, http://www.elysee.fr/elysee/elysee.fr/francais_archives/interventions/discours_et_declarations/2001/fevrier/allocution_de_m_jacques_chirac_president_de_la_republique_a_l_occasion_de_l_ouverture_du_forum_mondial_des_biotechnologies-lyon.3196.html; "Saddleback Presidential Candidates Forum," August 16, 2008, http://transcripts.cnn.com/TRANSCRIPTS/0808/16/se.02.html.

U.S.-based Ford Foundation. The idea of a fourteen-day cutoff point for research was first articulated by the EAB in 1979 and then incorporated into the Warnock committee report in the United Kingdom five years later. The pro-life movement developed most quickly and powerfully in the United States during the early 1980s and served as a catalytic example for antiabortion activists in the United Kingdom. The term "therapeutic cloning" was first coined in the United Kingdom and caught on in other countries. The debate over the Embryo Protection Law in Germany, with its strong anti-eugenic impetus, energized French research opponents. And Bush's August 2001 stem cell compromise—federally funded stem cell research, but only with cells already derived from embryos—served as a model of sorts for the German stem cell import law.

Just as often, however, transnational linkages served to reinforce the national character of the controversy. For example, French and German politicians denounced the prevalence of utilitarian thinking in American and British debates and criticized the term "pre-embryo" as a cynical effort to define the moral dilemmas of embryo research out of existence. Europeans expressed incomprehension in the face of the public-private distinction in the United States, which allowed the coexistence of drawn-out battles over government funding coupled with a laissez-faire attitude to research in the private sector. French, British, and German leaders distinguished the secular tenor of their bioethical debates from faith-filled American ones. And research supporters in the United Kingdom and France, when reminded of Germany's comprehensive ban on embryo research, balked at the idea of "taking lessons" from their ally and erstwhile enemy.

What about the constraints posed by international organizations on national debates? These remained weak over the entire period. The United Nations Educational, Scientific and Cultural Organization (UNESCO) engaged bioethical questions but served more as a discussion forum than as a governance institution. In the period from 2002 to 2005, the UN General Assembly took up the cloning issue but was unable to reach consensus on whether to endorse a comprehensive ban or prohibit its reproductive variant.[15] Even at the European level, international constraints were minimal. The Council of Europe's 1997 Biomedicine Convention addressed embryo research and other bioethical questions, but Germany rejected it as too lenient, Britain rejected it as too restrictive, and France signed but did not ratify it. Into the

---

15. Thomas Banchoff, "Religious Pluralism and the Politics of a Global Cloning Ban," in *Religious Pluralism, Globalization, and World Politics*, ed. Thomas Banchoff (Oxford: Oxford University Press, 2008), 275–96.

new century, the European Union wrangled over how to fund embryonic stem cell research but eventually decided to respect each member state's national laws. Europe, like the UN, remains a forum for debate about how to govern the ongoing revolution in the life sciences. But governance itself still resides predominantly at the national level.

An underlying reason for limited transnational and international constraints is the persistence of the nation-state as the key actor in world affairs, even in an era of globalization. On trade and monetary policy there is considerable international coordination and governance, particularly in the context of the European Union. However, value-driven issues such as abortion, euthanasia, and embryo research remain the almost exclusive preserves of nation-states. To be considered legitimate, decisions on divisive ethical issues must be reached by democratic institutions that are the focus of collective identity. Nation-states best meet that standard today. The French Council of State made this point in a 2009 report. International coordination on bioethical matters was fine as long as it did not undercut national law which, for France, was based on "fundamental principles" anchored in the "Declaration of the Rights of Man."[16]

New Scientific and Technological Frontiers

How different countries navigate future embryo politics will depend in large part on scientific and technological developments. The immediate focus of embryo politics over the next decade will likely remain stem cell research. Embryonic, adult, and IPS cell research all have the potential to revolutionize regenerative medicine. One decade into the new century, however, no one knows which will move most quickly and effectively from research in the laboratory to tissue replacement therapy in practice. As long as the competition is open, the arguments that took shape in 2006 through 2008 will likely persist. Some will insist on the parallel pursuit of multiple research programs, including embryonic stem cells and therapeutic cloning, and others will criticize the destruction of embryos in research and argue that IPS and adult stem cells should be the exclusive focus of attention.

Even if IPS cells should prove superior to embryonic stem cells, ethical and political controversy surrounding embryo research is unlikely to cease. Efforts to improve IVF techniques and combat infertility will involve experiments with embryos, as they have since the 1970s. And research on embryos,

---

16. Conseil d'Etat, *La révision des lois de bioéthique* (Paris: Conseil d'Etat, 2009), 105.

where it is permitted, will provide a window on human development during the first days and weeks after fertilization, filling knowledge gaps about the embryo's interaction with the environment and the origins of human disease. As stockpiles of frozen embryos from fertility clinics worldwide continue to grow, ethical controversy and policy struggles over when and whether they can be used in biomedical research will remain with us.

IPS technology might further increase the embryos available for experiments. Research made public in 2008–9 showed how somatic cells could be reprogrammed to become the equivalent of sperm and egg cells, a potential way to overcome egg shortages and create embryos more easily in the laboratory. Asked by the leading British scientific journal *Nature* in 2008 to look ahead on the thirtieth anniversary of the birth of Louise Brown, a leading developmental biologist speculated that "maybe 20–30 years from now we'll read in newspapers that someone made 20,000 embryos and studied their development and we'll decide it's OK."[17] Whether such technology proves feasible and whether or not it flourishes will depend on where the science goes, how the ethical problems are defined, and how they play out in national political contexts.

Two controversial areas moving onto the policy agenda are preimplantation genetic diagnosis and genetic enhancement. Each technology—one already in place, the other speculative—combines familiar questions about the moral status of the embryo and the alleviation of human suffering with broader controversies about human freedom, equality, and the future of evolution itself. The ethics and politics of each issue have begun to take shape in different ways on both sides of the Atlantic.

Preimplantation Genetic Diagnosis

Advances in human genetics and genomic analysis intersected with embryo research in the late 1980s to open up a new field of inquiry and practice—the screening of human embryos before their transfer to the womb. In 1990 a London-based research team led by Alan Handyside announced in *Nature* that they had determined the sex of embryos for several couples at risk of having children with diseases linked to the male chromosome. Only the female embryos were then implanted.[18] The procedure, which typically involved

---

17. Davor Solter quoted in Helen Pearson, "Making Babies: The Next 30 Years," *Nature* 454, no. 7202 (2008): 260.

18. Alan Handyside and E. H. Kontogianni, "Pregnancies from Biopsied Human Preimplantation Embryos Sexed by Y-Specific DNA Amplification," *Nature* 344 no. 6268 (1990): 768–70.

removing and testing cells from a three-day-old embryo, was subsequently extended beyond sex-linked disorders such as Duchenne muscular dystrophy, to single-gene diseases like cystic fibrosis and chromosomal abnormalities including Down syndrome. PGD got first sustained media attention in 2001, with a first "savior sibling" case in the United Kingdom involving parents' desire to screen embryos to insure the birth of a compatible tissue donor for a sick older child.

The possibility of genetic screening and selection of embryos had caught the attention of ethics committees and legislators before it became reality. In its 1985 report the German Benda Commission was open to the possibility of screening embryos for serious genetic diseases but warned that it might one day lead to the "eugenic selection of the embryos to be implanted as well as for the selection of the sex of the child desired." The restrictive 1990 Embryo Protection Law appeared to rule out PGD altogether.[19] In France, the CCNE's 1986 report on embryo research called for a moratorium on any "pre-transfer genetic diagnosis," fearing it "could lead to ethically reprehensible practices of standardising human reproduction for reasons of health or convenience."[20] The 1994 Bioethics Laws would allow for PGD only when a couple had a high probability of giving birth to a child with a severe genetic disease. The U.K. Human Fertilisation and Embryology Authority, created through 1990 legislation, permitted but carefully regulated the use of PGD in the years that followed.

In the United States, the technology was not yet on the horizon of the Ethics Advisory Board in 1979; fifteen years later, it was welcomed by the 1994 Human Embryo Research Panel as a way to screen for serious genetic diseases. In the meantime, PGD technology had begun to spread through the largely unregulated U.S. fertility industry. Around the turn of the century, a practice illegal in the United Kingdom, Germany, and France—embryo selection for sex for nonmedical reasons—was offered by more and more fertility clinics. In 1999 the ethics committee of a leading professional association, the American Society for Reproductive Medicine, issued nonbinding guidelines advising against PGD for sex selection. When in September 2001 the chair of the committee suggested that embryo selection for "family balancing"

Edwards had suggested the possibility of PGD for sex-linked diseases as early as 1971. See Robert G. Edwards and David J. Sharpe, "Social Values and Research in Human Embryology," *Nature* 231, no. 5298 (1971): 87–91.

19. Benda Commission, *Working Group on In Vitro Fertilisation,* 80.

20. CCNE, "Opinion on Embryo Research Aiming to Achieve Pre-Transfer Genetic Diagnosis for Which a Moratorium Was Declared in 1986," July 18, 1990, http://www.ccne-ethique.fr/docs/en/avis019.pdf.

might indeed be permissible, a media backlash ensued, including a critical editorial in the *New York Times*. The ethics committee affirmed its continued opposition to the practice, and the chair retreated, expressing doubt that "a couple's desire for gender variety in offspring is sufficient to outweigh the need to show special respect to embryos."[21] Despite these recommendations the practice proliferated. A 2006 study found that three quarters of the U.S.-based fertility clinics surveyed offered PGD services and that two-fifths of those offered a sex-selection option.[22]

No political drive for regulation has ensued. In a 2004 report the President's Council on Bioethics noted the absence of any "governmental body, state or federal, monitoring or regulating PGD."[23] Further controversies—such as an offer by a Los Angeles–based clinic in 2009 to select embryos based on hair and eye color—sparked outrage in the media but no sustained legislative action. In the meantime, ethical and policy debate proceeded on the other side of the Atlantic. In the United Kingdom, the HFEA launched a public consultation on PGD in 2005 and, the following year, approved its use in new areas, including testing for late-onset diseases such as breast and ovarian cancers. Parliament passed legislation outlawing PGD for nonmedical sex selection in 2008, confirming longstanding HFEA policy.[24] In January 2003 a slim majority of the German National Ethics Council came out in favor of PGD to prevent severe genetic diseases, provoking a barrage of criticism and revealing the lack of political interest in lifting the country's blanket prohibition. France continued to move cautiously. In a 2002 opinion the CCNE majority opposed extending the use of PGD beyond serious genetic diseases, but the 2004 Bioethics Law did approve the possibility of "savior siblings" in certain cases.[25]

As the science and technology of PGD improves, future ethical and political battles may be fought over efforts to select embryos on a wider variety of criteria. The ability to routinely and inexpensively decipher the genome of an embryo—only years away—will combine with increasing knowledge of the genetic contribution to human physical and behavioral characteristics,

---

21. "Choosing the Sex of Your Baby," *New York Times*, September 30, 2001.

22. Susannah Baruch, David Kaufman, and Kathy L. Hudson, "Genetic Testing of Embryos: Practices and Perspectives of U.S. IVF Clinics," *Fertility and Sterility* 89, no. 5 (2006): 1053–58.

23. President's Council on Ethics, *Reproduction and Responsibility: The Regulation of New Biotechnologies* (Washington, DC: President's Council on Bioethics, 2004), 102.

24. Human Fertilisation and Embryology Authority, *Outcome of the Public Consultation on Preimplantation Genetic Diagnosis* (London: Human Fertilisation and Embryology Authority, 2001).

25. Nationaler Ethikrat, *Genetic Diagnosis before and during Pregnancy* (Berlin: German National Ethics Council, 2003); CCNE, "Reflections concerning an Extension of Preimplantation Genetic Diagnosis," July 4, 2002, http://www.ccne-ethique.fr/docs/en/avis072.pdf.

giving parents more options. In 2010, on the twentieth anniversary of his breakthrough, Handyside suggested that "improved sequencing technologies and progress in identifying genetic variants that contribute to trait heritability will lead to increasingly accurate predictions." That knowledge could extend to "an embryo's future risk of diabetes, cancer, schizophrenia and other common diseases." It might also extend to traits that Handyside did not mention, such as sexual orientation, propensity to obesity or alcoholism, and characteristics including height, strength, intelligence, and memory. Most human characteristics have complex genetic and environmental bases, and embryo selection may fail to achieve its desired ends. In any case, the demand for PGD and its extension into new areas is likely to grow in the decades ahead—as will controversy surrounding it.

Genetic Enhancement

Future controversy surrounding PGD may intersect with the ethical and policy challenges posed by a more speculative frontier technology: genetic enhancement. The idea of improving the human race through scientific means, articulated by the eugenic movement of the first half of the twentieth century and discredited by Nazi racist policies, reemerged in a new guise after World War II with the discovery of the structure of DNA and the dramatic progress of molecular biology. During the 1960s, some leading scientists, including the American geneticist and Nobel laureate Joshua Lederberg, welcomed the prospect of "engineering of human development." Others were less sanguine. The Swiss zoologist Adolf Portmann saw humanity "on the brink of a dark contemporary era which envisions the biotechnological breeding of human beings." The prospect of humanity taking evolution into its own hands, most forcefully portrayed in Aldous Huxley's dystopian 1932 novel, *Brave New World,* was still far off. But it appeared to be moving closer.

The first fertilization of a human egg in the laboratory in 1968 provoked new speculation about the possibility of human genetic enhancement, as did the birth of Louise Brown a decade later.[26] In both these instances, media fascination with eugenics and the possibility of a new race of superhumans gradually subsided with the awareness of the huge scientific and technological barriers still to be overcome. It was one thing to alter the genetic makeup of single-celled organisms such as bacteria—a technology in place by the mid-1970s—but quite another to work with mammals or humans.

---

26. Robert L. Sinsheimer, "Genetic Engineering: The Modification of Man," *Impact of Science on Society* 20, no. 4 (1970): 280.

Understanding of the human genome was limited, and the technical obstacles to adding and deleting genes in a laboratory embryo were tremendous. Into the 1980s, national ethics committees and civil servants focused their attention on efforts to heal genetic diseases in body cells through somatic cell gene therapy. The more distant frontier of modifying germ cells and embryos capable of passing genetic changes to future generations occasioned little debate.

In the meantime, however, a series of quiet technological breakthroughs were bringing that frontier closer. The early 1980s saw the first successful inheritable genetic modifications in mice. The technology gradually spread to other mammals and was first demonstrated in sheep in 2000 and primates in 2001. Advances in cloning and stem cell manipulation were also critical. With the announcement of Dolly in 1997 and subsequent cloning of other mammals, scientists learned how to derive stem cells from embryos, to add or delete genes, and then observe and test the modified cells before cloning embryos with the desired characteristics. The future use of this technique as a possible way to modify humans was not lost on observers. In the wake of the first successful isolation of human embryonic stem cells in November 1998, a *Washington Post* story saw in them "a relatively simple method for creating 'designer' babies bearing specific genetic traits."[27]

While the perfection of any such methods remained decades away, national ethics committees touched on the possibility of genetic modification and enhancement relatively early. The charge to the EAB in 1978 noted public concerns about "selective breeding" and "attempts to control the genetic makeup of offspring," but the group did not take up those speculative issues.[28] One of the first sustained discussions goes back to 1979, when a group of Jewish, Protestant, and Roman Catholic leaders convinced President Jimmy Carter to put the issue on the agenda of the new President's Commission for the Study of Ethical Problems in Medicine and Biomedical and Behavioral Research. The commission's 1982 report, *Splicing Life,* focused mainly on the science and ethics of somatic gene therapy but also addressed genetic modification under the heading of "zygote therapy." It condemned the technology as unfeasible, unsafe, and ethically problematic— particularly if it were deployed not just to repair defects but also to enhance

27. "A Crucial Human Cell Is Isolated, Multiplied," *Washington Post,* November 6, 1998.

28. Joseph A. Califano, *Inside: A Public and Private Life* (New York: PublicAffairs, 2004), 350–51. Also quoted in "HEW Urged to Lift Ban on Test-Tube Birth Studies," *Washington Post,* September 16, 1978.

characteristics.[29] No federal legislation on genetic modification was passed over the next two decades, but the National Institutes of Health did make explicit in 1985 that it would not "at present entertain proposals for germ line alterations."[30]

In Europe, the Warnock committee report of 1984 mentioned genetic modification under the heading "prevention of genetic defects," noting it might one day be possible to "insert a replacement gene which will remedy" a defect in an embryo. Such modification raised fewer ethical problems than enhancement. "Public anxiety about these techniques centres, not so much on their possible therapeutic use, but on the idea of the deliberate creation of human beings with specific characteristics," the report noted. "This has overtones of selective breeding." There was no call for a ban on genetic modification because the techniques were "purely speculative." While the 1990 U.K. legislation did not mention the issue, subsequent HFEA regulations explicitly prohibited "altering the genetic structure of any cell while it forms part of an embryo."[31]

The discussion of genetic modification and enhancement was even more perfunctory in French and German ethics committees and government circles. The Benda Commission was outspoken about eugenic dangers in its 1985 report, noting the potential therapeutic applications of genetic modification but also that "measures have to be taken to avert the danger of man being manipulated by genetic engineers."[32] While the Embryo Protection Law of 1990 did not mention genetic modification as a possibility, its strictures on embryo research prohibited it in law and practice. In France, the CCNE's 1986 report warned of future "interventions defining human beings, which awaken or reawaken the spectre of eugenics." The committee's 1990 opinion called for a "formal prohibition of any attempt to perform germinal gene therapy."[33] And the 1994 Bioethics Laws altered the French civil code so as to prohibit "any eugenic practice which aims at organizing the selection of

---

29. President's Commission for the Study of Ethical Problems in Medicine and Biomedical and Behavioral Research, *Splicing Life: The Social and Ethical Issues of Genetic Engineering with Human Beings* (Washington, DC: U.S. Government Printing Office, 1982), 48. The report noted that without genetic diagnosis of embryos—a technology not yet established at the time—"the use of gene splicing as a 'treatment' seems dubious."

30. Quoted in Albert R. Jonsen, Robert M. Veatch, and LeRoy Walters, eds., *Source Book in Bioethics: A Documentary History* (Washington, DC: Georgetown University Press, 1998), 315.

31. Human Fertilisation and Embryology Authority, *Code of Practice*, 6th ed. (London: Human Fertilisation and Embryology Authority, 2003), 93.

32. Benda Commission, *Working Group on In Vitro Fertilisation*, 4.

33. CCNE, "Opinion on Gene Therapy," December 13, 1990, http://www.ccne-ethique.fr/docs/en/avis022.pdf.

persons," and stated that "there may be no alteration [of genetic characteristics] with a view to changing the descent of a person."[34]

The cloning and stem cell breakthroughs of 1997–98 and the deciphering of the human genome in the years that followed sparked some further reflection on genetic modification and enhancement. The most comprehensive treatment grew out of a working group set up by the American Association for the Advancement of Science consisting of scientists, ethicists, theologians, and policy analysts. After three years of deliberation and study, its report reached mainly negative conclusions. "Over a long period of time, germ line gene modification could be used to decrease the incidence of certain inherited diseases in the human gene pool currently causing great suffering," it noted. In the meantime, though, significant technical obstacles, safety issues, and ethical concerns remained: "Genes that are transmitted to future generations have the potential to bring about not only a medical, but also a social revolution, for they offer us the power to mold our children in a variety of novel ways."[35]

Future Paths of Embryo Politics

At the end of the first decade of the twenty-first century, embryo selection, modification, and enhancement technologies are at an early phase of development, as is the ethical and policy struggle around them. It is not too early, however, to sketch the emerging contours of controversy and how they both extend and break with post-1968 patterns. Knowing where we have been can help to map out and select possible futures.

By the mid-1980s, embryo politics had come to center on debates about the moral status of the embryo and the promise of biomedical research. The stem cell and cloning breakthroughs of 1997–98 and the rise of an ethic of healing strained, but did not dismantle, those terms of debate. Research proponents increasingly dismissed the relevance of the embryo's moral status, and opponents often refused to recognize the promise of embryonic stem cells. But even as the quality of public debate declined amid charges and countercharges, two core questions remained: When does fully human life begin and deserve protection? And under what conditions can embryos be created

---

34. *French Civil Code,* translated by Georges Rouhette with Ann Berton, Legisfrance.gouv.fr, February 21, 2004, http://www.legifrance.gouv.fr/html/codes_traduits/code_civil_textA.htm.

35. Mark S. Frankel and Audrey R. Chapman, *Human Inheritable Genetic Modifications: Assessing Scientific, Ethical, Religious, and Policy Issues* (Washington, DC: American Academy for the Advancement of Science, 2000), 3–4.

and destroyed to advance biomedical knowledge that might alleviate human suffering? How to combine respect for the embryo and solidarity with the sick remained a moral quandary, even if increasingly obscured by polemics and polarized policy debates.

PGD and genetic enhancement link back to this moral quandary as well. Both technologies raise questions about the moral status of the embryo as an object to be observed and discarded or, in the case of enhancement, manipulated. Both engage the possibility of a future reduction in suffering through the selection or engineering of embryos with better health and life chances. Not surprisingly, principled opponents of all embryo research such as the Catholic Church also tend to oppose all PGD and genetic engineering. The Vatican has already gone on record against both practices.[36] Many supporters of embryo, stem cell, and cloning research are more open to both technologies. The bioethicist Peter Singer, for example, has no principled objection to the selecting or manipulation of embryos, should it contribute to greater human flourishing.[37]

While the emerging debate about embryo selection and enhancement links back to established controversies, it also raises new questions about freedom, equality, and the future of human evolution that were less salient during the first few decades of embryo politics. One should be wary of generalization, because the fronts are still ill-defined and the selection and enhancement issues differ in important respects, but two broad camps are already taking shape.

For one camp, PGD and genetic enhancement represent a danger in the form of liberal eugenics that threaten human freedom, equality, and the integrity of the human species. In this optic, children selected on important traits or engineered for them would have a diminished sense of autonomy; greater parental power would reduce their experience of freedom. Moreover, uneven access to the technologies would reinforce existing social inequalities and marginalize the disabled, who would increasingly be stigmatized as "mistakes." Genetic enhancement technologies, if allowed to proceed, could alter the future of human evolution and culminate in the creation of a genetic caste system or even the splitting off of a new, superhuman species. Leading thinkers and commentators who have voiced some of these concerns include

---

36. See, most recently, *Instruction Dignitatis Personae on Certain Bioethical Questions.*

37. Peter Singer, "Shopping at the Genetic Supermarket," foreword to *The Ethics of Inheritable Genetic Modification: A Dividing Line?* ed. John E. J. Rasko, Gabrielle O'Sullivan, and Rachel A. Ankeny (Cambridge: Cambridge University Press, 2006), xiii–xxxi.

Leon Kass and Francis Fukuyama in the United States, Jürgen Habermas in Germany, and Jacques Testart in France.[38]

An opposing camp sees the new technologies as an occasion for hope, not fear. Some scholars question whether embryo selection or enhancement will reduce a child's sense of autonomy, given that parents already exercise tremendous power over the formation of their offspring. Others acknowledge the problem of unequal access to new technologies and the stigmatization of the disabled, but insist that the state can step in to close the access gap and guarantee the social and political equality of all its citizens. And they note earlier dramatic breaks in human biological and cultural evolution, feared at the time and now accepted, and ask whether humanity should not use the knowledge at its disposal to steer its course for the better. Among those who have taken up and developed one or more of these arguments are Ronald Green and Lee Silver in the United States, John Harris, Julian Savulescu, and Nick Bostrom in the United Kingdom, Peter Sloterdijk in Germany, and Bernard Debré in France.[39]

The clash between critics and supporters of these frontier technologies is now taking place more often at academic conferences than on national bioethics committees. The debate has yet to move into the media spotlight or onto the public agenda in any sustained fashion. Even at this early stage in the controversy, however, national histories and institutions are framing the issue. The legacy of Nazi eugenics is particularly salient in Germany, where Sloterdijk's favorable speculations on genetic selection brought down a storm of criticism from Habermas and others. In France, debates between Testart, Frydman, and others revolve around the negative legacy of eugenics and its relationship to France's positive revolutionary and Enlightenment tradition. In the United States and the United Kingdom, where eugenics has

---

38. Leon R. Kass, *Life, Liberty, and the Defense of Dignity: The Challenge for Bioethics* (San Francisco: Encounter Books, 2002); Francis Fukuyama, *Our Posthuman Future: Consequences of the Biotechnology Revolution* (New York: Farrar, Straus and Giroux, 2002); Jürgen Habermas, *The Future of Human Nature* (Cambridge: Polity, 2003); Jacques Testart, *Des hommes probables: De la procréation aléatoire à la reproduction normative* (Paris: Seuil, 1999).

39. Ronald Michael Green, *Babies by Design: The Ethics of Genetic Choice* (New Haven: Yale University Press, 2007); Lee M. Silver, *Remaking Eden: Cloning and Beyond in a Brave New World* (New York: Avon Books, 1997); John Harris, *Enhancing Evolution: The Ethical Case for Making Better People* (Princeton: Princeton University Press, 2007); Julian Savulescu and Nick Bostrom, *Human Enhancement* (Oxford: Oxford University Press, 2009); Peter Sloterdijk, *Regeln für den Menschenpark: Ein Antwortschreiben zu Heideggers Brief über den Humanismus* (Frankfurt am Main: Suhrkamp, 1999); Bernard Debré, *La grande transgression: L'homme génétiquement modifié* (Neuilly-sur-Seine, Fr.: Lafon, 2000). Debré has expressed support for "an individualized eugenics, synonymous with liberty, framed within a law that prohibits any state eugenics." See his debate with Christine Boutin in "Clonage thérapeutique: Progrès ou danger?" *L'Express*, January 19, 2006.

less historical resonance, supporters of the new technologies are more numerous and vocal. A "transhumanist" movement, committed to improving the physical and mental capacities of human beings through technology, has emerged in both countries.[40] In the United States, in particular, the absence of clear national regulation of PGD and genetic enhancement technologies has encouraged a more free-wheeling debate.

What can be gleaned from the first four decades of embryo politics as lessons for the next four, and beyond? Two stand out: widely different policy responses to the same scientific and technological breakthroughs are possible; and serious ethical reflection and contestation can inform those responses.

The history of embryo politics shows the decisive role of the state in the governance of research and its trajectory. The scientific community governs itself in key respects by validating new knowledge through peer review. Its own competitive dynamics drive inquiry into new domains, including the development of human life from its earliest stages. However, governments can and do set limits on what is permitted and, through funding mechanisms, they shape the evolution of research agendas. Over four decades, the leading Atlantic scientific powers provided legal frameworks encompassing what can and cannot be done with embryos in the laboratory. State governance will continue to matter going forward. The routine selection of embryos for positive physical and mental traits will almost certainly take place somewhere in the world at some point, as will efforts at human genetic enhancement. But whether such research and practices take hold in particular countries will depend on political struggles and policy outcomes.

The divergent responses of the United States, United Kingdom, Germany, and France to scientific and technological revolutions during the first four post-1968 decades suggests a variety of national approaches going forward, ranging from the restrictive to the liberal. It is possible to criminalize all experiments with embryos, as in Germany and—through 2004—in France; to regulate research at the national level, as in Britain; or to have different policies for the public and private sectors, as in the United States. Of course, elected leaders cannot simply look abroad for policy models. Their own national historical legacies, institutions, and electoral and interest group politics constrain the options at their disposal. Still, awareness of the choices made in other national contexts can enrich the policy debate by suggesting a wider range of alternatives.

---

40. More recently, transhumanists have preferred the label "humanity+." See, for example, http://www.humanityplus.org/.

The history of embryo politics also shows how serious ethical reflection can inform that policy debate and its outcomes. In the decades after 1968, advances in IVF and embryo research challenged academics, practitioners, and policymakers to puzzle through moral dilemmas concerning the protection of life and obligations to the sick. Some supporters of IVF as an infertility treatment wrestled with whether to support the embryo research necessary to make it safe and effective. Supporters of infertility-related experiments later had to decide for or against the destruction of embryos for other research programs, including stem cells and regenerative medicine. Some generally opposed to embryo research asked whether surplus IVF embryos destined to die in any case might not be used in pursuit of worthy biomedical goals. At the same time, those who rejected the deliberate creation of embryos for research as an illicit instrumentalization of human life were confronted with therapeutic cloning as a possible means to advance regenerative medicine. Each of these developments provided new occasion to draw on philosophical and religious resources to puzzle through difficult ethical trade-offs.

At the turn of the century, as embryo politics grew more polarized, pro- and antiresearch positions hardened and the quality of ethical debate declined. That trend need not persist into the future. The four decades covered in this book provide many examples of public reflection on complex moral dilemmas. Given the policy challenges that lie ahead we will need to build on that legacy. The problem of the moral status of the embryo will always be with us, as will the imperative to alleviate suffering and promote human flourishing. The prospect of genetic selection and engineering raise new and momentous questions about human freedom, equality, and the future of evolution.

We are called to take up those questions and decide where we come down, as individuals and as members of national political communities—through an open and critical exchange of ethical perspectives on new developments. Given the stakes for the human future, science and technology that touch the beginning of human life must be governed. We may not make the right decisions. But we should make them our own.

❦ Bibliography

Abbott, Alison. "Stem Cell Research in Doubt as Funders Clash with Government." *Nature* 411, no. 6834 (2001): 119–20.

Abel, Olivier. "Biologie et éthique." *Etudes théologiques et réligieuses* no. 2 (1987): 198–208.

Académie des sciences de l'Institut de France and Académie Nationale de Médecine (French Academy of Sciences and National Academy of Medicine). "Recommandations de l'Académie des sciences et de l'Académie Nationale de Médecine relatives à l'utilisation de cellules souches embryonnaires humaines." June 10, 2002. http://www.academie-sciences.fr/actualites/textes/cellules_souches_10_06_02.pdf.

Académie Nationale de Médecine. "Communiqué concernant le projet de loi relatif à la bioéthique." January 8, 2002.

Agence de la biomedicine (French Biomedicine Agency). *Bilan d'application de la loi de bioéthique du 6 août 2004*. Paris: Agence de la biomédecine, 2008.

All-Party Parliamentary Pro-Life Group. "Response of the All-Party Parliamentary Pro-Life Group to the HGAC/HFEA Consultation Paper 'Cloning Issues in Reproduction, Science and Medicine'." April 1998.

American Association for the Advancement of Science. "President Bush's Stem Cell Policy: A Statement of the American Association for the Advancement of Science." August 17, 2001. http://www.aaas.org/spp/cstc/docs/01–08-17_stemstmt.htm.

American Fertility Society. "Ethical Considerations of the New Reproductive Technologies." In *Source Book in Bioethics: A Documentary History*. Edited by Albert R. Jonsen, Robert M. Veatch, and LeRoy Walters, 358–68. Washington, DC: Georgetown University Press, 1998.

Annas, George J. "Ethics Committees: From Ethical Comfort to Ethical Cover." *Hastings Center Report* 21, no. 3 (1991): 18–21.

———. "Why We Should Ban Human Cloning." *New England Journal of Medicine* 339, no. 2 (1998): 122–25.

Annas, George J., Arthur Caplan, and Sherman Elias. "The Politics of Human-Embryo Research: Avoiding Ethical Gridlock." *New England Journal of Medicine* 334, no. 20 (1996): 1329–32.

———. "Stem Cell Politics, Ethics and Medical Progress." *Nature Medicine* 5, no. 12 (1999): 1339–41.

Annas, George J., and Sherman Elias. "Politics, Morals and Embryos." *Nature* 431, no. 7004 (2004): 19–20.

Assemblée Nationale (French National Assembly). *Compte rendu intégral*. November 19, 1992.

——. *Compte rendu intégral*. November 20, 1992.

——. *Compte rendu intégral*. April 7, 1994.

——. *Compte rendu intégral*. April 13, 1994.

——. *Compte rendu intégral*. April 14, 1994.

——. *Compte rendu intégral*. January 15, 2002.

——. *Compte rendu intégral*. January 16, 2002.

——. *Compte rendu intégral*. January 17, 2002.

——. *Compte rendu intégral*. January 22, 2002.

——. *Compte rendu intégral*. December 9, 2003.

——. *Compte rendu de l'audition publique ouverte a la presse*. November 29, 2007. http://www.assemblee-nationale.fr/13/rap-off/i1325-tII.asp.

——. *"Projet de loi relatif à la bioéthique."* June 20, 2001. http://www.assemblee-nationale.fr/11/projets/pl3166.asp.

——. *Rapport d'information sur la bioéthique*. Paris: Assemblée nationale, 1992.

——. *Rapport fait au nom de la commission spéciale sur le projet de loi relatif à la bioéthique*. Paris: Assemblée nationale, 2002.

Association Française contre les Myopathies (French Muscular Dystrophy Association). Letter to National Assembly deputies. Manuscript. January 24, 2003.

Association of Medical Research Charities. "Stem Cell Research: AMRC Responds to Donaldson Report and Government Response." Press release, August 16, 2000.

Association of Medical Research Charities and Genetic Interest Group. "Letter to the Prime Minister about the Creation of Hybrid Embryos for Research." April 5, 2007. http://www.amrc.org.uk/tabs_news-2007_letter-to-the-prime-minister-about-the-creation-of-hybrid-embryos-for-research.

Atlan, Henri, Marc Augé, Mireille Delmas-Marty, Roger-Pol Droit, and Nadine Fresco. *Le clonage humain*. Paris: Editions du Seuil, 1999.

Banchoff, Thomas. "Path-Dependence and Value-Driven Issues: The Comparative Politics of Stem Cell Research." *World Politics* 57, no. 2 (2005): 200–30.

——. "Religious Pluralism and the Politics of a Global Cloning Ban." In *Religious Pluralism, Globalization, and World Politics*. Edited by Thomas Banchoff, 275–96. Oxford: Oxford University Press, 2008.

——. "Stem Cell Politics, Religious and Secular: The United States and France Compared." In *Democracy and the New Religious Pluralism*. Edited by Thomas Banchoff, 301–21. Oxford: Oxford University Press, 2007.

Barth, Hermann. "Rechtfertigung durch Heilungshoffnungen? Einige gute Gründe gegen das sogenannte therapeutische Klonen." February 2, 2005. http://www.ekd.de/vortraege/barth/050202_barth_klonen.html.

Baruch, Susannah, David Kaufman, and Kathy L. Hudson. "Genetic Testing of Embryos: Practices and Perspectives of U.S. IVF Clinics." *Fertility and Sterility* 89, no. 5 (2006): 1053–58.

Baylis, Françoise, and Carolyn McLeod. "The Stem Cell Debate Continues: The Buying and Selling of Eggs for Research." *Journal of Medical Ethics* 33, no. 12 (2007): 726–31.

Benda Commission. *Working Group on In Vitro Fertilisation, Genom Analysis, and Gene Therapy Report*. Bonn: Federal Ministry for Research and Technology, 1985.

Bernard, Charles, and Alain Claeys. *Rapport d'information de la mission d'information commune préparatoire au projet de loi de révision des lois "bioéthiques" de juillet 1994.*

Vol. 2. *Auditions.* Paris: Office parlementaire d'évaluation des choix scientifiques et technologiques, 2001.

Bioindustry Association. "BIA Welcomes Donaldson Recommendations on Cell Nuclear Replacement." Press release, August 30, 2000.

Biotechnology Industry Organization. "BIO Supports Bans on Cloning Humans, Seeks Medical Research Protection." Press release, June 7, 1997. http://www.bio.org/news/pressreleases/newsitem.asp?id=1997_0607_01.

Birke, Lynda, Susan Himmelweit, and Gail Vines. *Tomorrow's Child: Reproductive Technologies in the 90s.* London: Virago Press, 1990.

Blank, Robert H. *Regulating Reproduction.* New York: Columbia University Press, 1990.

Bock, Gregory, and Maeve O'Connor, eds. *Human Embryo Research—Yes or No?* London: Tavistock, 1986.

Böckle, Franz, ed. *Der Umstrittene Naturbegriff: Person, Natur, Sexualität in der kirchlichen Morallehre.* Düsseldorf: Patmos-Verlag, 1987.

Bonnicksen, Andrea L. *In Vitro Fertilization: Building Policy from Laboratories to Legislatures.* New York: Columbia University Press, 1989.

Bowker, J. W. "Religions and the Status of the Embryo." In *Human Embryo Research—Yes or No?* Edited by Gregory Bock and Maeve O'Connor, 164–79. London: Tavistock, 1986.

British Medical Association Working Group on In-Vitro Fertilisation. "Appendix VI: Interim Report on Human In Vitro Fertilisation and Embryo Replacement and Transfer." *British Medical Journal* 286, no. 6377 (1983): 1594–95.

Brown, Eric B. "The Dilemmas of German Bioethics." *New Atlantis* no. 5 (2004): 37–53.

Bulger, Ruth Ellen, Elizabeth Meyer Bobby, Harvey V. Fineberg, and Institute of Medicine (U.S.) Committee on the Social and Ethical Impacts of Developments in Biomedicine. *Society's Choices: Social and Ethical Decision Making in Biomedicine.* Washington, DC: National Academy Press, 1995.

Bulger, Ruth Ellen, Elizabeth Heitman, and Stanley Joel Reiser. *The Ethical Dimensions of the Biological Sciences.* New York: Cambridge University Press, 1993.

Bundesärztekammer (German Medical Association). "Beschlussprotokoll des 100. Deutschen Ärztetages." May 27–30, 1997. http://www.bundesaerztekammer.de/downloads/beschlussprotokoll_100_daet_eisenach_1997.pdf.

——. "Beschlussprotokoll des 104. Deutschen Ärztetages vom 22.–25. Mai 2001 in Ludwigshafen: Forschung mit humanen embryonalen Stammzellen." May 2001. http://www.bundesaerztekammer.de/page.asp?his=0.2.23.2618.2619.2626.

Bundesministerium der Justiz (Federal Ministry of Justice). "Bundesjustizministerin Zypries beim Humboldt-Forum 'Vom Zeugen zum Erzeugen? Verfassungsrechtliche und rechtspolitische Fragen der Bioethik': Wir brauchen eine Spezifikation der Werte." Press release, October 29, 2003.

——. "Gesetz zur Sicherstellung des Embryonenschutzes im Zusammenhang mit Einfuhr und Verwendung menschlicher embryonaler Stammzellen." *Bundesgesetzblatt Jahrgang 2002,* no. 42. June 29, 2002. http://www.bmbf.de/pub/stammzellgesetz.pdf.

Bundespräsidialamt (Office of the Federal President). "Wird Alles Gut?—Für Einen Fortschritt Nach Menschlichem Maß." Press release, May 18, 2001. http://

www.bundespraesident.de/Reden-und-Interviews/Reden-Johannes-Rau-, 11070.41073/Wird-alles-gut-Fuer-einen-Fort.htm?global.back=.

Bundesregierung (Federal Government). "Rede von Bundeskanzler Gerhard Schröder anlässlich der Verleihung der Ehrendoktorwürde der Universität Göttingen." Press release, June 14, 2005. http://www.bundesregierung. de/Content/DE/Bulletin/2001__2005/2005/06/__Anlagen/nr-58-1858077,property=publicationFile.pdf.

Bundestag (German Parliament). *Antwort der Bundesregierung auf die grossen Anfragen der Abgeordneten Frau Dr. Hickel und der Fraktion Die Grünen, Drucksache 10/1153.* Bonn: Deutscher Bundestag, 1984.

——. *Ausschuss für Bildung, Forschung und Technikfolgenabschätzung, 34. Sitzung, 09. Mai 2007. Protokoll 16/34.* Berlin: Deutscher Bundestag, 2007.

——. *Gesetz für eine menschenfreundliche Medizin—Gesetz zur Änderung des Stammzellgesetzes, Drucksache 16/7982.* Berlin: Deutscher Bundestag, 2008.

——. *Gesetz zur Änderung des Stammzellgesetzes, Drucksache 16/7981.* Berlin: Deutscher Bundestag, 2008.

——. *Kabinettbericht zur künstlichen Befruchtung beim Menschen, Drucksache 11/1856.* Bonn: Deutscher Bundestag, 1988.

——. *Keine Änderung des Stichtages im Stammzellgesetz—Adulte Stammzellforschung fördern, Drucksache 16/7985.* Berlin: Deutscher Bundestag, 2008.

——. "Keine verbrauchende Embryonenforschung: Import humaner embryonaler Stammzellen grundsätzlich verbieten und nur unter engen Voraussetzungen Zulassen." *Drucksache 14/8102.* Berlin: Deutscher Bundestag, 2002.

——. "Schutz der Menschenwürde angesichts der biomedizinischen Möglichkeiten— Kein Import embryonaler Stammzellen." *Drucksache 14/8101.* Berlin: Deutscher Bundestag, 2002.

——. "Verantwortungsbewusste Forschung an embryonalen Stammzellen für eine ethisch hochwertige Medizin." *Drucksache 14/8103.* Berlin: Deutscher Bundestag, 2002.

——. *Verbot des Klonens von Menschen. Drucksache 13/7243.* Berlin: Deutscher Bundestag, 1997.

——. *Verhandlungen des deutschen Bundestages. Stenographischer Bericht,* ser. 10 (January 17, 1985).

——. *Verhandlungen des deutschen Bundestages. Stenographischer Bericht,* ser. 11 (March 21, 1987).

——. *Verhandlungen des deutschen Bundestages,* ser. 11 (February 25, 1988).

——. *Verhandlungen des deutschen Bundestages,* ser. 11 (December 8, 1989).

——. *Verhandlungen des deutschen Bundestages,* ser. 11 (October 23, 1990).

——. *Verhandlungen des deutschen Bundestages,* ser. 11 (October 24, 1990).

——. *Verhandlungen des deutschen Bundestages,* ser. 11 (November 29, 2000).

——. *Verhandlungen des deutschen Bundestages,* ser. 14 (May 31, 2001).

——. *Verhandlungen des deutschen Bundestages,* ser. 14 (January 30, 2002).

——. *Verhandlungen des deutschen Bundestages,* ser. 14 (January 31, 2002).

——. *Verhandlungen des deutschen Bundestages,* ser. 16 (April 11, 2008).

——. *Zweiter Zwischenbericht der Enquête-Kommission Recht und Ethik der modernen Medizin. Teilbericht Stammzellforschung. Drucksache 14/7546.* Berlin: Deutscher Bundestag, 2001.

Bundesverband der Pharmazeutischen Industrie (German Pharmaceutical Industry Association). "Embryonenforschung erst nach Experimenten an Säugetieren und adulten Stammzellen." Press release, January 24, 2002.

Bundesverfassungsgericht (Federal Constitutional Court). *BVerfGE 39, 1— Schwangerschaftsabbruch I*. February 25, 1975. http://www.servat.unibe.ch/dfr/bv039001.html.

———. *2 BvF 2/90*. May 28, 1993. http://www.bverfg.de/entscheidungen/fs19930528_2bvf000290en.html.

Burd, Stephen. "House Unit Votes to Bar Federal Funds for Research on Embryos." *Chronicle of Higher Education* 42, no. 43 (July 5, 1996): A24.

Butler, Declan. "Ethics Bill Prompts Second Thoughts among Scientists." *Nature* 367, no. 6460 (1993): 209.

———. "France Is Urged to Loosen Ban on Embryo Research." *Nature* 387, no. 6630 (1997): 218.

Cahill, Lisa Sowle. "The Embryo and the Fetus: New Moral Contexts." *Theological Studies* 54, no. 1 (1993): 124–42.

Cahill, Lisa Sowle, and Margaret A. Farley. *Embodiment, Morality, and Medicine*. New York: Springer, 1995.

Califano, Joseph A. *Inside: A Public and Private Life*. New York: PublicAffairs, 2004.

Callahan, Daniel. "Promises, Promises: Is Embryonic Stem-Cell Research Sound Public Policy?" *Commonweal*, January 14, 2005, 12–14.

———. "The Puzzle of Profound Respect." *Hastings Center Report* 25, no. 1 (1995): 39–40.

Capron, Alexander M. "An Egg Takes Flight: The Once and Future Life of the National Bioethics Advisory Commission." *Kennedy Institute of Ethics Journal* 7, no. 1 (1997): 63–80.

Carmen, Ira H. *Politics in the Laboratory: The Constitution of Human Genomics*. Madison: University of Wisconsin Press, 2004.

Charo, R. Alta. "The Hunting of the Snark: The Moral Status of Embryos, Right-to-Lifers, and Third World Women." *Stanford Law and Policy Review* 6, no. 2 (1995): 11–37.

Chartier, Michel, Georges David, Jean Michaud, Joseph Moingt, Berard Quelquejeu, Claude Sureau, Charles Thibault, and Paul Valadier. *Aux débuts de la vie: Des catholiques prennent position*. Paris: Editions la découverte, 1990.

Church of England. *Report of Proceedings: General Synod, February 1985*. London: Church House, 1985.

———. *Report of Proceedings: General Synod, July 2003*. London: Church House, 2003.

Church of England Board for Social Responsibility. *Abortion and the Church: What Are the Issues?* London: Church House, 1993.

———. *Human Fertilisation and Embryology: The Response of the Board for Social Responsibility of the General Synod of the Church of England to the DHSS Report of the Committee of Inquiry*. London: Church of England, 1984.

———. *Personal Origins*. London: Church House, 1985.

———. "Warnock Evidence." Manuscript. February 24, 1983.

Church of England Mission and Public Affairs Council. *Embryo Research: Some Christian Perspectives*. London: Church House, 2003.

——. "Response from the Church of England Mission and Public Affairs Council to the Call for Evidence from the Joint Committee on the Draft Human Tissue and Embryos Bill." June 2007. http://www.cofe.anglican.org/info/socialpublic/science/hfea/humantissue.pdf.

Claeys, Alain. *Rapport sur les recherches sur le fonctionnement des cellules humaines.* Paris: Office parlementaire d'évaluation des choix scientifiques et technologiques, 2006.

Claeys, Allain, and Claude Huriet. *Rapport sur l'application de la Loi no. 94–654 du 29 juillet 1994. Audition.* Paris: Office parlementaire d'évaluation des choix scientifiques et technologiques, 1999.

——. *Rapport sur le clonage, la thérapie cellulaire et l'utilisation thérapeutique des cellules embryonnaires.* Paris: Office parlementaire d'évaluation des choix scientifiques et technologiques, 2000.

Claeys, Alain, and Jean Leonetti. *Rapport d'information fait au nom de la mission d'information sur la révision des lois de bioéthique. Auditions.* Paris: Assemblée nationale, 2010.

Coghlan, Andy. "Are Human-Animal 'Cybrids' Really Possible?" *New Scientist* 195, no. 2621 (2007): 15.

Cohen, Cynthia B. *Renewing the Stuff of Life: Stem Cells, Ethics, and Public Policy.* Oxford: Oxford University Press, 2007.

Comité Consultatif National d'Ethique (National Consultative Ethics Committee). "Opinion on Embryo Research Aiming to Achieve Pre-Transfer Genetic Diagnosis for Which a Moratorium Was Declared in 1986." July 18, 1990. http://www.ccne-ethique.fr/docs/en/avis019.pdf.

——. "Opinion on the Establishment of Collections of Human Embryo Cells and Their Use for Therapeutic or Scientific Purposes." March 11, 1997. http://www.ccne-ethique.fr/docs/en/avis053.pdf.

——. "Opinion on Ethical Problems Arising out of Artificial Reproductive Techniques." October 23, 1984. http://www.ccne-ethique.fr/docs/en/avis003.pdf.

——. "Opinion on Gene Therapy." December 13, 1990. http://www.ccne-ethique.fr/docs/en/avis022.pdf.

——. "Opinion on the Preliminary Draft Revision of the Laws on Bioethics." January 18, 2001. http://ccne-ethique.fr/docs/en/avis067.pdf.

——. "Opinion on Research and Use of In-Vitro Human Embryos for Scientific and Medical Purposes." December 15, 1986. http://www.ccne-ethique.fr/docs/en/avis008.pdf.

——. "Opinion on Sampling of Dead Human Embryonic and Fetal Tissue for Therapeutic, Diagnostic, and Scientific Purposes." May 22, 1984. http://www.ccne-ethique.fr/docs/en/avis001.pdf.

——. "Re-examination of the Law on Bioethics." June 25, 1998. www.ccne-ethique.fr/docs/en/avis060.pdf.

——. "Reflections concerning an Extension of Preimplantation Genetic Diagnosis." July 4, 1992. http://www.ccne-ethique.fr/docs/en/avis072.pdf.

Commission nationale consultative des droits de l'homme (National Consultative Commission on Human Rights). "Avis portant sur l'avant-projet de loi tendant à la révision des lois relatives à l'ethique biomédicale." January 25, 2001. http://www.cncdh.fr/IMG/pdf/01.01.25_Avis_Ethique_biomedicale_.pdf.

———. "Avis portant sur la révision des lois de 1994 sur la bioéthique." June 29, 2000. http://www.cncdh.fr/article.php3?id_article=262.

———. "Avis sur les sciences de la vie et Droits de l'Homme." September 21, 1989. http://www.cncdh.fr/article.php3?id_article=276.

Committee on the Biological and Biomedical Applications of Stem Cell Research. "Stem Cells and the Future of Regenerative Medicine." Washington, DC: National Academy Press, 2002.

Conférence des évêques de France (French Bishops' Conference). "L'embryon humain n'est pas une chose." June 21, 2001. http://www.cef.fr/catho/espacepresse/communiques/2001/commu20010625embryon.php.

———. "Pas d'exception au respect dû à l'embryon humain." January 27, 2003. http://www.eglise.catholique.fr/conference-des-eveques-de-france/texteset-declarations/pas-dexception-au-respect-du-a-lembryon-humain-.html.

"Confused Comment on Warnock." *Nature* 312, no. 5993 (1984): 389.

Congregation for the Doctrine of the Faith. *Instruction Dignitatis Personae on Certain Bioethical Questions.* December 12, 2008. http://www.vatican.va/roman_curia/congregations/cfaith/documents/rc_con_cfaith_doc_20081208_dignitas-personae_en.html#_ftn36.

———. *Instruction on Respect for Human Life in Its Origin and on the Dignity of Procreation: Replies to Certain Questions of the Day.* February 22, 1987. http://www.vatican.va/roman_curia/congregations/cfaith/documents/rc_con_cfaith_doc_19870222_respect-for-human-life_en.html.

Congressional Research Service. *Genetic Engineering: Evolution of a Technological Issue.* Washington, DC: Government Printing Office, 1972.

Conseil constitutionnel. "Décision no. 94–343/344 DC du 27 juillet 1994." http://www.conseil-constitutionnel.fr/conseil-constitutionnel/francais/les-decisions/acces-par-date/decisions-depuis-1959/1994/94–343/344-dc/decision-n-94-343-344-dc-du-27-juillet-1994.10566.html.

Conseil d'Etat. *Les lois de la bioéthique: Cinq ans après.* Paris: La Documentation française, 1999.

———. *La révision des lois de bioéthique.* Paris: La Documentation française, 1999.

———. *Sciences de la vie: De l'éthique au droit.* Paris: La Documentation française, 1988.

Conseil National de L'Ordre des Médecins. "Révision des lois de bioéthique." *Bulletin de l'Ordre National des Médecins* (July 1998).

Cook-Deegan, Robert M. *The Gene Wars: Science, Politics, and the Human Genome.* New York: Norton, 1994.

Curran, Charles E. *Moral Theology: A Continuing Journey.* Notre Dame, IN: University of Notre Dame Press, 1982.

Davies, David. "Embryo Research." *Nature* 320, no. 6059 (1986): 208.

Debré, Bernard. *La grande transgression: L'homme génétiquement modifié.* Neuilly-sur-Seine, Fr.: Lafon, 2000.

Democratic Party. "The Democratic Party Platform of 2000." August 14, 2000. http://www.presidency.ucsb.edu/ws/index.php?pid=29612.

"Deputies Endorse Research on Human Stem Cells, Set Budget Priorities." *Episcopal Press and News*. August 2, 2003. http://www.episcopalarchives.org/cgi-bin/ENS/ENSpress_release.pl?pr_number=2003–188-ADeputies.

Deutsche Bischofskonferenz (German Bishops' Conference). "Erklärung des Vorsitzenden der Unterkommission Bioethik der Deutschen Bischofskonferenz, Bischof Dr. Gebhard Fürst, zum Votum des Nationalen Ethikrates vom 29. November 2001." Press release, November 30, 2001. http://www.alt.dbk.de/aktuell/meldungen/2903/index.html.

———. "Erklärung des Vorsitzenden der Deutschen Bischofskonferenz, Erzbischof Dr. Robert Zollitsch, zur Debatte über das Stammzellgesetz am 11.04.2008." Press release, April 10, 2008. http://www.dbk.de/nc/funktionen/suche/?tx_s olr[q]=zollitsch+stammzellgesetz&id=69.

Deutsche Forschungsgemeinschaft (German Research Foundation). "DFG Puts Forward New Recommendations for Stem Cell Research." Press release, November 10, 2006.

———. "Empfehlungen der Deutschen Forschungsgemeinschaft zur Forschung mit menschlichen Stammzellen." Press release, May 3, 2001. http://www.dfg.de/aktuell/stellungnahmen/dokumentation_1.html.

———. *Forschungsfreiheit: Ein Plädoyer für bessere Rahmenbedingungen der Forschung in Deutschland*. Weinheim, Ger.: VCH, 1996.

———. "Statement des DFG-Präsidenten, Professor Ernst-Ludwig Winnacker, zum Klonen menschlicher Embryozellen." Press release, January 1999. http://www.dfg.de/download/pdf/dfg_im_profil/reden_stellungnahmen/archiv_download/emb_klon_stat_99.pdf.

Deutscher Multiple Sklerose Gesellschaft (German Multiple Sclerosis Society). "Zur Bedeutung der Stammzellen: Forschung für die Therapie der Multiplen Sklerose." Press release, July 2001.

Dickson, David. "France Introduces Bioethics Law." *Science* 243, no. 4896 (1989): 1284.

Doerflinger, Richard M. "Public Comment: NIH Human Embryo Research Panel." February 22, 1994. http://www.usccb.org/prolife/issues/bioethic/embryo/rd20294.shtml.

———. "Testimony of Richard M. Doerflinger on Behalf of the Committee for Pro-Life Activities, United States Conference of Catholic Bishops before the Subcommittee on Labor, Health and Human Services, and Education Senate Appropriations Committee Hearing on Stem Cell Research." July 18, 2001. http://www.usccb.org/prolife/issues/bioethic/stemcelltest71801.htm.

Donceel, Joseph. "Immediate Animation and Delayed Hominization." *Theological Studies* 31, no. 1 (1970): 76–105.

Dunstan, Gordon. "The Moral Status of the Human Embryo: A Tradition Recalled." *Journal of Medical Ethics* 10, no. 1 (1984): 38–44.

Dyson, Anthony Oakley, and John Harris. *Experiments on Embryos*. New York: Routledge, 1990.

Edwards, Robert G. "The Bumpy Road to Human In Vitro Fertilisation." *Nature* 7, no. 10 (2001): 1091–94.

———. "The Case for Studying Human Embryos and Their Constituent Tissues In Vitro." In *Human Conception In Vitro*. Edited by Robert G. and Jean M. Purdy Edwards, 371–87. London: Academic Press, 1982.

———. "IVF and the History of Stem Cells." *Nature* 413, no. 6854 (2001): 349–51.

———. *Life before Birth: Reflections on the Embryo Debate.* New York: Basic Books, 1989.

———. "Stem Cells Today: Origin and Potential of Embryo Stem Cells." *Reproductive Biomedicine Online* 8, no. 3 (2004): 275–306.

Edwards, Robert G., Barry D. Bavister, and Patrick C. Steptoe. "Early Stages of Fertilization In Vitro of Human Oocytes Matured In Vitro." *Nature* 221, no. 5181 (1969): 632–35.

Edwards, Robert G., and Patrick Christopher Steptoe. *A Matter of Life: The Story of a Medical Breakthrough.* New York: Morrow, 1980.

Eser, Albin, Wolfgang Frühwald, Ludger Honnefelder, Hubert Markl, Johannes Reiter, Widmar Tanner, and Ernst-Ludwig Winnacker. *Klonierung beim Menschen: Biologische Grundlagen und ethisch-rechtliche Bewertung.* June 1997. http://www.freidok.uni-freiburg.de/volltexte/3691/pdf/Eser_Klonierung_beim_Menschen.pdf.

Etats généraux de la bioéthique. "Rapport final: Etats généraux de la bioéthique." July 1, 2009. http://www.etatsgenerauxdelabioethique.fr/uploads/rapport_final.pdf.

Ethics Advisory Board. *Report and Conclusions: HEW Support of Research Involving Human In Vitro Fertilization and Embryo Transfer.* Washington, DC: Department of Health, Education, and Welfare, 1979.

Etzioni, Amitai. *Genetic Fix: The Next Technological Revolution.* New York: Macmillan, 1973.

Evangelische Kirche in Deutschland (Evangelical Church in Germany). "Im Geist der Liebe mit dem Leben umgehen." *EKD-Texte 71,* August 2002. http://www.ekd.de/EKD-Texte/44633.html.

———. "CDU und EKD Sprachen über Bioethik und Zuwanderungspolitik." Press release, June 1, 2001. http://www.ekd.de/bioethik/5228.html.

———. "Der menschliche Embryo ist keine bloße Biomasse." Press release, December 7, 2001. http://ekd.de/presse/pm124_2001_stammzellen.html.

———. "Der Schutz menschlicher Embryonen darf nicht eingeschränkt werden: Erklärung des Rates der EKD zur aktuellen bioethischen Debatte." Press release, May 22, 2001. http://www.ekd.de/presse/5220.html.

———. "Kirchen Schreiben an Bundestagsabgeordnete." Press release, January 17, 2002. http://www.ekd.de/print.php?file=/presse/pm6_2002_kirchenbrief_mdbs_menschenschutz.html.

———. "Klonen ist ein Irrweg." Press release, September 13, 2004. http://www.ekd.de/bioethik/presse/pm167_2004_klonen_ekd_dbk.html.

———. "Klonen ist nicht zu verantworten." Press release, February 13, 2004. http://www.ekd.de/presse/pm21_2004_klonen.html.

———. "Lockerung der Stammzellforschung von Bischof Huber befürwortet." Press release, February 11, 2008. http://www.ekd.de/aktuell_presse/news_2008_02_11_1_rv_sz_interview_stammzellen.html.

———. *Von der Würde menschlichen Lebens: Eine Handreichung der EKD zur ethischen Urteilsbildung.* Hannover: Evangelische Kirche in Deutschland, 1985.

———. "Zur Achtung vor dem Leben: Maßstäbe für Gentechnik und Fortpflanzungsmedizin." November 6, 1987. http://www.ekd.de/EKD-Texte/achtungvordemleben_1987.html.

Evangelical Church in Germany and German Bishops' Conference. "Gott ist ein Freund des Lebens: Herausforderungen und Aufgaben beim Schutz des Lebens." November 30, 1989. http://www.ekd.de/EKD-Texte/44678. html.

Evans, John Hyde. *Playing God?: Human Genetic Engineering and the Rationalization of Public Bioethical Debate.* Chicago: University of Chicago Press, 2002.

Fagniez, Pierre-Louis. *Cellules souches et choix éthiques.* Paris: Assemblée nationale, 2006.

———. *Rapport fait au nom de la commission des affaires culturelles, familiales et sociales sur le projet de loi, adopté par le Sénat, relatif à la bioéthique.* Paris: Assemblée nationale, 2003.

Fédération protestante de France (Protestant Federation of France). "A propos du clonage: Eléments de débat et de réflexion." November 15, 2001. http://www.protestants.org/?id=1731.

———. "Révision des lois bioéthiques en 2001." November 2000. http://www.protestants.org/index.php?id=1961.

———. "Le temps est venu de réviser les lois de bioéthique." January 12, 2003. http://www.protestants.org/docpro/doc/1146.htm.

Ferree, Myra Marx, William Anthony Gamson, Jürgen Gerhards, and Dieter Rucht. *Shaping Abortion Discourse: Democracy and the Public Sphere in Germany and the United States.* Cambridge, U.K.: Cambridge University Press, 2007.

Fink, Simon. "Politics as Usual or Bringing Religion Back In? The Influence of Parties, Institutions, Economic Interests, and Religion on Embryo Research Laws." *Comparative Political Studies* 41, no. 12 (2008): 1631–56.

Fletcher, Joseph. "Ethical Aspects of Genetic Controls: Designed Genetic Changes in Man." *New England Journal of Medicine* 285, no. 14 (1971): 776–83.

———. *The Ethics of Genetic Control: Ending Reproductive Roulette.* Garden City, NJ: Anchor Books, 1974.

Ford, Norman M. *When Did I Begin?: Conception of the Human Individual in History, Philosophy, and Science.* Cambridge: Cambridge University Press, 1988.

Fox, Renée C., Judith P. Swazey, and Judith C. Watkins. *Observing Bioethics.* Oxford: Oxford University Press, 2008.

France Biotech. "France Biotech souhaite que la recherche médicale sur les cellules souches et le clonage thérapeutique puisse se développer en France avec une réglementation stricte." Press release, January 10, 2002.

Frankel, Mark S., and Audrey R. Chapman. *Human Inheritable Genetic Modifications: Assessing Scientific, Ethical, Religious, and Policy Issues.* Washington, DC: American Academy for the Advancement of Science, 2000.

French, Andrew J., Catharine A. Adams, Linda S. Anderson, John R. Kitchen, Marcus R. Hughes, and Samuel H. Wood. "Development of Human Cloned Blastocysts Following Somatic Cell Nuclear Transfer with Adult Fibroblasts." *Stem Cells* 26, no. 2 (2008): 485–93.

French Civil Code. Translated by Georges Rouhette with Ann Berton. Legisfrance. gouv.fr. February 21, 2004. http://www.legifrance.gouv.fr/html/codes_traduits/code_civil_textA.htm.

Frew, Andreas. "Congressional Murder Most Foul: Report from the Heady Heights of Capitol Hill." *New Scientist* 144, no. 1949 (1994): 67–68.

Frydman, Rene. *Dieu, la medecine, et l'embryon*. Paris: Éditions Odile Jacob, 1999.

Fukuyama, Francis. *Our Posthuman Future: Consequences of the Biotechnology Revolution*. New York: Farrar, Straus and Giroux, 2002.

Galston, William A. *Public Matters: Essays on Politics, Policy and Religion*. Lanham, MD: Rowman and Littlefield, 2005.

"Genetic Engineering in Man: Ethical Considerations." *Journal of the American Medical Association* 220, no. 5 (1972): 721.

Gerhardt, Volker. "Vom Zellhaufen zur Selbstachtung: Warum Nida-Ruemelins Definition des Menschen richtig ist." *Focus*, January 22, 2001.

Goodwin, Jeff, James M. Jasper, and Francesca Polletta. *Passionate Politics: Emotions and Social Movements*. Chicago: University of Chicago Press, 2001.

Gottweis, Herbert, Brian Salter, and Cathy Waldby. *The Global Politics of Human Embryonic Stem Cell Science: Regenerative Medicine in Transition*. Basingstoke, UK: Palgrave Macmillan, 2009.

Green, Ronald Michael. *Babies by Design: The Ethics of Genetic Choice*. New Haven: Yale University Press, 2007.

——. *The Human Embryo Research Debates: Bioethics in the Vortex of Controversy*. New York: Oxford University Press, 2001.

Grobstein, Clifford. "External Human Fertilization." *Scientific American* 240, no. 6 (1979): 57–67.

Grobstein, Clifford, Michael Flower, and John Mendeloff. "External Human Fertilization: An Evaluation of Policy." *Science* 222, no. 4620 (1983): 127–33.

Gros, François, and Gérard Huber, eds. *Vers un anti-destin? Patrimoine génétique et droits de l'humanité*. Paris: Éditions Odile Jacob, 1992.

Grossman, Edward. "The Obsolescent Mother: A Scenario." *Atlantic* 227, no. 5 (1971): 39–50.

Gunning, Jennifer, and Veronica English. *Human In Vitro Fertilization: A Case Study in the Regulation of Medical Innovation*. Aldershot, UK: Dartmouth 1993.

Habermas, Jürgen. *The Future of Human Nature*. Cambridge, UK: Polity, 2003.

Hadlington, Simon. "British Government Hedges Bets on Embryo Research." *Nature* 330, no. 6147 (1987): 409.

Haldane, J. B. S. *Daedalus; or, Science and the Future*. New York: E. P. Dutton and Company, 1924.

Hall, Peter A., and Rosemary C. R. Taylor. "Political Science and the Three New Institutionalisms." *Political Studies* 44 (1996): 936–57.

Hall, Stephen S. *Merchants of Immortality: Chasing the Dream of Human Life Extension*. New York: Houghton Mifflin, 2003.

——. "President's Bioethics Council Delivers." *Science* 297, no. 5613 (2002): 322–24.

Handyside, Alan, and E. H. Kontogianni. "Pregnancies from Biopsied Human Preimplantation Embryos Sexed by Y-Specific DNA Amplification." *Nature* 344, no. 6268 (1990): 768–70.

Häring, Bernard, and Gabrielle L. Jean. *Medical Ethics*. Slough, UK: St. Paul Publications, 1972.

Harris, John. *Enhancing Evolution: The Ethical Case for Making Better People*. Princeton: Princeton University Press, 2007.

——. "The Ethical Use of Human Embryonic Stem Cells in Research and Therapy." In *A Companion to Genethics*. Edited by Justine Burley and John Harris, 158–74. Malden, MA: Blackwell 2002.

——. "In Vitro Fertilization: The Ethical Issues." *Philosophical Quarterly* 33, no. 132 (1983): 217–37.

——. "Stem Cells, Sex, and Procreation." *Cambridge Quarterly of Healthcare Ethics* 12, no. 4 (2003): 353–71.

Henig, Robin Marantz. *Pandora's Baby: How the First Test Tube Babies Sparked the Reproductive Revolution.* Boston: Houghton Mifflin, 2004.

Hill, Thomas E. *Respect, Pluralism, and Justice: Kantian Perspectives.* Oxford: Oxford University Press, 2000.

Hoffman, David I., Gail L. Zellman, C. Christine Fair, Jacob F. Mayer, Joyce G. Zeitz, William E. Gibbons, and Thomas G. Turner, Jr. "Cryopreserved Embryos in the United States and Their Availability for Research." *Fertility and Sterility* 79, no. 5 (2003): 1063–69.

Höfling, Wolfram. "Verfassungsrechtliche Aspekte der Verfügung über menschliche Embryonen und 'humanbiologisches Material." May 2001. http://www.bund estag.de/gremien/medi/medi_gut_hoe.pdf.

Holden, Constance. "Random Samples." *Science* 295, no. 5562 (2002): 2009.

Holden, Constance, and Gretchen Vogel. "Cell Biology: A Seismic Shift for Stem Cell Research." *Science* 319, no. 5863 (2008): 560–63.

Holland, Suzanne, Karen Lebacqz, and Laurie Zoloth. *The Human Embryonic Stem Cell Debate: Science, Ethics, and Public Policy.* Cambridge: MIT Press, 2001.

The Holy Synod of the Orthodox Church in America. "Embryonic Stem Cell Research in the Perspective of Orthodox Christianity." October 17, 2001. http://www.oca.org/Docs.asp?ID=50&SID=12.

Honecker, Martin. "Embryonenschutz aus ethischer Sicht." *Reproduktionsmedizin* 18, no. 2 (2002): 58–60.

Huber, Wolfgang. "Ethik und Demokratie." June 19, 2004. http://www.kinder krankenhausseelsorge.de/vortraege/huber/04_06_19_huber_katholikentag.html.

——. "Wissenschaft Verantworten: Überlegungen Zur Ethik der Forschung." July 14, 2006. http://www.ekd.de/vortraege/2006/060714_rv_heidelberg.html.

"Human Cloning Requires a Moratorium, Not a Ban." *Nature* 386, no. 6620 (1997): 1.

Human Genetics Advisory Commission and Human Fertilisation and Embryology Authority. *"Cloning Issues in Reproduction, Science and Medicine."* Human Genetics Advisory Commission (December 1998). http://www.dh.gov. uk/prod_consum_dh/groups/dh_digitalassets/@dh/@ab/documents/ digitalasset/dh_104395.pdf.

——. "Cloning Issues in Reproduction, Science and Medicine." Human Genetics Advisory Commission (January 2008). http://www.dh.gov.uk/prod_ consum_dh/groups/dh_digitalassets/@dh/@ab/documents/digitalasset/ dh_104394.pdf.

Human Fertilisation and Embryology Authority. *Code of Practice,* 6th ed. London: Human Fertilisation and Embryology Authority, 2003.

——. *Outcome of the Public Consultation on Preimplantation Genetic Diagnosis.* London: Human Fertilisation and Embryology Authority, 2001.

Hwang, Woo Suk, Young June Ryu, Jong Hyuk Park, Eul Soon Park, Eu Gene Lee, Ja Min Koo, Hyun Yong Jeon, Byeong Chun Lee, Sung Keun Kang, Sun Jong Kim, Curie Ahn, Jung Hye Hwang, Ky Young Park, Jose B. Cibelli, and Shin Yong Moon. "Evidence of a Pluripotent Human Embryonic Stem Cell Line Derived from a Cloned Blastocyst." *Science* 303, no. 5664 (2004): 1669–74.

Hwang, Woo Suk, Sung Il Roh, Byeong Chun Lee, Sung Keun Kang, Dae Kee Kwon, Sue Kim, Sun Jong Kim, Sun Woo Park, Hee Sun Kwon, Chang Kyu Lee, Jung Bok Lee, Jin Mee Kim, Curie Ahn, Sun Ha Paek, Sang Sik Chang, Jung Jin Koo, Hyun Soo Yoon, Jung Hye Hwang, Youn Young Hwang, and Ye Soo Park. "Patient-Specific Embryonic Stem Cells Derived from Human SCNT Blastocysts." *Science* 308, no. 5729 (2005): 1777–83.

Isasi, Rosario M., and Bartha M. Knoppers. "Mind the Gap: Policy Approaches to Embryonic Stem Cell and Cloning Research in 50 Countries." *European Journal of Health Law* 13, no. 1 (2006): 9–25.

"IVF Remains in Legal Limbo." *Nature* 327, no. 6118 (1987): 87.

Jaenisch, Rudolph. "Human Cloning: The Science and Ethics of Nuclear Transplantation." *New England Journal of Medicine* 351, no. 27 (2004): 2787–91.

Jakobovits, Immanuel. *Jewish Medical Ethics: A Comparative and Historical Study of the Jewish Religious Attitude to Medicine and Its Practice.* New York: Philosophical Library, 1959.

Jasanoff, Sheila. *Designs on Nature: Science and Democracy in Europe and the United States.* Princeton: Princeton University Press, 2005.

Jepson, Rick. "Ensoulment: Stem Cells, Cloning, and the Beginning of Life." *Sunstone* 147 (October 2007): 69–71.

John Paul II. "Address of His Holiness John Paul II to the Leaders in Catholic Health Care." September 14, 1987. http://www.vatican.va/holy_father/john_paul_ii/speeches/1987/september/documents/hf_jp-ii_spe_19870914_organiz-sanitarie-cattoliche_en.html.

——. "Address of John Paul II to Members of the Pontifical Academy of Sciences." October 23, 1982. http://www.vatican.va/holy_father/john_paul_ii/speeches/1982/october/documents/hf_jp-ii_spe_19821023_pont-accademia-scienze_en.html1982.

——. "Address of Pope John Paul II to the President of the United States of America, H. E. George Walker Bush." July 23, 2001. http://www.vatican.va/holy_father/john_paul_ii/speeches/2001/documents/hf_jp-ii_spe_20010723_president-bush_en.html.

Johnson, Martin H., Sarah B. Franklin, Matthew Cottingham, and Nick Hopwood. "Why the Medical Research Council Refused Robert Edwards and Patrick Steptoe Support for Research on Human Conception in 1971." *Human Reproduction* 25, no. 9 (2010): 2157–74.

Jonas, Hans. *Technik, Medizin und Ethik: Zur Praxis des Prinzips Verantwortung.* Frankfurt: Suhrkamp, 1987.

Jones, Alun, and Walter F. Bodmer. *Our Future Inheritance: Choice or Chance?* London: Oxford University Press, 1974.

Jones, David Albert. *The Soul of the Embryo: An Enquiry into the Status of the Human Embryo in the Christian Tradition.* New York: Continuum, 2004.

Jones, David. "A Theologian's Brief: On the Place of the Human Embryo within the Christian Tradition and the Theological Principles for Evaluating Its Moral Status." *Ethics and Medicine: An International Journal of Bioethics* 17, no. 3 (2001): 143–54.

Jonsen, Albert R. *The Birth of Bioethics.* New York: Oxford University Press, 1998.

Jonsen, Albert R., Robert M. Veatch, and LeRoy Walters, eds. *Source Book in Bioethics: A Documentary History.* Washington, DC: Georgetown University Press, 1998.

Jospin, Lionel. "Allocution de Monsieur Lionel Jospin, Premier ministre, devant le Comité consultatif national d'éthique pour les sciences de la vie et de la santé." November 28, 2000. http://infodoc.inserm.fr/inserm/ethique.nsf/93723852 0af658aec125704b002bded2/dfa9bb7b3ffbafccc12570a500515047.

———. "Allocution en clôture du colloque Biovision sur la politique de développement des biotechnologies, à Lyon (Rhône)." March 29, 1999. http://lesdiscours.vie-publique.fr/pdf/993000885.pdf.

Kahn, Axel. "Clone Mammals... Clone Man." *Nature* 387, no. 6635 (1997): 754.

Kass, Leon R. *Life, Liberty, and the Defense of Dignity: The Challenge for Bioethics.* San Francisco: Encounter Books, 2002.

———. "Making Babies: The New Biology and the 'Old' Morality." *Public Interest* 26, (1972): 18–56.

———. "The New Biology: What Price Relieving Man's Estate?" *Science* 174, no. 4011 (1971): 779–88.

———. *Toward a More Natural Science: Biology and Human Affairs.* New York: Free Press, 1985.

———. "The Wisdom of Repugnance." In *The Ethics of Human Cloning.* Edited by Leon Kass and James Q. Wilson, 3–60. Washington, DC: AEI Press, 1998.

Katznelson, Ira. "Structure and Configuration in Comparative Politics." In *Comparative Politics: Rationality, Culture, and Structure.* Edited by Mark I. Lichbach and Alan S. Zuckerman, 81–111. Cambridge: Cambridge University Press, 1997.

Keller, Rolf, Hans-Ludwig Günther, and Peter Kaiser Keller. *Embryonenschutzgesetz: Kommentar zum Embryonenschutzgesetz.* Stuttgart: Kohlhammer, 1992.

Kiessling, Anne A. "In the Stem-Cell Debate, New Concepts Need New Words." *Nature* 412, no. 6844 (2001): 255.

Kleiner, Kurt. "Clinton U-Turn on Embryo Research." *New Scientist* 144, no. 1957 (1994): 6–7.

Knowles, Lori P., and Gregory E. Kaebnick. *Reprogenetics: Law, Policy, and Ethical Issues, Bioethics.* Baltimore: Johns Hopkins University Press, 2007.

Korobkin, Russell, and Stephen R. Munzer. *Stem Cell Century: Law and Policy for a Breakthrough Technology.* New Haven: Yale University Press, 2007.

Lansac, Jacques. "French Law Concerning Medically Assisted Reproduction." *Human Reproduction* 11, no. 9 (1996): 1843–47.

Lanza, Robert P., et al. "Science over Politics." *Science* 283, no. 5409 (1999): 1849–50.

Latham, Melanie. *Regulating Reproduction: A Century of Conflict in Britain and France.* Manchester, U.K.: University of Manchester Press, 2002.

Lebacqz, Karen. "On the Elusive Nature of Respect." In *The Human Embryonic Stem Cell Debate: Science, Ethics, and Public Policy.* Edited by Suzanne Holland, Karen Lebacqz, and Laurie Zoloth, 149–62. Cambridge: MIT Press, 2001.

Lenoir, Noëlle. *Aux frontières de la vie: Une éthique biomédicale à la française.* Paris: La Documentation française, 1991.

Luker, Kristin. *Abortion and the Politics of Motherhood.* Berkeley: University of California Press, 1985.

MacKinnon, Barbara. *Human Cloning: Science, Ethics, and Public Policy.* Urbana: University of Illinois Press, 2000.

Mahoney, James. "Path Dependence in Historical Sociology." *Theory and Society* 29 (2000): 507–48.

Mahoney, John. *Bio-ethics and Belief: Religion and Medicine in Dialogue.* London: Sheed and Ward, 1984.

Maienschein, Jane. *Whose View of Life? Embryos, Cloning, and Stem Cells.* Cambridge: Harvard University Press, 2003.

Markl, Hubert. "Freiheit, Verantwortung, Menschenwürde: Warum Lebenswissenschaften mehr sind as Biologie." June 22, 2001. http://www.mpg.de/pdf/jahrbuch_2001/jahrbuch2001_009_024.pdf.

Marshall, Eliot. "Human Embryo Research: Clinton Rules Out Some Studies." *Science* 266, no. 5191 (1994): 1634–35.

——. "Rules on Embryo Research Due Out." *Science* 265, no. 5175 (1994): 1024–26.

Mattei, Jean-François. "Bioéthique—Audition de M. Jean-François Mattei, ministre de la santé, de la famille et des personnes handicapées." December 12, 2002. http://www.senat.fr/commission/soc/soc021214.html#toc9.

——. *La vie en questions, pour une éthique biomédicale.* Paris: La Documentation française, 1993.

——. "Vers une révision des lois 'bioéthiques'?" In *Les lois bioéthiques à l'épreuve des faits: Réalités et perspectives.* Edited by Briggitte Feuillet-Le Mintier, 330–41. Paris: Presses Universitaires de France, 1999.

McCormick, Richard A. *The Critical Calling: Reflections on Moral Dilemmas since Vatican II.* Washington, DC: Georgetown University Press, 2006.

——. "The Ethical and Religious Challenges of Reproductive Technology." *Cambridge Quarterly of Healthcare Ethics* 8 (1999): 547–56.

——. "Life in the Test Tube." *New York Times,* August 6, 1978, E17.

——. "Who or What Is the Preembryo?" *Kennedy Institute of Ethics Journal* 1, no. 1 (1991): 1–15.

McGee, Glenn, and Arthur A. Caplan. "The Ethics and Politics of Small Sacrifices in Stem Cell Research." *Kennedy Institute of Ethics Journal* 9, no. 2 (1999): 151–58.

McHugh, Paul R. "Zygote and 'Clonote': The Ethical Use of Embryonic Stem Cells." *New England Journal of Medicine* 351, no. 3 (2004): 209–11.

McLaren, Anne. "Embryo Research." *Nature* 320, no. 6063 (1986): 570.

——. "Research on the Human Conceptus and Its Regulation in Britain Today." *Journal of the Royal Society of Medicine* 83, no. 4 (1990): 209–13.

McLaughlin, Loretta. *The Pill, John Rock, and the Church: The Biography of a Revolution.* Boston: Little, Brown, 1982.

"The Meaning of Life." *Nature* 412, no. 6844 (2001): 255.

Medical Research Council. "Research Related to Human Fertilisation and Embryology: Statement by the Medical Research Council." *British Medical Journal* 285, no. 6353 (1982): 1480.

Meilaender, Gilbert. *Neither Beast nor God: The Dignity of the Human Person.* New York: Encounter Books, 2009.

——. "The Point of a Ban: Or, How to Think about Stem Cell Research." *Hastings Center Report* 31, no. 1 (2001): 9–16.

Meyer, Michael J., and Lawrence J. Nelson. "Respecting What We Destroy: Reflections on Human Embryo Research." *Hastings Center Report* 31, no. 1 (2001): 16–23.

Monroe, Kristen R., Ronald Baker Miller, and Jerome S. Tobis. *Fundamentals of the Stem Cell Debate: The Scientific, Religious, Ethical, and Political Issues.* Berkeley: University of California Press, 2008.

Mooney, Christopher Z., ed. *The Public Clash of Private Values: The Politics of Morality Policy.* New York: Chatham House, 2001.

Mulkay, Michael. *The Embryo Research Debate: Science and the Politics of Reproduction.* Cambridge: Cambridge University Press, 1997.

National Bioethics Advisory Commission. *Cloning Human Beings: Report and Recommendations of the National Bioethics Advisory Commission.* Rockville, MD: National Bioethics Advisory Commission, 1997.

——. *Ethical Issues in Human Stem Cell Research.* Rockville, MD: National Bioethics Advisory Commission, 1999.

National Council of Churches. *Genetic Science for Human Benefit.* New York: NCCCUSA, 1986.

Nationaler Ethikrat (German National Ethics Council). *Cloning for Reproductive Purposes and Cloning for the Purposes of Biomedical Research.* Berlin: German National Ethics Council, 2004.

——. *Genetic Diagnosis before and during Pregnancy.* Berlin: German National Ethics Council, 2003.

——. *Opinion on the Import of Human Embryonic Stem Cells.* Berlin: German National Ethics Council, 2001.

——. *Wortprotokoll: Niederschrift über den öffentlichen Teil der Sitzung, 23. September 2004.* Berlin: Nationaler Ethikrat, 2004.

National Institutes of Health. "NIH Publishes Draft Guidelines for Stem Cell Research." Press release, December 1, 1999. http://www.nih.gov/news/pr/dec99/od-01.htm.

——. *Report of the Human Embryo Research Panel.* Vol. 1. Bethesda, MD: National Institutes of Health, 1994.

Nisbet, Matthew C. "The Polls—Trends: Public Opinion about Stem Cell Research and Human Cloning." *Public Opinion Quarterly* 68, no. 1 (2004): 131–54.

Norman, Colin. "IVF Research Moratorium to End?" *Science* 241, no. 4864 (1988): 405–6.

Nuffield Council on Bioethics. "Stem Cell Therapies: The Ethical Issues." April 2000.

Nussbaum, Martha Craven. *Frontiers of Justice: Disability, Nationality, Species Membership.* Cambridge: Harvard University Press, 2006.

Office of Technology Assessment. *Biomedical Ethics in U.S. Public Policy.* Washington, DC: U.S. Government Printing Office, 1993.

O'Leary, Don. *Roman Catholicism and Modern Science: A History.* London: Continuum, 2007.

O'Mahony, Patrick J. *A Question of Life: Its Beginning and Transmission.* London: Continuum, 1990.

Palca, Joseph. "Doing Things with Embryos." *Hastings Center Report* 25, no. 1 (1995): 5.

——. "New Watchdogs in Washington." *Hastings Center Report* 23, no. 2 (1994): 5.

——. "A Word to the Wise." *Hastings Center Report* 22, no. 4 (1994): 5.

Paul VI. *Humanae Vitae: On the Regulation of Birth.* July 25, 1968. http://www.vatican.va/holy_father/paul_vi/encyclicals/documents/hf_p-vi_enc_25071968_humanae-vitae_en.html.

Pearson, Helen. "Early Embryos Can Yield Stem Cells . . . and Survive." *Nature* 442, no. 7105 (2006): 858.

——. "Making Babies: The Next 30 Years." *Nature* 454, no. 7202: 260–62.

Perry, Daniel. "Patients' Voices: The Powerful Sound in the Stem Cell Debate." *Science* 287, no. 5457 (2000): 1423.

Peters, Ted. "Embryonic Stem Cells and the Theology of Dignity." In *The Human Embryonic Stem Cell Debate: Science, Ethics, and Public Policy.* Edited by Suzanne Holland, Karen Lebacqz, and Laurie Zoloth, 127–39. Cambridge: MIT Press, 2001.

Pierson, Paul. "Increasing Returns, Path Dependence, and the Study of Politics." *American Political Science Review* 94, no. 2 (2000): 251–67.

Pierson, Paul, and Theda Skocpol. "Historical Institutionalism in Contemporary Political Science." In *Political Science: The State of the Discipline.* Edited by Ira Katznelson and Helen V. Milner, 693–721. New York: Norton, 2002.

Polanyi, Michael. "The Republic of Science: Its Political and Economic Theory." *Minerva* 1, no. 1 (1962), 54–73.

Polkinghorne, John. "Therapeutic Uses of Cell Nuclear Replacement." 2000. http://www.cofe.anglican.org/info/socialpublic/science/hfea/cnr.pdf2000.

Pontifical Academy for Life. "Declaration on the Production and the Scientific and Therapeutic Use of Human Embryonic Stem Cells." August 25, 2000. http://www.vatican.va/roman_curia/pontifical_academies/acdlife/documents/rc_pa_acdlife_doc_20000824_cellule-staminali_en.html.

——. "Reflections on Cloning." June 25, 1997. http://www.vatican.va/roman_curia/pontifical_academies/acdlife/documents/rc_pa_acdlife_doc_30091997_clon_en.html.

Potts, Malcolm, Peter Diggory, and John Peel. *Abortion.* Cambridge: Cambridge University Press, 1977.

Présidence de la République (Presidency of the Republic). "Allocution de M. Jacques Chirac Président de la République à l'occasion de l'ouverture du forum mondial des biotechnologies." Press release, February 8, 2001.

———. "Allocution de M. François Mitterrand, Président de la République, à l'occasion de la mise en place du Comité consultatif national d'éthique pour les sciences de la vie et de la santé." Press release, December 2, 1983. http://lesdiscours. vie-publique.fr/pdf/837208100.pdf.

———. "Allocution de M. Jacques Chirac Président de la République à l'occasion de l'ouverture du forum mondial des biotechnologies." Press release, February 8, 2001.

———. "Visite en France de Sa Sainteté le pape Benoît XVI: Allocution de M. Le Président de la République Française." September 12, 2007. http://www.ely see.fr/president/les-actualites/discours/2008/visite-en-france-de-sa-saintete-le-pape-benoit-xvi.2085.html.

President's Commission for the Study of Ethical Problems in Medicine and Biomedical and Behavioral Research. *Splicing Life: A Report on the Social and Ethical Issues of Genetic Engineering with Human Beings.* Washington, DC: U.S. Government Printing Office, 1982.

President's Council on Bioethics. *Alternative Sources of Pluripotent Stem Cells: A White Paper.* Washington, DC: President's Council on Bioethics, 2005.

———. "Human Cloning and Human Dignity: An Ethical Inquiry." Washington, DC: President's Council on Bioethics, 2002.

———. *Reproduction and Responsibility: The Regulation of New Biotechnologies.* Washington, DC: President's Council on Bioethics, 2004.

Press Office of Senator Sam Brownback, "Brownback Applauds New Stem Cell Advances." Press release, November 20, 2007. http://brownback.senate.gov/pressapp/record.cfm?id=287831.

Prime Minister's Office. "Speech by the U.K. Prime Minister, Mr. Tony Blair, at the European Bioscience Conference." November 20, 2000. http://www.mon santo.co.uk/news/ukshowlib.phtml?uid=4104.

Rahner, Karl. "The Problem of Genetic Manipulation." In *Theological Investigations: Writings of 1965–1967.* New York: Crossroad, 1976.

Ramsey, Paul. *Fabricated Man: The Ethics of Genetic Control.* New Haven: Yale University Press, 1970.

———. "Shall We 'Reproduce'?: The Medical Ethics of In Vitro Fertilization." *Journal of the American Medical Association* 220, no. 10 (1972): 1346–50.

Randerson, James. "The Battle over Stem Cells." *New Scientist* 184, no. 2468 (2004): 23.

Rawls, John. *A Theory of Justice.* Cambridge: Harvard University Press, 1971.

Republican Party. "Republican Party Platform of 1976." August 18, 1976. http://www.presidency.ucsb.edu/ws/index.php?pid=25843.

———. "Republican Party Platform of 1980." July 15, 1980. http://www.presidency.ucsb.edu/ws/index.php?pid=25844.

———. "Republican Platform 2000." July 31, 2000. http://www.pbs.org/newshour/bb/election/july-dec00/platform4.html.

Ricard, Jean-Pierre. "Pas d'exception au respect dû à l'embryon humain." January 27, 2003. http://www.eglise.catholique.fr/conference-des-eveques-de-france/textes-et-declarations/pas-dexception-au-respect-du-a-lembryon-humain-.html.

Robertson, John A. "Ethics and Policy in Embryonic Stem Cell Research." *Kennedy Institute of Ethics Journal* 9, no. 2 (1999): 109–36.

——. "Symbolic Issues in Embryo Research." *Hastings Center Report* 25, no. 1 (1995): 37–38.

Roe v. Wade. 410 U.S. 113, 93 S.Ct. 705, 35 L.Ed.2nd 147 (1973).

Royal Society. "Whither Cloning?" Press release, January 1, 1998. http://royalsociety. org/Whither-Cloning.

Royal College of Obstetricians and Gynaecologists. *Report of the RCOG Ethics Committee on In Vitro Fertilization and Embryo Replacement or Transfer.* London: Chamelion Press, 1983.

Rozenberg, Jacques J. *Bioethical and Ethical Issues Surrounding the Trials and Code of Nuremberg: Nuremberg Revisited.* Lewiston, NY: Edwin Mellen Press, 2003.

Ruse, Michael, and Christopher A. Pynes. *The Stem Cell Controversy: Debating the Issues.* Amherst, NY: Prometheus Books, 2003.

Sacred Congregation for the Doctrine of the Faith. "Declaration on Procured Abortion." November 18, 1974. http://www.vatican.va/roman_curia/con gregations/cfaith/documents/rc_con_cfaith_doc_19741118_declaration-abortion_en.html.

"Saddleback Presidential Candidates Forum." August 16, 2008. http://transcripts. cnn.com/TRANSCRIPTS/0808/16/se.02.html.

Savulescu, Julian, and Nick Bostrom. *Human Enhancement.* Oxford: Oxford University Press, 2009.

Schockenhoff, Eberhard. "Die Ethik des Heilens und die Menschenwürde" In *Gattungsethik—Schutz für das Menschengeschlecht?* Edited by Matthias Kaufmann and Lukas Sosoe, 343–73. Frankfurt am Main: Lang, 2005.

Schröder, Gerhard. "Der neue Mensch." *Die Woche,* December 20, 2000.

Schröder, Richard. "Die Forschung an embryonalen Stammzellen: Argumentationstypen und ihre Voraussetzungen. Erweiterte Fassung eines Vortrags im Tübinger Stift am 20.2.2002." February 20, 2002. http://www2.hu-berlin. de/theologie/schroeder/bioethiktueb.pdf.

Science et foi: Colloque, 1er février 1992. Paris: Centurion, 1992.

Seeber, David. "Die neuen Techniken menschlicher Fortpflanzung." *Herder Korrespondenz* 40, no. 3 (1986): 143–47.

Sen, Amartya Kumar, and Bernard Arthur Owen Williams. *Utilitarianism and Beyond.* Cambridge: Cambridge University Press, 1982.

Sénat (French Senate). *Auditions du 10 Novembre 1999.* November 10, 1999. http:// www.senat.fr/rap/r99–238-2/r99–238-24.html.

——. "Audition de M. Jean-François Mattei, ministre de la santé, de la famille et des personnes handicapées." December 12, 2002. http://www.senat.fr/commission/ soc/soc021214.html#toc9.

Sérusclat, Franck. *Sciences de la vie et droits de l'Homme: Bouleversement sans contrôle ou législation à la française.* Paris: Office parlementaire d'évaluation des choix scientifiques et technologiques, 1992.

Sève, Lucien. *Pour une critique de la raison bioéthique.* Paris: Jacob, 1994.

Shannon, Thomas A., and Allan B. Wolter. "Reflections on the Moral Status of the Pre-Embryo." *Theological Studies* 51, no. 4 (1990): 603–26.

Sharpe, David J., and Robert G. Edwards. "Social Values and Research in Human Embryology." *Nature* 231, no. 5298 (1971): 87–91.

Sicard, Didier. "Réflexions sur le progrès en médecine." *Contrepoint Philosophique.* October 2004. http://www.contrepointphilosophique.ch/Ethique/Sommaire/ProgresEnMedecine.html?Article=ProgresEnMedecine.htm.

Silver, Lee M. *Remaking Eden: Cloning and Beyond in a Brave New World.* New York: Avon Books, 1997.

Singer, Peter. *Embryo Experimentation.* Cambridge: Cambridge University Press, 1990.

———. "Shopping at the Genetic Supermarket." Foreword to *The Ethics of Inheritable Genetic Modification: A Dividing Line?* Edited by John E. J. Rasko, Gabrielle O'Sullivan, and Rachel A. Ankeny, xiii–xxxi. Cambridge: Cambridge University Press, 2006.

———. "On Being Silenced in Germany." *New York Review of Books* 38, no. 14 (1991): 36–42.

Singer, Peter, and Helga Kuhse. *Unsanctifying Human Life: Essays on Ethics.* Oxford: Blackwell, 2002.

Singer, Peter, and Deane Wells. *Making Babies: The New Science and Ethics of Conception.* New York: C. Scribner's Sons, 1985.

Sinsheimer, Robert L. "Genetic Engineering: The Modification of Man." *Impact of Science on Society* 20, no. 4 (1970): 279–91.

Sloterdijk, Peter. *Regeln für den Menschenpark: Ein Antwortschreiben zu Heideggers Brief über den Humanismus.* Frankfurt am Main: Suhrkamp, 1999.

———. "Rules for the Human Zoo: A Response to the Letter on Humanism." *Environment and Planning D: Society and Space* 27, no. 1 (2009): 12–28.

Sofres. *Les attitudes de l'opinion publique en France, Allemagne, Grande-Bretagne et aux Etats-Unis à l'égard de la science.* Paris: Sofres, 2001.

Southern Baptist Convention. "Resolution on Abortion and Infanticide." May 1982. http://www.sbc.net/resolutions/amResolution.asp?ID=20.

———. "Resolution on Human Cloning." June 21, 2001. http://www.sbc.net/resolutions/amResolution.asp?ID=572.

———. "Resolution on Human Embryonic and Stem Cell Research," June 1999, http://www.sbc.net/resolutions/amResolution.asp?ID=620.

Steinbock, Bonnie. "Ethical Issues in Human Embryo Research." In *Papers Commissioned for the NIH Human Embryo Research Panel,* 27–50. Bethesda, MD: National Institutes of Health, 1994.

———. *Life before Birth: The Moral and Legal Status of Embryos and Fetuses.* New York: Oxford University Press, 1992.

Stevens, M. L. Tina. *Bioethics in America: Origins and Cultural Politics.* Baltimore: Johns Hopkins University Press, 2000.

Stith-Coleman, Irene. *Human Embryo Research.* Washington, DC: Congressional Research Service, 1998.

Svea, Luise Hermann. *Policy Debates on Reprogenetics.* Frankfurt: Campus Verlag, 2009.

"Synod OKs Federally-Funded Embryonic Stem Cell Research." *United Church News.* July 11–17, 2001. http://www.ucc.org/ucnews/julaug01/synod-oks-federally-funded.html.

Taguieff, Pierre-André. "L'espace de la bioéthique: Esquisse d'une problématisation." *Res Publica* 21 (1995): 30–37.

Tatalovich, Raymond, and Byron W. Daynes, eds. *Moral Controversies in American Politics: Cases in Social Regulatory Policy.* Armonk, NY: M. E. Sharpe, 1998.

Tauer, Carol A. "Embryo Research and Public Policy: A Philosopher's Appraisal." *Journal of Medicine and Philosophy* 22, no. 5 (1997): 423–39.

———. "The Tradition of Probabilism and the Moral Status of the Early Embryo." *Theological Studies* 45, no. 1 (1984): 3–33.

Testart, Jacques. *Des hommes probables: De la procréation aléatoire à la reproduction normative.* Paris: Seuil, 1999.

———, ed. *Le magasin des enfants.* Paris: Editions François Bourin, 1990.

———. *L'oeuf transparent.* Paris: Flammarion, 1986.

Thelen, Kathleen. "Historical Institutionalism in Comparative Politics." *Annual Review of Political Science* 2 (1999): 369–404.

Thomson, James A., Joseph Itskovitz-Eldor, Sander S. Shapiro, Michelle A. Waknitz, Jennifer J. Swiergiel, Vivienne S. Marshall, and Jeffrey M. Jones. "Embryonic Stem Cell Lines Derived from Human Blastocysts." *Science* 282, no. 5391 (1998): 1145–47.

Trounson, Alan, and Linda Mohr. "Human Pregnancy Following Cryopreservation, Thawing and Transfer of an Eight-Cell Embryo." *Nature* 305, no. 5936 (1983): 707–9.

Turney, Jon. *Frankenstein's Footsteps: Science, Genetics, and Popular Culture.* New Haven: Yale University Press, 1998.

United Kingdom. Department of Health. *Government Response to the Recommendations Made in the Chief Medical Officer's Expert Group Report.* London: Her Majesty's Stationery Office, 2000.

———. Department of Health. *Review of the Human Fertilisation and Embryology Act.* London: Her Majesty's Stationery Office, 2006.

———. "Speech by Lord Warner, Parliamentary Under-Secretary of State in the Lords, 19 May 2004: Launch of UK Stem Cell Bank." Press release, May 19, 2004. http://collections.europarchive.org/tna/20060802142310/dh.gov.uk/en/News/Speeches/Speecheslist/DH_4084091.

———. *Stem Cell Research: Medical Progress with Responsibility.* August 16, 2000. http://www.dh.gov.uk/en/Publicationsandstatistics/Publications/PublicationsPolicyAndGuidance/DH_4065084.

———. Department of Health and Social Security. *Report of the Committee of Inquiry into Human Fertilisation and Embryology.* London: Her Majesty's Stationery Office, 1984.

———. House of Commons. Science and Technology Committee. *Government Proposals for the Regulation of Hybrid and Chimera Embryos.* London: Her Majesty's Stationery Office, 2007.

———. House of Lords. "Stem Cell Research." Sessional Papers, 2001–02. Stem Cell Research Committee. Vol. 1. February 27, 2002. http://www.publications.parliament.uk/pa/ld/ldstem.htm.

———. *Parliamentary Debates.* Commons, 5th ser., vol. 954 (July 25, 1978).

———. *Parliamentary Debates.* Commons, 6th ser., vol. 21 (March 30, 1982).

———. *Parliamentary Debates.* Commons, 6th ser., vol. 64 (July 18, 1984).

——. *Parliamentary Debates.* Commons, 6th ser., vol. 68 (November 23, 1984).

——. *Parliamentary Debates.* Commons, 6th ser., vol. 73 (February 15, 1985).

——. *Parliamentary Debates.* Commons, 6th ser., vol. 171 (April 23, 1990).

——. *Parliamentary Debates.* Commons, 6th ser., vol. 356 (November 17, 2000).

——. *Parliamentary Debates.* Commons, 6th ser., vol. 357 (December 15, 2000).

——. *Parliamentary Debates.* Commons, 6th ser., vol. 475 (May 12, 2008).

——. *Parliamentary Debates.* Commons, 6th ser., vol. 476 (May 19, 2008).

——. *Parliamentary Debates.* Lords, 6th ser., vol. 513 (December 7, 1989).

——. *Parliamentary Debates.* Lords, 6th ser., vol. 621 (January 22, 2001).

——. *Parliamentary Debates.* Lords, Written Answers, 6th ser., vol. 621 (February 1, 2001).

United Methodist Church. "Resolution 3182: Human Cloning." In *The Book of Resolutions of the United Methodist Church.* Nashville: United Methodist Publishing House, 2008. http://www.umc.org/site/apps/nlnet/content2.aspx?c =lwL4KnN1LtH&b=4951419&content_id={5C125586-247C-45DE-8063-EEC128BC5F89}&notoc=1.

United States Conference of Catholic Bishops. "Catholic Bishops Criticize Bush Policy on Embryo Research." Press release, August 9, 2001. http://www.usccb.org/comm/archives/2001/01–142.shtml.

U.S. Congress. *Congressional Record.* 104th Cong., 2nd sess., 1996. Vol. 142, no. 102.

——. *Congressional Record.* "Human Cloning Prohibition Act—Motion to Proceed." 105th Cong., 2d sess., 1998. Vol. 144, pt. 10.

——. U.S. House of Representatives. Committee on Science, Subcommittee on Technology. "Biotechnology and the Ethics of Cloning: How Far Should We Go?" March 5, 1997. http://commdocs.house.gov/committees/science/hsy064170.000/hsy064170_0.HTM.

Vanderpool, Harold Y., ed. *The Ethics of Research Involving Human Subjects: Facing the 21st Century.* Frederick, MD: University Pub. Group, 1996.

Varmus, Harold. *The Art and Politics of Science.* New York: Norton, 2009.

Verband Forschender Arzneimittelhersteller (Association of Research-Based Pharmaceutical Companies). "Forschung mit humanen Stammzellen." Press release, April 30, 2001.

Verspieren, Patrick. "Les fécondations artificielles: A propos de l'Instruction romaine sur 'le don de la vie.'" *Etudes* 366, no. 5 (1987): 607–19.

Vogel, Gretchen. "Korean Team Speeds Up Creation of Cloned Human Stem Cells." *Science* 308, no. 5725 (2005): 1096–97.

Vogel, Gretchen, and Constance Holden. "Nuclear Transfer: Still on the Table." *Science* 319, no. 5863 (2008): 563.

Wadman, Meredith. "U.S. Biologists Adopt Cloning Moratorium." *Nature* 389, no. 6649 (1997): 319.

Walgate, Robert. "Human Embryology: France Seeks Policy in Haste." *Nature* 313, no. 6005 (1985): 728.

——. "French Scientist Makes a Stand." *Nature* 323, no. 6087 (1986): 385.

Walter, Jennifer K., and Eran P. Klein. *The Story of Bioethics: From Seminal Works to Contemporary Explorations.* Washington, DC: Georgetown University Press, 2003.

Walters, LeRoy. "Human Embryonic Stem Cell Research: An Intercultural Perspective." *Kennedy Institute of Ethics Journal* 14, no. 1 (2004): 3–38.

Warnock, Mary. *Nature and Mortality: Recollections of a Philosopher in Public Life.* London: Continuum, 2003.

Waters, Brent, and Ronald Cole-Turner. *God and the Embryo: Religious Voices on Stem Cells and Cloning.* Washington, DC: Georgetown University Press, 2003.

Watson, James. "Moving toward the Clonal Man." *Atlantic* 227, no. 5 (1971): 50–53.

Weissman, Irving. "Medicine: Politic Stem Cells." *Nature* 439 (2006): 145–47.

Wellcome Trust. "Wellcome Trust Interim Position Statement on Stem Cell Research." Press release, October 2000.

White House Press Office. "Bush Calls on Senate to Back Human Cloning Ban." Press release, April 10, 2002. http://georgewbush-whitehouse.archives.gov/news/releases/2002/04/20020410–4.html.

——. "Remarks by President Bush and Senator Kerry in Second 2004 Presidential Debate." Press release, October 9, 2004. http://georgewbush-whitehouse.archives.gov/news/releases/2004/10/20041009-2.html.

——. "Remarks by the President on Cloning." Press release, March 4, 1997.

——. "Remarks by the President on Stem Cell Research." Press release, August 9, 2001. http://bioethics.georgetown.edu/pcbe/reports/stemcell/appendix_b.html.

——. "Remarks by the President to the American Association for the Advancement of Science." Press release, February 13, 1998. http://clinton6.nara.gov/1998/02/1998-02-13-remarks-by-the-president-to-aaas.html.

——. "Signing of Stem Cell Executive Order and Scientific Integrity Presidential Memorandum." Press release, March 9, 2009. http://www.whitehouse.gov/the_press_office/Remarks-of-the-President-As-Prepared-for-Delivery-Signing-of-Stem-Cell-Executive-Order-and-Scientific-Integrity-Presidential-Memorandum/.

——. "Statement by Press Secretary on Human Stem Cell Research." Press release, July 14, 1999. http://archives.clintonpresidentialcenter.org/?u=071499-statement-by-press-secretary-on-human-stem-cell-research.htm.

——. "To the Congress of the United States." Press release, June 9, 1997. http://clinton3.nara.gov/New/Remarks/Mon/19970609–15987.html.

Yamanaka, Shinya, and Kazutoshi Takahashi. "Induction of Pluripotent Stem Cells from Mouse Embryonic and Adult Fibroblast Cultures by Defined Factors." *Cell* 126, no. 4 (2006): 663–76.

Young, Emma. "Human Embryos Created for Cell Harvest." *New Scientist.com,* July 11, 2001. http://www.newscientist.com/article/dn997.

Yoxen, Edward. "Historical Perspectives on Human Embryo Research." In *Experiments on Embryos.* Edited by Anthony Oakley Dyson and John Harris, 27–41. London: Routledge, 1990.

Zook, Jim. "House Unit Votes to Bar Federal Funds for Research on Embryos." *Chronicle of Higher Education* 41, no. 6 (July 5, 1996): A33.

INDEX

CPSIA information can be obtained at www.ICGtesting.com
Printed in the USA
BVOW032146050613

322577BV00004B/10/P

9 780801 478819